Medical Statistics
A Practical Approach

Medical
Statistics
A Practical Approach

Tze-San Lee

Western Illinois University, USA

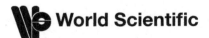 **World Scientific**

NEW JERSEY · LONDON · SINGAPORE · BEIJING · SHANGHAI · HONG KONG · TAIPEI · CHENNAI · TOKYO

Published by

World Scientific Publishing Co. Pte. Ltd.

5 Toh Tuck Link, Singapore 596224

USA office: 27 Warren Street, Suite 401-402, Hackensack, NJ 07601

UK office: 57 Shelton Street, Covent Garden, London WC2H 9HE

British Library Cataloguing-in-Publication Data
A catalogue record for this book is available from the British Library.

MEDICAL STATISTICS
A Practical Approach

ISBN 978-981-121-751-7 (hardcover)
ISBN 978-981-121-842-2 (paperback)
ISBN 978-981-121-752-4 (ebook for institutions)
ISBN 978-981-121-753-1 (ebook for individuals)

For any available supplementary material, please visit
https://www.worldscientific.com/worldscibooks/10.1142/11752#t=suppl

Printed in Singapore

Preface

This book is based upon the lecture notes I gave when I was invited to teach a course in biostatistics offered by the School of Public Health, Zhejiang University in China to international students who enrolled in the MSBG program during the 2012 summer session.

There are a total of 13 chapters. The topics and their arrangement were determined from my own experience gained from teaching for over 20 years. I believe that the content of this book will contain the necessary statistical techniques needed to understand the majority of articles appearing in medical literature. Overall, the emphasis is focused on practical applications, so the mathematical derivation of the statistical method have been largely omitted. This book could be used as a text and/or reference book for the undergraduate, residency training, or for continuing medical education.

Chapter 0 gives an introduction on two general questions: what medical statistics is and why doctors need to study it. Chapter 1 presents the concept of a random variable and elementary estimation formulas in descriptive statistics. Chapter 2 distinguishes the theoretical from the empirical probabilities, and examines applications of sensitivity and specificity in epidemiology. Chapter 3 introduces classic random variables with their probability distributions and how to use them to model real world problems. Basic notions of inferential statistics is covered in Chap. 4. A comparison between means/variances is provided in Chap. 5. Inference on proportions is studied in Chap. 6, correlation/regression is covered in Chap. 7, and nonparametrical methods are studied in Chap. 8. Chapter 9 discusses various ways for determination of the sample sizes that are required in investigations. Design of observational/experimental studies and types of bias are covered in Chap. 10. Chapter 11 presents how to conduct inference for contingency tables, whereas Chap. 12 shows how to analyze the survival data. References are attached as a last section in each chapter.

I would like to thank my many colleagues and students throughout my careers who have given me enlightened discussions, suggestions and feedbacks. I would also like to thank my wife and children for their understanding and support of my endeavors.

T-S Lee,
Atlanta, Georgia

Contents

Table of Figures

List of Notations

0 Introduction

Statistics is intrinsically different from mathematics. Mathematics adopts the method of deduction, but statistics uses the method of induction. The primary function of statistics is to gather and assess data rigorously and critically. Yet, statistics is not a science, rather it is a technology.[4] As a result, statistical significance is not equivalent to scientific significance. Thus, statistics is not an easy subject to comprehend and apply.

As far as understanding the subject of statistics, there are three levels.[3] The first level is for the individual. Statistics provides the base for understanding the issues that affect our role as citizens in a democracy. The second level is for professions such as medicine, economics and science, where data interpretation and analysis are a necessary part of one's work. According to the third level, there are professional statisticians ranging from data gatherers to pure mathematicians.

0.1 What is Medical Statistics?

Statistics is neither mathematics nor probability; nevertheless, both mathematics and probability are used to lay down a solid foundation of statistics. It is the subject to deal with all kinds of data, primarily to draw statistical inference from the sample data about certain aspects or characteristic of the given population. Random variables play the central role in statistics, while data is the life blood of random variables.

First, a population must be specified. The population used here is a generic term, and does not necessarily need to refer to human population. It is just a set of elements and could be anything. A few examples are people, animals used in the laboratory, or stocks on the New York Stock Exchange. Second, a random variable must be defined, namely, on what aspect of the population we are interested in studying. One example may be the effectiveness of a new drug in curing a disease. Third, we need to collect a set of sample data on the defined random variable. By using the terminology in college algebra, a random variable is a function that maps the population (the domain) to the data (the range). A formal definition of a random variable is defined in the next chapter (see Definition 1.1.1). Note that unlike mathematics, there is a real-world price to collect the data.

Depending the nature of the data, we thus have all kinds of applied statistics. If the statistical method is applied to analyze the medical data, the subject is called medical statistics. Similarly, if the same method is used to deal with the economic data, the subject is then called the economic statistics. With a minor adjustment, the statistical method could be applied basically to any kind of data. There is no definite minimum amount of knowledge of statistics that doctors need for the correct diagnosis. In any case, my hope is including medical statistics in the undergraduate curriculum will lead all doctors to be better equipped to cope with quantitative information in its various guises.[2]

0.2 Why A Need To Study Medical Statistics?

For any physician today to work in the 21st century[5] it is required to acquire full knowledge of a medical specialty and to be challenged throughout his/her years of practice to keep pace with the expansion of science and technology in that specialty. To respond to the patient's personal concerns and problems requires a general professional education. However, this is beyond the scope of this book.

At a minimum physicians and medical students are rquired to study the subject of medical statistics in medical school for the following reasons[1]:

(i) Given the widespread use of statistical techniques in medicine, no one can do it without understanding the fundamentals of statistics;

(ii) The planning, conduct and interpretation of much of medical research are becoming increasingly relied on statistical methodology;

(iii) Even if they do not carry out research themselves, doctors need to read and interpret the published research of others. One of the most important skills a physician should have is the ability to critically analyze original contributions to the medical literature.

(iv) Basic science and clinical education should be integrated so that students can develop abilities to incorporate scientific concepts and principles into solving clinical problems.

References

1. Altman DG, Bland JM. (1991) Improving doctor's understanding of statistics. *J R Statist Soc A* **154**: 223–267.
2. Appleton DR. (1990) What statistics should we teach medical undergraduates and graduates? *Stat Med* **9**: 1013–1021.
3. Bodmer WF. (1985) Understanding statistics. *J R Statist Soc A* **148**: 69–81.
4. Healy MJR. (1978) Is statistics a science? *J R Statist Soc A* **141**: 385–393.
5. The GPEP Report. (1984) *Physicians for the Twenty-First Century*. Association of American Medical Colleges, Washington, DC.

1 Descriptive Statistics

In this chapter we are going to learn the notion of random variables illustrated by some concrete real-world examples. Also, let us learn how to collect the sample data of high quality. By using concrete examples let me point out that the sample selection bias can easily cripple the quality of the sample data. Finally, I will show how to use the sample data to estimate the population parameter of the probability distribution associated with a random variable.

1.1 Random Variables

We are living in the era of information. Constantly, we are bombarded by all kinds of information. To assess these information intelligently, we need to be proficient in using the statistical instruments. Since random variables are the central figure in statistics, we need to firmly grasp the intrinsic meaning of random variables. In terms of the concept of function in mathematics, a random variable is formally defined as follows.

Definition 1.1.1. A random variable (or "r.v.") X is a function that maps the population onto the data, namely,

$$X: \{\text{the population}\} \to \{\text{the data}\}. \tag{1.1.1}$$

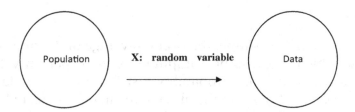

Fig. 1.1-1. Definition of a random variable X.

Remarks

1. Even though a random variable is a function, we do not use the symbol of little letter "f" as was followed in college algebra. Instead, a capital letter "X" is used here to denote a random variable conventionally (Fig. 1.1-1).

2. For practicality, a random variable is not as abstract as it appears. It oftentimes refers specifically to an aspect of the population. For example, if the population is taken as people living in the United States (US), and we are interested in the weight or height of all individuals in the population, we could let two random variables (or "r.v.s") X and Y denote his/her weight and height, respectively. By using a physical check-up, the information on his/her weight/height can be measured precisely. By using Eq. (1.1.1), they can be expressed as, for instance, X(Jim) = 185 pounds and Y(Jim) = 6 feet 1 inch, X(Mary) = 130 pounds and Y(Mary) = 5 feet 6 inches.

3. After the data of the entire population is collected, the probability distribution of the r.v. X will emerge if the data is grouped into many tiny intervals and their frequencies are plotted. A random variable has its own unique probability distribution, and vice versa. Hence, the terms of a random variable and its probability distribution are used interchangeably without mentioning.

Definition 1.1.2. Two important parameters associated with a probability distribution of the r.v. X are its mean (μ_X) and its variance (σ_X^2).

Remarks

1. The mean of X is simply the overall-average of the population data, which can also be computed as the expected value of X, provided that the probability distribution of X is known, namely, $\mu_X = E(X)$. Graphically, the mean of X is located at the center of the distribution if the distribution is symmetric about its mean.

2. The variance of X is a measure of the overall-spread of the population data about the center of the distribution, which can be calculated by using the expected value, namely, $\sigma_X^2 = E[(X - \mu_X)^2]$.

3. μ_X and σ_X^2 are supposed to be constants. However, they are often unknown in practical applications. Hence, we need to collect the sample data, which is a subset of the population data, to estimate these unknown parameters. The issue concerning us is how accurate these estimators are. Well, it depends on the quality of the collected sample data. The quality of the sample data depends on what sampling technique is used as will be covered in the next section.

1.2   The Medical Sampling Technique

Before addressing the statistically sounding strategy, let me first mention some poorly executed sampling examples.

A. *Examples of Biased Samples*

Example 1.2A-1. Sample size too small[17]

In many textbooks it is claimed that the decrease in the weight of the heart is relatively smaller than that in the voluntary muscles if an adult animal is starved. This claim is mainly based on a poorly designed experiment in which only two cats were used — one starved and one well-fed. After a period of experiment it was found that the heart of the starved cat lost 2.6% of its weight, while the voluntary muscles lost 30.5% of their weight. This superficial observation was quoted in a textbook as a matter of fact. Unfortunately, this fact is not true. As a result, the inference drawn from this experiment is misleading.

Remarks

1. Since the sample size is way too small, no sampling error was taken into consideration. The accuracy of any statistical inference depends on the sample errors. The larger the sample size, the smaller the sampling error.
2. How to determine the adequate sample size will be studied in Chap. 9.

Example 1.2A-2. Unrepresentative sample

In Britain it was widely believed that its population suffers from deteriorating physique. This impression was drawn from the claim that of every five men offering to enlist in the Army, only two were found to be effective soldiers after two years. A committee was set up to consider the validity of this claim. Finally, it concluded in a report that little evidence of progressive physical deterioration was found, but the men voluntarily offering to enlist at that time were not representative of the population as a whole.

Example 1.2A-3. A poorly-designed case-control study

The effects of propranolol in the acute phase of myocardial infarction was assessed by comparing two similar groups of patients in which only one group received propranolol.[14] Patients admitted to hospital with a history suggestive of myocardial infarction within the preceding 24 hours were altered in receiving propranolol in addition to the usual treatment, while the other patients were treated in an identical fashion except that no propranolol was administered.

Among 91 patients (68 males and 23 females), 45 patients received propranolol (treatment group) and 46 did not (control group). In the control group, 29 (63% = 29/46) patients survived and 16 (35% = 16/46) died, while in the treatment group 38 (84% = 38/45) patients survived and 7 (16% = 7/45) died. A conclusion was drawn that propranolol was effective because the mortality of the control group was 2.5 times that of the treatment group and the difference was statistically significant at the level of 2.5%.

Remarks

1. The sampling plan to collect the sample data is poorly designed, because patients were not randomly assigned to the control or the treatment group; rather they were assigned to receive propranolol based on the order of their admission to hospital.
2. A properly designed case-control study was carried out as shown in Example 1.3-4. The inference drawn was that the difference in the mortality between the two groups was not statistically significant.

Example 1.2A-4. Hospital samples

In order to obtain enough cases for a satisfactory conclusion, a researcher might carry out his research on patients having a specific disease who were associated with a certain risk factor in a hospital. A control group is a group of patients from the same hospital who were without this risk factor. If the probability that a person entered hospital differed according to whether he had the disease and risk factor, then the hospital population would not reflect the true incidence of these two factors (disease and risk) and would give a false picture on the problem under investigation. The conclusion is simply an artifact, regardless of how carefully the sample is selected.

Remarks

1. Similarly, inference that is drawn from post-mortem records is more likely to be biased. See Berkson[1] for concrete examples.
2. The problem arose mainly because the sampling probability was not the same between two groups. In fact, when

observations are collected so that the probability of selection is not independent of the outcome variable, it always results in biased sampling, namely, the collected data are not random samples. This is a very important issue in sampling, called the sample selection bias, which will be further covered in Sec. 10.5.

B. *Random Sampling/Assignment*

The principle of randomization is the minimal requirement that has to be applied to assure the quality of the collected data. That is, the simplest precaution against bias in sampling/assignment is to take the sample or assign subjects to treatment "at random". Besides, depending on classification of the sample size, it is classified as the fixed or random sample size. For the case of the fixed sample size, the sample size is determined *a priori* before the collection. Of course, there are criteria on how large the sample size is needed (see Chap. 9). For the case of a random sample size, it is determined sequentially according to the criterion of Wald's sequential analysis.[16]

Let us consider the case of fixed sample size first. Basically, random sampling is a process of selection that assures that every element of the population has the same probability of being selected. There are many different sampling strategies one can employ depending on the need of practical application. The following strategy is the most basic one.

Definition 1.2.1. A sample is said to be a simple random sample (SRS) if each member of the population has the same probability of being selected to be included in the sample.

Remarks

1. If the population is finite, which has only N members, each member is then labeled by the number from 1 to N. Thus, if a SRS of size n is desired, one could use the table random digits to choose these n members from the population.

2. Ordinarily, a SRS is chosen by the selection without replacement. This guarantees that no two members in the SRS are the same.

Sometimes auxiliary information can be used to stratify the population into several subpopulation (or strata). This leads to the following sampling plan.

Definition 1.2.2. A stratified sample is a sample plan that consists of selecting a SRS from each strata.

Remark

The estimation formula for the population mean and variance using the stratified sampling strategy is given in Chap. 6 of Ref. 9.

Definition 1.2.3. There are two types of cluster sampling:

(i) A simple one-stage cluster sampling is a strategy that selects a SRS from clusters and then includes all units in the selected clusters into the sample.
(ii) A simple two-stage cluster sampling is a strategy that consists of two stages; at the first stage clusters are selected by the SRS and then listing units within each selected cluster are selected by another SRS to be included finally in the sample.

Remarks

1. A simple one-stage cluster sampling is treated in Chap. 9 of Ref. 9.
2. A simple two-stage cluster sampling is treated in Chap. 10 of Ref. 9.

1.3 Examples of Random Variables

Depending on the measurement scale for collecting the data, random variables are classified into two categories: (1) categorical (nominal or ordinal) and (2) numerical (discrete or continuous) (see Definitions 1.3.1 and 1.3.2). In this section we are going to present them in terms of concrete examples.

Definition 1.3.1. A categorical r.v. X is said to be nominal if its data are not ordered; otherwise, it is said to be ordinal.

Definition 1.3.2. A numerical r.v. X is said to be discrete if its data are not real numbers, but only comprised of nonnegative integers; otherwise it is called continuous.

Remark

For types of random variables, please see Examples 1.3-1 to 1.3-6.

Example 1.3-1. Top 10 cancer deaths in the US[15]

Consider the population in the United States (US). Let a r.v. X be defined as the top 10 cancer deaths. Their rates in 2012 are collected that are given in the following table.

Remarks

1. Table 1.3-1 is adapted from the United States Cancer Statistics Report. The original table has additional information that is broken down by race.[15]
2. Note that cancer is not the leading cause of death, but merely the No. 2 cause of deaths. The other nine top causes of disease deaths are ranked accordingly: (1) heart disease, (2) chronic lower respiratory diseases, (3) stroke, (4) unintentional injuries, (5) Alzheimer's disease, (6) diabetes, (7) nephritis, nephrotic syndrome, (8) influenza and pneumonia, and (9) suicide.[12]
3. All ten r.v.s, FEBR, PROS, LUBR, CORE, COUT, URBL, MESK, NHLY, KRPS and THRD, in this example are nominal.
4. For convenience, we sometimes use numbers to express that the selected individual has the described cancer. For instance, $X = FEBR = 1$ (or "Yes") means that the selected woman died of breast cancer; otherwise $X = FEBR = 0$ (or "No"). $Pr(X = FEBR = 1) = 0.001222$ is interpreted in two ways: (i) the mortality of females is 1222 per one million people, or; (ii) the probability

Table 1.3-1.   The Probability Distribution of Top 10 Cancer Deaths in the US Population — All Races

Cancer Sites (X)	Rate (Pr(X = 1))
Female breast (FEBR)	0.001222
Prostate (PROS)	0.001053
Lung and bronchus (LUBR)	0.000604
Colon and rectum (CORE)	0.000389
Corpus and uterus, NOS (COUT)	0.000257
Urinary bladder (URBL)	0.000202
Melanomas of the skin (MESK)	0.000199
Non-Hodgkin lymphoma (NHLY)	0.000185
Kidney and renal pelvis (KRPS)	0.000159
Thyroid (THRD)	0.000143

that a randomly selected female who dies of breast cancer is 0.001222 (see Chap. 2 for the interpretation by using the concept of probability).

5. Incidentally, all the probabilities in Table 1.3-1 can be interpreted as a number per 100,000 people. For example, $Pr(X = FEBR = 1) = 0.001222$ means that there are 1222 deaths that are attributed to breast cancer per one million females.

Example 1.3-2. Framingham Heart Study

Because President Roosevelt died of a sudden stroke on 12 April 1945, the US Public Health Service began to ponder how to tackle the issue of reducing the mortality of coronary heart disease (CHD) in the general population. A better idea is to conduct a longitudinal cohort study, that is, to select a group of people who are free of the disease and to do a follow-up to see what happens to this cohort many years thereafter.

Framingham, a small college town lying 21 miles west of Boston, was selected in mid-1947 to conduct such a study. It has a population of 28,800. To avoid selecting people who are either too young or too old, the age of people included in the cohort was restricted to lie between 30 and 62 years old. The study was established during the period 1948 to 1950.[4]

Of the 6507 persons selected at random, 4469 persons aged 30 to 62, which comprised the sample population, came in for medical examination. Another group of 740 volunteers was also included. Although the sample population and the volunteer groups differ in some minor particulars, none of these differences present any problem in the analysis. Hence, they were combined. From this number 5127 persons (2283 men and 2844 women) who were free of CHD were chosen as the study cohort. Details on employing the systematic sampling strategy on selecting the sample population is described in Ref. 4.

In a 1961 article (see Ref. 6) it was found that the incidence of CHD was marked differently in the "sex by age" categories (Table 1.3-2). The overall incidence of CHD for men is about 2.5 times of that for women. By taking age into consideration, there is a 13 times difference between men and women in the younger age group (30–44). However, in the older age group (45–62) there is only a twofold difference in the ratio of men to women.

Remarks

1. Table 1.3-2 is adapted from Table 3B that was given in Ref. 6.
2. All risk factors are nothing but random variables. As far as their type is concerned, CHD and SEX are nominal, whereas Age and BP are continuous.

Table 1.3-2. Six-year Incidence Rate of New CHD by Age and Sex

Age at Entry	Incidence Rate
Men	0.0548 (=125/2283)
30–44	0.0249 (=31/1246)
45–62	0.0906 (=94/1047)
Women	0.0214 (=61/2844)
30–44	0.0019 (=3/1543)
45–62	0.0446 (=58/1301)

3. A later study finds more risk factors for cardiovascular disease (CVD)[5]: a history of CVD (HCVD), diabetes (DIAB), smoking (SMOK), blood pressure (BP), and blood lipid concentrations (BLC).

Example 1.3-3. Occupational hazard: Radiation poisoning study[7]

The tragedy of female dial painters attributed to radiation poison is probably the first widely known incident of occupational hazards. Because it was a well-paying job, many young women were attracted to work in the dial-painting industry in the US. Unaware of radium poisoning, a common practice adopted by dial painters was to tip the brushes with their lips in order to provide a fine point for painting. The luminous material usually contained $10\,\mu\text{Ci}$ per gram. As a result, dial painters were exposed to an intake of radium into their bodies. Several years after leaving the plant, the former dial painters began developing a variety of mysterious medical problems. The most common symptoms experienced were horrible teeth and jaw problems. For a most readable story of this deadly glow tragedy see Mullner's book.[11]

The study population is a cohort of 4337 females employed in the US radium-dial industry, which is maintained by the CHR at ANL. This is exactly the same cohort as that of Rowland *et al.*,[13] except that this cohort was enlarged because of extra effort to collect additional subjects after 1976. Ever since data has been consolidated in the CHR at ANL, all located subjects have been followed for vital status since 1967. Death certificates were obtained as soon as the CHR had knowledge of any deaths and is coded (8th International Classification of Diseases) by the National Center for Health Statistics. Usually, an attempt is made to contact all living subjects annually by mail. Subjects would be contacted by telephone if they do not respond. Details of any follow-up method, follow-up period, dose measurement, and others are given in Argonne's internal report. After excluding those with unknown

Table 1.3-3. Rates of Mortality, Bone- and Head Cancer Among the US Female Radium Dial Workers Whose Status are Known till the End of 1984[7]

Group	No.	Mortality	Rate of Bone Sarcoma $(\Pr(X = x))$	Rate of Head Carcinoma $(\Pr(Y = y))$
Measured (=1)	1884	474	(=46/1884)	(=19/1884)
Unmeasured (=0)	1804	656	(=18/1804)	(=5/1804)

birth dates or no social security numbers, only 3688 cases were usable (Table 1.3-3).

Example 1.3-4. Lung cancers and smoking[18]

Although there is some evidence of a greater than average risk in some occupations to develop lung cancer, these occupations could not account for the general increase in pulmonary cancer. It is thought of interest to select a particular population group that is homogeneous economically, with little occupational exposure to respiratory irritants and with equal access to diagnostic facilities. Physicians are believed to represent such a group. Wynder & Cornfield[18] has reported a study on the exposure to tobacco and other possible respiratory irritants on 63 physicians with lung cancer and 133 physicians with cancers in areas where respiratory irritants are not believed to play a part. Among these 133 physicians, 43 cases were of cancer to the stomach and kidney, 45 cases were of cancer to the colon and lymphoma, and 45 cases were cancer of the bladder, leukemia and sarcoma. The data in Table 1.3-4 are taken from Cornfield[3] who only used 43 cases and from those suffering from cancer of the stomach and kidney as a control group. The nonsmoker was defined to be a person who smoked the equivalent of less than one cigarette a day. We are interested in testing whether the data concerning the smoking status in Table 1.3-4 for both cases and controls are misclassified.

Table 1.3-4.   The Mortality Rates of Physicians With and Without Lung Cancers

Smoking Status	Lung Cancer Patients $(X = x)$	$\Pr(X = x)$	Controls $(Y = y)$	$\Pr(Y = y)$
Smoker (=1)	60	0.952 (=60/63)	32	0.744 (=32/43)
Nonsmokers (=0)	3	0.048 (=3/63)	11	0.256 (=11/43)

Remark

Note that, conventionally, we use X (or Y) = 1 if a physician is a smoker; X (or Y) = 0 otherwise, though both X and Y are nominal.

Example 1.3-5. A multicenter study on the effectiveness of using propranolol in treating patients of acute myocardial infarction

Physicians from 10 centers participated in the trial.[18] Patients included those who presented a history of acute myocardial infarction within the preceding 24 hours. The diagnosis, which was confirmed as soon as possible after admission, required meeting any two of the following criteria: characteristic clinical presentation, electrocardiogram changes of recent infarction (pathological Q-waves and ST/T changes), or evidence of acute ischemia (ST/T wave only), elevation of serum-glutamic-oxaloacetic-aminase (SGOT), serum-lactate-dehydrogenase (SLDH), or above normal serum-hydroxybutyric-dehydrogenase (SMBD) for the hospital.

Of the 226 patients who entered the trial, 31 were withdrawn, leaving 195 (155 men and 40 women) for analysis. Twenty mg of Propranolol ("Inderal") or an identical placebo was given orally every 6 hours for 28 days. The study was double-blinded with random allocation of patients to the placebo or treated group. Anticoagulants were given according to the normal practice for

Table 1.3-5. Mortality Rates for the Placebo and Treated Group

Group	Death Rate $(Pr(X = x))$
Treated (=1)	15% (=15/100)
Placebo (=0)	12.6% (=12/95)

each physician. The mortality rates for the placebo and treated group were obtained as given in Table 1.3-5.

Example 1.3-6. A controlled trial on using streptomycin to treat tuberculosis[10]

In 1946 no controlled trial of using streptomycin in treating pulmonary tuberculosis had been undertaken. For research purposes the Committee of the British Medical Research Council decided to use a part of the small supply of streptomycin provided by the US to be employed in a rigorously planned investigation with concurrent controls.

The first patient was admitted in January 1947. By September 1947, 109 patients had been accepted and no more were admitted to this trial. Two patients died within the preliminary observation week. Of the remaining 107 patients, 55 had been allocated to the streptomycin group and 52 to the control group. Determination of whether a patient would be treated by streptomycin and bed-rest (S cases) or by bed-rest alone (C cases) was made by reference to a statistical series based on random sampling numbers drawn up for each sex at each center. The details are given in Ref. 10.

The general trend of results during the course of the trial was followed via the monthly reports from the center. The analysis of results up to six months after the patient's admission is given in Table 1.3-6.

Differences between the S- and C-groups leave no room for doubt. The most outstanding difference is in the category of "considerable improvement" in which 20 patients of the S-group

Table 1.3-6. Assessment of Radiological Appearance on Six Months as Compared with that of Admission

Radiological Assessment (RASS)	S-group	C-group
Considerable improvement (: +2)	0.51 (=28/55)	0.08 (=4/52)
Moderate or slight improvement (: +1)	0.18 (=10/55)	0.25 (=13/52)
No material change (: 0)	0.04 (=2/55)	0.06 (=3/52)
Moderate or slight deterioration (: −1)	0.09 (=9/55)	0.23 (=12/52)
Considerable deterioration (: −2)	0.11 (=6/55)	0.11 (=6/52)
Deaths (: −3)	0.07 (=4/55)	0.27 (=14/52)
Total	1.0	1.0

and only 4 of the C-group were considerably improved. The probability that such a difference occurs by chance is less than one in a million.

Remarks

1. Table 1.3-6 is taken from Table II in Ref. 10.
2. The r.v. RASS in Table 1.3-6 is ordinal. For convenience, we oftentimes use integers to denote the ordered categories, as shown in the parenthesis of column 1 in Table 1.3-6.
3. The test for significance between two proportions will be covered in Chap. 6.

1.4   The Frequency Distribution of the Sample Data

Generally speaking, the population data of a random variable is rarely available. Hence, the most we can do is to collect the sample data, which is a subset of the population data. In principle, the sample data has to be collected with high quality by using the sound sampling technique described in Sec. 1.2.

The sample data has two ways of usage: (i) to construct the frequency distribution of the random variable and (ii) to use them in estimating the value of the unknown population parameters

(μ_X and σ_X^2) of the probability distribution corresponding to the given r.v. X.

A. Constructing the Frequency Distribution

A guiding procedure for constructing the frequency distribution is given as follows:

Step 1. Depending on the sample size, the number of class intervals is chosen so that the average number of observations in each class is at least five;

Step 2. The limits for each class interval must agree with the accuracy of the data;

Step 3. Class intervals of equal width are preferred;

Step 4. The first and the last class interval must contain the smallest and largest observation. Also, class intervals must be mutually exclusive, yet all inclusive.

Step 5. Tally the data into each of the class interval and convert the absolute frequency into the relative frequency.

Remarks

1. Open-ended class interval should be avoided.
2. Use the histogram to display the distribution graphically.

Example 1.4-1. Forced expiratory volume in one second (FEV1)

The data of FEV1 values of 57 medical students are given as follows[2]:

4.47, 3.1, 4.5, 4.9, 3.5, 4.14, 4.32, 4.8, 3.1, 4.68, 4.47, 3.57, 2.85, 5.1, 5.2, 4.8, 5.1, 4.3, 4.7, 4.08, 3.48, 4.2, 3.7, 5.3, 4.71, 4.1, 4.3, 3.39, 3.69, 4.44, 5, 4.5, 4.2, 4.16, 3.7, 3.83, 3.9, 4.47, 3.3, 5.43, 3.42, 3.6, 3.2, 4.56, 4.78, 3.6, 3.96, 3.19, 2.85, 3.04, 3.78, 3.75, 4.05, 3.54, 4.14, 2.98, 3.54.

(a) Find the frequency distribution for the above data set.
(b) Display the frequency distribution graphically.

Solution

(a) Let us follow the guiding procedure described above. The sample size is only 57.

Step 1. Since the average number of observations in each interval should be at least 5, the number of class intervals is at most 11 (=57/5 = 11.4).

Step 2. Let us say that we are interested in only taking eleven intervals. Thus, the equal width of the class interval is determined by using the distance between the largest and the smallest observation divided by 11 as follows:

$$(5.43 - 2.85)/11 = 0.235.$$

Therefore, we use the equal width to be 0.24.

Step 3. Since the first interval has included the smallest observation and the last interval, the largest observation, the frequency distribution is accordingly constructed as follows:

For convenience, we use the positive integers to represent the class intervals accordingly, that is, $X = 1$ means $X = 2.75 - 2.99$, $X = 2$ means $X = 3.00 - 3.24$, and so on.

(b) There are two ways to display Table 1.4-1 graphically: (i) the histogram (Fig. 1.4-1) and (ii) the frequency polygon (Fig. 1.4-2).

Remarks

1. The frequency distribution will be different. It depends on the number of class intervals chosen and the interval width determined. See Exercise 1.6-1 in Sec. 1.6.
2. If the population data are available, we can choose a sufficiently small interval width. Then either the histogram or the polygon will become approximately a continuous curve

Table 1.4-1.   The Frequency Distribution of the FEV1 Data

FEV1 (X = j)	Tally	Absolute Frequency	Relative Frequency $p_j = \Pr(X = j)$
2.75–2.99	///	3	0.053 (=3/57)
3.00–3.24	/////	5	0.088 (=5/57)
3.25–3.49	////	4	0.07 (=4/57)
3.50–3.74	///// ////	9	0.158 (=9/57)
3.75–3.99	/////	5	0.088 (=5/57)
4.00–4.24	///// ///	8	0.14 (=8/57)
4.25–4.49	///// //	7	0.123 (7/57)
4.50–4.74	///// /	6	0.105 (=6/57)
4.75–4.99	////	4	0.07 (=4/57)
5.00–5.24	////	4	0.07 (=4/57)
5.25–5.49	//	2	0.035 (=2/57)
Total		57	1.0

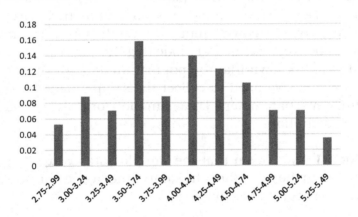

Fig. 1.4-1.   The histogram of FEV1.

that represents the underlying probability distribution of the population data.

B. *Estimation of the Population Parameters*

For a continuous r.v. X, the plot of its probability distribution will be a continuous curve, e.g., the normal random variable in

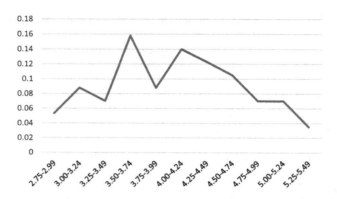

Fig. 1.4-2.   The frequency polygon of FEV1.

Sec. 3.3. Thus, its center can be measured by three parameters: (i) mean (μ_X), (ii) median (med_X) and (iii) mode (mod_X). If the curve is symmetric, these three parameters will reduce to a single parameter. However, if the curve is not symmetric, these three parameters are located differently on the data axis. The median always lies between mean and mode (Fig. 1.4-3).

As it is well-known that the population data for the r.v. X are rarely available, we need to collect the sample data to estimate these unknown parameters. The estimation formula is given in the following definition.

Definition 1.4.1.   Given that the sample data $\{x_1, x_2, \ldots, x_n\}$ are collected from the r.v. X, then the sample mean, median and mode are given, respectively, as follows:

(i) The sample mean (μ_X)

  (a) Ungrouped data

$$\bar{x} = \frac{\sum_{i=1}^{n} x_i}{n}.$$
(1.4.1)

  (b) Grouped data

$$\bar{x}_g = \sum_{j=0}^{k} p_j m_j,$$
(1.4.2)

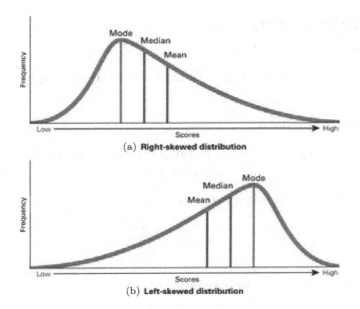

(a) **Right-skewed distribution**

(b) **Left-skewed distribution**

Fig. 1.4-3. **The location of mean, median, and mode of a skewed curve.**

where $\{p_j\}$ and $\{m_j\}$ represent the relative frequency (or $p_j = \Pr(X = j)$) and the midpoint in the jth class interval, and k is the total number of class intervals.

(ii) The sample median ($\widehat{med}_X$)

   (a) Ungrouped data

     Assume that the sample data are re-arranged in an ordered way so that $x_{[1]} \leq x_{[2]} \leq \cdots \leq x_{[n]}$. Then the sample median is given by

$$\widehat{med}_x = \begin{cases} x_{\left[\frac{n+1}{2}\right]}, & \text{if } n \text{ is odd;} \\ \dfrac{x_{[n/2]} + x_{[n/2]+1}}{2}, & \text{if } n \text{ is even.} \end{cases} \qquad (1.4.3)$$

   (b) Grouped data

     $\widehat{med}_{g,X}$ = the data point x_{med} so that the relative frequency of either

$$X \leq x_{med} \quad \text{or} \quad X \geq x_{med} \text{ is } 0.5. \qquad (1.4.4)$$

(iii) The sample mode $(\widehat{mod}_X)$

   (a) Ungrouped data

$$\widehat{mod}_X = \text{the data point has the largest frequency.}$$

(1.4.5)

   (b) Grouped data

$$\widehat{mod}_{g,X} = \text{the midpoint of the class interval that has the largest frequency.}$$

(1.4.6)

(iv) The sample geometric mean $(\bar{x}_{GM})$

$$\bar{x}_{GM} = \sqrt[n]{\prod_{i=1}^{n} x_i}.$$

(1.4.7)

(v) The sample harmonic mean $(\bar{x}_{HM})$

$$\bar{x}_{HM} = \left(\sum_{i=1}^{n} x_i^{-1} / n \right)^{-1}.$$

(1.4.8)

Remarks

1. For a nominal random variable, Eq. (1.4.1) reduces the sample proportion $(\hat{p})$. Note that the population proportion (p) is the key parameter in Bernoulli or Binomial random variable (see Chap. 3).
2. For the sample of a continuous r.v. X, the sample mode estimator does not exist if all the sample data values are distinct.
3. For some random variables used in environmental science, it is deemed appropriate to take the logarithmic transformation first before analyzing the data, say, let $Y = \log(X)$. Then the sample mean of Y is just the harmonic mean of X. For a proof see Exercise 1.6-3.
4. For some random variables we need to take the reciprocal transformation first, say, let $Z = X^{-1}$. Then the sample mean of Z is just the harmonic mean of X. For a proof see Exercise 1.6-4.

5. Since the sample geometric or harmonic mean are seldom employed, the formula for the grouped data is not listed here.

To measure the spread of the probability distribution of X, there are three population parameters that could accomplish this duty: (i) "Mean Deviation" (md_X), (ii) "Variance" (var_X) or "Standard Deviation" (sd_X), or (iii) Interquartile Range (IQR_X). Their sample estimators are given in the following definition.

Definition 1.4.2. Assume that the sample data $\{x_1, x_2, \ldots, x_n\}$ are collected from the continuous r.v. X, then the sample mean deviation, sample variance or sample standard deviation, and sample interquartile range are given, respectively, as follows:

(i) The sample mean deviation $(\widehat{md}_X)$

  (a) Ungrouped data

$$\widehat{md}_X = \frac{\sum_{i=1}^n |x_i - \bar{x}|}{n}. \tag{1.4.9}$$

  (b) Grouped data

$$\widehat{md}_{g,X} = \sum_{j=1}^k p_j |m_j - \bar{x}_g|, \tag{1.4.10}$$

  where m_j and $\bar{x}_g$ denote the midpoint in the jth class interval and the sample mean for the grouped data.

(ii) The sample variance (s_X^2)

  (a) Ungrouped data

$$\widehat{var}_X \equiv s_X^2 = \frac{\sum_{i=1}^n (x_i - \bar{x})^2}{n-1}. \tag{1.4.11}$$

(b) Grouped data

$$\widehat{var}_X \equiv s_{g,X}^2 = \sum_{j=1}^{k} p_j (m_j - \bar{x}_g)^2, \qquad (1.4.12)$$

where $p_j = \Pr(X = j)$.

In addition, the sample standard deviation (s_X) is just the positive square root of the sample variance.

(iii) The sample interquartile range ($\widehat{IQR}_X$)

$$\widehat{IQR}_X = x_{75\%} - x_{25\%}, \qquad (1.4.13)$$

where $x_{25\%}$ and $x_{75\%}$ represent the 25th (or 1st quartile) and 75th (or 3rd quartile) percentile of the sample data distribution.

Remarks

1. The sample standard deviation is also referred to as the standard error of the sample mean.
2. The denominator n − 1 of Eq. (1.4.11) has an interpretation in terms of "degrees of freedom". Originally, a random sample $\{x_1, x_2, \ldots, x_n\}$ of size n has n degrees of freedom since they provide n independent pieces of information about the r.v. X. But, n sample deviations $d_i (\equiv x_i - \bar{x})$, $i = 1, \ldots, n$ has only n − 1 degrees of freedom since they provide only n − 1 rather than n independent pieces of information. See Exercise 1.6-7 for a proof.
3. For the ungrouped data, we sometimes cannot find the exact 25th or 75th percentile of X. Instead, we use the closest approximation to substitute for them (Example 1.4-3). However, there is a better way to find them by using the notion of order statistics in Chap. 8 (Example 8.1-1). The concept of the $100p^{th}$ percentile will be covered formally in Chap. 3.

Example 1.4-2

Find the sample (i) mean, (ii) median and (iii) mode for (a) the ungrouped data given in Example 1.4-1, and (b) the grouped data in Table 1.4-1.

Solution

(a) (i) By using Eq. (1.4.1), the sample mean is given by

$$
\begin{aligned}
\bar{x} = (&4.47 + 3.1 + 4.5 + 4.9 + 3.5 + 4.14 + 4.32 + 4.8 + 3.1 \\
&+ 4.68 + 4.47 + 3.57 + 2.85 + 5.1 + 5.2 + 4.8 + 5.1 \\
&+ 4.3 + 4.7 + 4.08 + 3.48 + 4.2 + 3.7 + 5.3 + 4.71 \\
&+ 4.1 + 4.3 + 3.39 + 3.69 + 4.44 + 5 + 4.5 + 4.2 + 4.16 \\
&+ 3.7 + 3.83 + 3.9 + 4.47 + 3.3 + 5.43 + 3.42 + 3.6 \\
&+ 3.2 + 4.56 + 4.78 + 3.6 + 3.96 + 3.19 + 2.85 + 3.04 \\
&+ 3.78 + 3.75 + 4.05 + 3.54 + 4.14 + 2.98 + 3.54)/57 \\
= \;&4.060702.
\end{aligned}
$$

(ii) Let us use the stem-and-leaf technique to rearrange the data in an ordered way. The idea is to separate each observation into two parts: stem and leaf. Then, collect the stems together to plot accordingly on the left side and the leaves on the right side of a vertical line. In this data set, the integer part is chosen as the stem with the decimal part as the leaf. First, we have only four stems: 2, 3, 4 and 5. Then, we list them on the left side and then put the leaf of each observation one-by-one behind their stem on the right side, as follows:

Second, let us order the leaves behind each stem in Fig. 1.4-4.

Since the sample size 57 is an odd number, the median is the 29th term in Fig. 1.4-5. There are 3 and 23 terms behind stems 2 and 3, respectively. Accordingly, the

```
2| 85 85 98
3| 10 50 10 57 48 70 39 69 70 83 90 30 42 60 20 60 96 19
       04 78 75 54 54
   4| 47 50 90 14 32 80 68 47 80 30 70 08 20 71 10 30 44 50
       20 16 47 56 78 05 14
   5| 10 20 10 30 00 43
```

Fig. 1.4-4.   A stem-and leaf plot of the FEV1 data.

```
2| 85 85 98
3| 04 10 10 19 20 30 39 42 48 50 54 54 57 60 60 69 70 70
       75 78 83 90 96
   4| 05 08 10 14 14 16 20 20 30 30 32 44 47 47 47 50 50 56
       68 70 71 78 80 80 90
   5| 00 10 10 20 30 43
```

Fig. 1.4-5.   An ordered stem-and leaf plot of the FEV1 data.

29th term is the 3rd term behind stem 4. Therefore, the sample median is 4.10.

(iii) From the ordered stem-and-leaf in Fig. 1.4-5 we note that the data values 2.85, 3.10, 3.54, 3.60, 3.70, 4.14, 4.20, 4.30, 4.50, 4.80 and 5.10 all have the frequency 2, whereas the data value 4.47 has the frequency three, which is the largest. Hence, the sample mode is 4.47.

(b)   (i) By putting the midpoint in Table 1.4-1 we have
By multiplying the entries in column 2 with that of column 5, the sample mean of Eq. (1.4.2) for the grouped data of Table 1.4-1 is given by the last entry in column 4, namely,

$$\bar{x}_g = 4.06175.$$

(ii) After adding the relative frequency in the class intervals from 2.75–2.99 to 3.75–3.99 in Table 1.4-1 we have the sum to be 0.457. The deviation from the half of the total probability 0.5 is 0.043 (=0.5–0.457). By assuming the relative frequency in the class interval 4.00–4.24 is evenly distributed, we then calculate the sample median

Table 1.4-2. Calculation of the Sample Mean for the Grouped Data

FEV1	Relative Frequency (p_j)	Midpoint (m_i)	$m_j \times p_j$
2.75–2.99	0.053 (=3/57)	2.87	0.15211
3.00–3.24	0.088 (=5/57)	3.12	0.27456
3.25–3.49	0.07 (=4/57)	3.37	0.2359
3.50–3.74	0.158 (=9/57)	3.62	0.57196
3.75–3.99	0.088 (=5/57)	3.87	0.34056
4.00–4.24	0.14 (=8/57)	4.12	0.5768
4.25–4.49	0.123 (=7/57)	4.37	0.53751
4.50–4.74	0.105 (=6/57)	4.62	0.4851
4.75–4.99	0.07 (=4/57)	4.87	0.3409
5.00–5.24	0.07 (=4/57)	5.12	0.3584
5.25–5.49	0.035 (=2/57)	5.37	0.18795
Total	1.0		4.06175

by using Eq. (1.4.4) as follows:

$$\widehat{med}_{g,X} = 4.00 + \frac{0.043}{0.14} \times 0.24 = 4.0737143 \approx 4.074.$$

(iii) The largest frequency in Table 1.4-1 is 9 of the class interval 3.50–3.74. By using Eq. (1.4.7), the sample mode for Table 1.4-1 is given by the midpoint of the interval 3.50–3.74, namely,

$$\widehat{mod}_{g,X} = \frac{3.50 + 3.74}{2} = 3.62.$$

Example 1.4-3

Find the sample (i) mean deviation, (ii) standard deviation and (iii) interquartile range, respectively, for (a) the ungrouped data in Example 1.4-1, and (b) the grouped data in Table 1.4-1.

Solution

(a)   (i) By using Eq. (1.4.9) we have

$$\widehat{md}_X = (|4.47 - 4.060702| + |3.1 - 4.060702|$$
$$+ |4.5 - 4.060702| + |4.9 - 4.060702|$$
$$+ |3.5 - 4.060702| + \cdots + |4.14 - 4.060702|$$
$$+ |2.98 - 4.060702| + |3.54 - 4.060702|)/57$$
$$= 0.562419.$$

(ii) By using Eq. (1.4.11) we have

$$\widehat{var}_X \equiv s_X^2 = (4.47 - 4.060702)^2 + (3.1 - 4.060702)^2$$
$$+ (4.5 - 4.060702)^2 + (3.5 - 4.060702)^2 + \cdots$$
$$+ (4.14 - 4.060702)^2 + (2.98 - 4.060702)^2$$
$$+ (3.54 - 4.060702)^2]/(57 - 1)$$
$$= 4.133214.$$

Therefore, $s_X = \sqrt{s_X^2} = \sqrt{4.133214} = 2.033031 \approx 2.033$.

(iii) The total number of 57 observations divides the x-axis into 58 subintervals. By assuming that the areas for each subinterval are the same and the total area under the probability distribution curve is one, we have, by using Fig. 1.4-4, that the 14th, 15th, 43rd and 44th terms are the 24.1^{th} (=14/58), 25.4^{th} (=15/58), 74.1^{th} (=43/58) and 75.4^{th} (=44/58) percentile, namely,

$$x_{24.1\%} = 3.54, x_{25.4\%} = 3.54, x_{74.1\%} = 4.50, x_{75.4\%} = 4.56.$$

As a result, the sample interquartile range is given by using Eq. (1.4.13)

$$\widehat{IQR}_X = x_{75.4\%} - x_{25.4\%} = 4.56 - 3.54 = 1.02.$$

(b) (i) By using Eq. (1.4.10) we have from Table 1.4-2

$$\widehat{md}_{g,X} = 0.053 \times |2.87 - 4.06175| + 0.088$$
$$\times |3.12 - 4.06175| + 0.07 \times |3.37 - 4.06175|$$
$$+ 0.158 \times |3.62 - 4.06175| + 0.088$$
$$\times |3.87 - 4.06175| + 0.14 \times |4.12 - 4.06175|$$
$$+ 0.123 \times |4.37 - 4.06175| + 0.105$$
$$\times |4.62 - 4.06175| + 0.07 \times |4.87 - 4.06175|$$
$$+ 0.07 \times |5.12 - 4.06175| + 0.035$$
$$\times |5.37 - 4.06175| = 0.56226 \approx 0.562.$$

(ii) By using Eq. (1.4.12), we have

$$\widehat{var}_{g,X} \equiv s_{g,X}^2 = 0.053 \times (2.87 - 4.06175)^2 + 0.088$$
$$\times (3.12 - 4.06175)^2 + 0.07 \times (3.37 - 4.06175)^2$$
$$+ 0.158 \times (3.62 - 4.06175)^2 + 0.088$$
$$\times (3.87 - 4.06175)^2 + 0.14 \times (4.12 - 4.06175)^2$$
$$+ 0.123 \times (4.37 - 4.06175)^2 + 0.105$$
$$\times (4.62 - 4.06175)^2 + 0.07 \times (4.87 - 4.06175)^2$$
$$+ 0.07 \times (5.12 - 4.06175)^2 + 0.035$$
$$\times (5.37 - 4.06175)^2 = 0.449794.$$

Therefore, $s_{g,X} = \sqrt{0.449794} = 0.670667 \approx 0.67$.

(iii) We assume that the probability is evenly distributed over each class interval. First, we note that the 25th and 75th percentiles lie in the class interval of 3.50–3.74 and 4.50–4.74, respectively. Second, by using the linear interpolation technique we get

$$x_{25\%} = 3.50 + 0.24 \times \frac{0.25 - (0.053 + 0.088 + 0.07)}{0.158} \approx 3.559,$$

and

$$x_{75\%} = 4.50 + 0.24 \times \frac{0.75 - (0.053 + 0.088 + \cdots + 0.123)}{0.105}$$

$$\approx 4.569.$$

Thus, we have by using Eq. (1.4.13)

$$\widehat{IQR}_X = x_{75\%} - x_{25\%} = 4.569 - 3.559 = 1.01.$$

Remarks

1. If the readers are not familiar with the linear interpolation technique, please see Chap. 11 in my book on college algebra.[8]
2. Please compare the result here in (a) (iii) with that of Example 8.1-1.

1.5   Exercises

1. Redo Example 1.4-1 with the class interval as 2.50–2.99, 3.00–3.49, 3.50–3.99,..., and 5.00–5.49.
2. Show that n sample deviations are not independent by showing that the sum of n sample deviations is zero, namely, $\sum_{i=1}^{n}(x_i - \bar{x}) = 0$.
3. Let $Y = \log(X)$, where X be a positive random variable. Show that the sample mean of Y is the geometric mean of X, namely, $\bar{y} = \bar{x}_{GM}$.
4. Let $Z = X^{-1}$, where X is a positive random variable. Show that the sample mean of Z is the harmonic mean of X, namely, $\bar{z} = \bar{x}_{HM}$.

References

1. Berkson J. (1946) Limitations of the application of fourfold table analysis to hospital data. *Biometrics* **2**: 47–51.
2. Bland M. https:\\www-users.york.ac.uk/~mb55/datasets/fev57.dct.
3. Cornfield J. (1956) A statistical problem arising from the retrospective studies. *Proc Third Brkeley on Math Statist and Prob* **4**: 135–148.

4. Dawber TR, Meadors GF, Moore FE. (1951) Epidemiological approaches to heart disease: The Framingham Study. *Am J Public Health* **41**: 279–286.
5. Kannel WB. (2000) The Framingham Study: Its 50-year legacy and future promise. *J Atheroscler Thromb* **6**: 60–66.
6. Kannel WB, Dawber TR, Kagan A, *et al.* (1961) Factors of risk in the development of coronary heart disease — Six-year follow-up experience: The Framingham Study. *Ann Intern Med* **55**: 33–50.
7. Lee T-S. (2012) A Poisson regression model with interaction for female radium dial workers. *J Mod Appl Stat Methods* **11**: 233–241.
8. Lee T-S. (2015) *College Algebra: Historical Notes.* Applied Math Press, Lilburn, Georgia.
9. Levy PS, Lemeshow S. (1991) *Sampling of Populations: Methods and Applications.* Wiley, New York.
10. Streptomycin treatment of pulmonary tuberculosis (1948). *Br Med J* October 30, 769–782.
11. Mullner R. (1999) *Deadly Glow: The Radium Dial Worker Tragedy.* American Public Health Association, Washington, DC.
12. QuickStats: Number of deaths from 10 leading causes — National vital statistics system, United States, 2010 (2013). Morbidity and Mortality Weekly Report (MMWR), March 1, **62**: 155.
13. Rowland RE, Stehney AF, Lucas HF. (1978) Dose-response relationships for female radium workers. *Radiat Res* **76**: 368–383.
14. Snow PJD. (1965) Effect of propranolol in myocardial infarction. *Lancet* **286**: 551–553.
15. United States Cancer Statistics: Top 10 Cancer Sites (2012). https://nccd.cdc.gov/uscs/toptencancers.aspx.
16. Wald A. (1947) *Sequential Analysis.* Dover Publications, Inc., New York.
17. White C. (1953) Sampling in medical research. *Br Med J* **12**: 1284–1288.
18. Wynder EL, Cornfield J. (1953) Cancer of the lung in physicians. *New Engl J Med* **248**: 441–444.

Chapter **2** **Probability**

2.0 A Brief History of Probability

According to legend the notion of probability began in 1654 when B Pascal (1623–1662, French) solved two problems and then wrote to P de Fermat (1601–1665, French). However, in fine details this is inaccurate. Still, like so many persisting legends, the story of 1654 encapsulates the truth. The decade around 1660 was the birth time of probability. Why was it not earlier?

The seed of probability was "chance" (or "randomness"). The word of chance was, indeed, seeded much earlier than 1654 in the Eastern/Western culture. On one hand, stories about dicing occur frequently in Indian literature. Indian mathematical texts, dated about the end of the ninth century AD, contained a rich source of exercises in probability. On the other hand, deciding by lot is familiar in the Talmud, the Old Testament in the Bible. Although early probability calculations are few in number, a short list includes:

(i) Calculations for the throw of three dice in a poem in Latin, probably written in France in the 13th century;
(ii) Solution to the problem of points for two players and equally likely outcomes in an early 15th-century Italian manuscript;
(iii) Written discussions concerning the problem of points by Italian Mathematicians G Cardano (1501–1576), L Pacioli (1447–1517), GF Peverone and N Tartaglia (1500–1557) between 1490 and 1605;
(iv) Calculations on card and dice games by G Cardano; and

■ 34

(v) Calculation of probability of the sum of the points on throwing three dice shown by G Galilei (1564–1642, Italian).

From this list it shows that the idea of numerical discussion and evaluation of chances was present in Europe, at least from the 13th century.

But then what is new about the era of 1660? The duality of probability, the degree of belief warranted by evidence and stable long-run frequencies in repeated trials finally blossomed.[8] Since then it has continued to blossom into many areas: insurance and annuities in the 17th century, theory of measurements in the 18th century, biometrics in the 19th century, and agricultural and medical experiments in the 20th century.

2.1 Mathematical/Statistical Probability

Regardless of whether we like it or not, we are facing all kinds of uncertainty in our daily life. Probability is just a numerical number to assess rationally the degree of certainty regarding the occurrence of an event. A rudimentary definition is given as follows.

Definition 2.1.1. Let E be an event that is comprised of (observable, yet unpredictable) favorite outcomes. Then the probability of E, denoted by $Pr(E)$, is a nonnegative number between 0 and 1, namely, $0 \leq Pr(E) \leq 1$.

Remarks

1. If $Pr(E) = 0$, then E is called the impossible event, while E is the certain event if $Pr(E) = 1$.
2. "Probability" is intrinsically different from "possibility". Probability is a precise numerical quantity, whereas possibility is a vague qualitative concept.
3. There are two ways of calculating the probability of an event: (i) theoretical (or mathematical) and (ii) empirical (or statistical). Theoretically, there are two schools that differ on

calculation: (i) Bernoulli's relative frequency, and (ii) Laplace's equipossibility assumption. Empirically, the statistical probability is data-dependent, which is calculated by basing it on the collected data. In this book, the probability we are referring to is the statistical one. For a calculation on mathematical probability, see Chap. 19 in Ref. 10.

A useful notion in medical statistics that is alternative to probability is the odds given in the following definition.

Definition 2.1.2. The odds of an event E, denoted by od(E), is defined as

$$od(E) = Pr(E)/(1 - Pr(E)). \qquad (2.1.1)$$

Remarks

1. If E denotes the event of a rare disease, $od(E) = Pr(E)$.
2. The odds ratio that is the ratio of the odds for two binary random variables is an important index for testing whether these two random variables are independent. See Chap. 11 for details.

To measure the disease frequency, the following two terminologies are useful:

Definition 2.1.3. Let E be an event of the occurrence of a disease. Then the prevalence of E in a population is defined as the proportion of people who have a disease, that is,

$$Prevalence\,(\%) = \frac{\#\ of\ people\ with\ disease}{\#\ of\ people\ in\ the\ population} \times 100\%.$$

$$(2.1.2)$$

Remarks

The prevalence of E is also called the risk of E in epidemiology.

Definition 2.1.4. Let E be an event of the occurrence of a disease. Then the incidence of E is defined as the proportion of the number of new cases of disease that develop over time in the population, that is,

$$\text{Incidence of E} = \frac{\text{\# of new cases of disease}}{\text{population without disease at baseline}} \times 100\%.$$

(2.1.3)

or

$$\text{Incidence of E} = \frac{\text{\# of new cases of disease}}{\text{person time at risk}} \times 100\%.$$

(2.1.4)

Example 2.1-1

Suppose that a school authority was trying to find out the proportion of the school's students with anxiety disorder. A standardized test for anxiety disorder was administered to 200 second-year medical students. As a result of this test, 16 met the definition of anxiety disorder. What is the prevalence of anxiety disorder among second-year medical students?

Solution

By using Eq. (2.1.2), the prevalence is given by $(16/200) \cdot 100\% = 8\%$.

Example 2.1-2

Assume that there are 400 medical students at Z-University in January 2011, and 6 new cases of influenza develop from January to March. What is the incidence of influenza infection among Z-University medical students during the 3-month period from January to March 2011?

Solution

By using Eq. (2.1.4), we have

$$\text{Incidence} = 6\,\text{cases}/(400\,\text{students} \times 3\,\text{months})$$

$$= 6\,\text{cases}/1200\,\text{person} - \text{months}$$

$$= 0.005 \text{ cases/person} - \text{months}$$

$$= 5 \text{ cases per } 1000 \text{ person} - \text{months.}$$

Example 2.1-3

The Charlottesville Blood Pressure Survey[3] was started in January 1974. A total of 12,371 persons aged 15 or over were screened. The screening was conducted by students of the University of Virginia Medical Center. Staff physicians conducted regular sessions to instruct the screeners how to interview, administer questionnaires and measure blood pressure. Blood pressure was measured with an aneroid sphygmomanometer and a stethe in the right arm of the subject, who is at rest in the sitting position for five minutes at each of his/her three consecutive visits one week apart.

The criteria for hypertension was defined as the diastolic blood pressure (DBP) $\geq$ 90 mm Hg if the person's age was $<$ 55 years, or DBP $\geq$ 100 mm Hg if the person's age was $\geq$ 55 years. Because blood-pressure readings were measured more than once, hypertension was further classified as "sustained" if all three blood-pressure readings were elevated or "labile" if one or more, but not all three including the home blood-pressure reading, were elevated.

Comparing with four previous studies with only one blood-pressure measurement (Table 2.1-1), the prevalence of the Charlottesville study is the lowest (12.5%), very close to that of the Alameda study (13%).

Remarks

1. After taking multiple repeated readings into consideration, the prevalence of the Charlottesville study is lowered further to 6.8%. It is possible that a small decrease is due to the effect of regression towards the mean when the samples are reevaluated (see Sec. 7.1).
2. Another reasonable explanation for the decrease in blood pressure with subsequent measurements is that the baseline blood pressure is shifting in adolescents and young adults.[3]

Table 2.1-1. The Prevalence of 5 Studies

Location	Year	No. of Patients	No. of Visits	Prevalence*
Baldwin County	1962	3,084	1	0.175
National Health Survey	1960–1962	6,672	1	0.152
Alameda County	1966	2,495	1	0.13
Atlanta community	1970	5,947	1	0.281
Charlottesville community	1974	12,371	1	0.125
			≥3	0.068

*The hypertension of a patient is defined as his/her systolic/diastolic blood pressure ≥160/95 mm Hg.

2.2 Basic Laws For Probability

For more than one event, some operational rules for probability are needed. Let E and F be two events. Thus, three operational rules are given as follows.

Theorem 2.2.1. *Let E and F be two events that are subsets of the outcome space S.*

(i) *Complementary Rule*

$$Pr(E^c) = 1 - Pr(E), \qquad (2.2.1)$$

where $E^c (= S \backslash E)$ is the complement of E.

(ii) *Addition Rule*

$$Pr(E \cup F) = Pr(E) + Pr(F) - Pr(E \cap F). \qquad (2.2.2)$$

or if E and F are disjoint, then Eq. (2.2.2) is reduced to

$$Pr(E \cup F) = Pr(E) + Pr(F). \qquad (2.2.3)$$

(iii) *De Morgan's Law*

$$Pr[(E \cup F)^c] = Pr(E^c \cap F^c). \qquad (2.2.4)$$

Remarks

1. The complement of E is sometimes denoted by other symbols like E' or $\overline{E}$.
2. The proof of Theorem 2.2.1 can be found in Ref. 10; hence it is omitted here.

2.3   Conditional Probability

Whenever additional information is known, it can be incorporated into the calculation of the probability of an event through the concept of conditional probability, given as follows.

Definition 2.3.1.   Assume that event F has occurred. Then the conditional probability of E given F, denoted by Pr(E|F), is defined as

$$Pr(E|F) = Pr(E \cap F) / Pr(F). \tag{2.3.1}$$

If E and F are independent, then Eq. (2.3.2) is reduced to

$$Pr(E|F) = Pr(E). \tag{2.3.2}$$

Remarks

1. By multiplying the denominator of the right side of Eq. (2.3.1) to the left side, we end up with a new operational rule to add it to Theorem 2.2.1, that is,

   (iv) **Multiplication Rule**

   $$Pr(E \cap F) = Pr(E|F) \times Pr(F), \tag{2.3.3}$$

   If E and F are independent, then Eq. (2.3.3) is reduced to

   $$Pr(E \cap F) = Pr(E) \times Pr(F). \tag{2.3.4}$$

2. Given that F has occurred, the conditional probability Pr(E|F) is usually greater than the unconditional probability Pr(E). However, Eq. (2.3.2) implies that the conditional probability equals the unconditional one, provided that E and F are independent.

3. In terms of Bayesian terminology, the conditional probability is called the posterior probability of E, while the unconditional probability $Pr(E)$ is called the prior probability of E.

Theorem 2.3.1 (Bayes' theorem). *Assume that the sample space S is decomposed as the union of two disjoint events E_1 and E_2. Then,*

$$Pr(E_1|F) = \frac{Pr(F|E_1)Pr(E_1)}{Pr(F|E_1)Pr(E_1) + Pr(F|E_2)Pr(E_2)}. \tag{2.3.5}$$

Remarks

1. Equation (2.3.5) could be extended accordingly so that S is the union of k ($k \geq 3$) mutually disjoint events $\{E_j\}, j = 1, 2, \ldots, k$.
2. If we are interested in evaluating the degree of evidence provided by the collected data to test the hypothesis, an index called the "Bayes factor" is used to measure it. Let H and D denote the null hypothesis and the evidence supplied by the data. Thus, the Bayes factor is defined by

$$BF(D) = Pr(D|H) / Pr(D|H^c). \tag{2.3.6}$$

The right side of Eq. (2.3.6) is interpreted as the likelihood that the null hypothesis is true based on the evidence supplied by the collected data. An interesting relationship between the prior and posterior odds that the null hypothesis is true is obtained by applying Eqs. (2.1.1) and (2.3.1) as follows:

$$od(H|D) = \frac{Pr(H|D)}{Pr(H^c|D)} = \frac{Pr(D|H)}{Pr(D|H^c)} \times \frac{Pr(H)}{Pr(H^c)}$$

$$= BF(D) \times od(H). \tag{2.3.7}$$

Equation (2.3.7) implies that the posterior odds of the hypothesis equals the product of the Bayes factor and the prior odds of the hypothesis.

  More will be said in Chap. 4.

Example 2.3-1

Assume that roughly 6% of pregnant women attending a pre-natal clinic at a large urban hospital have bacteriuria (bacteria in the urine). Furthermore, assume that 30% of bacteriuria and 1% of non-bacteriuria pregnant women proceed to develop pyelonephritis. With the knowledge that a pregnant woman has developed pyelonephritis, what is the probability that she had bacteriuria?

Solution

Let E_1 and E_2 denote whether a woman has and does not have bacteriuria, respectively; and F be the occurrence of pyelonephritis. Thus, we have from the given information

$$Pr(E_1) = 0.06, \quad Pr(E_2) = 1 - 0.06 = 0.94,$$
$$Pr(F|E_1) = 0.3, \quad \text{and} \quad Pr(F|E_2) = 0.01.$$

By using Eq. (2.3.5), we have

$$Pr(E_1|F) = (0.3 \times 0.06)/(0.3 \times 0.06 + 0.01 \times 0.94) = 0.66.$$

Hence, the (conditional) probability that she had bacteriuria, given that she has developed pyelonephritis, is 0.66.

2.4 Sensitivity and Specificity

In screening a large population for a disease, the used diagnostic test is never 100% certain. This leads to the following notion for assessing its accuracy. The eight elements of a proper clinical evaluation of a diagnostic test is given in Ref. 7.

Definition 2.4.1. Let two binary random variables D and T denote the disease and diagnostic test, respectively. Assume that the sample data are cross-classified into Table 2.4-1.

Table 2.4-1. The Result of a Diagnostic Test for a Disease

Test Result (T)	Disease Status (D)		Total
	Present (= 1)	Absent (= 0)	
Positive (= 1)	a	b	a + b
Negative (= 0)	c	d	c + d
Total	a + c	b + d	n = a + b + c + d

Then the (estimated) sensitivity (Se), specificity (Sp), probabilities of false-positives (α) and -negatives (β) are defined, respectively, by

$$Se = Pr(T = 1|D = 1) = a/(a + c), \qquad (2.4.1)$$

$$Sp = Pr(T = 0|D = 0) = d/(b + d), \qquad (2.4.2)$$

$$\alpha = Pr(T = 1|D = 0) = b/(b + d), \qquad (2.4.3)$$

and

$$\beta = Pr(T = 0|D = 1) = c/(a + c). \qquad (2.4.4)$$

Remarks

1. Equation (2.4.1) is the conditional probability that the test truly detects the diseased, hence it represents the diagnostic ability of the test to detect diseases, whereas Eq. (2.4.2) is the conditional probability that the test truly detects the nondiseased; as a result, it represents the power of the test for detecting nondiseased. Also, it can be shown (see Exercise 2.5-1) that $Se = 1 - \beta$ and $Sp = 1 - \alpha$.

2. Incidentally, Eqs. (2.4.3) and (2.4.4) are also called errors of the first and second kind corresponding to the type I and II errors in Neyman's theory of hypothesis testing, which is covered in Chap. 4.

3. For a fixed sample size n, there is an inverse relationship between Se and Sp (see Fig. 2.4-1). Generally, β is the less important error to avoid. In practical applications, the physician

decides what is the acceptable level of α. For example, α might be established to be as small as 0.01 (or 1%) or even less for tuberculosis, whereas the physician might tolerate the level of α to be as high as 0.10 (or 10%) for bronchial asthma (see Example 2.4-2).

4. In epidemiology, there are two other measures, which are the positive predictive value (PPV) and negative predictive value (NPV). They are defined by:

$$PPV = Pr(D = 1|T = 1) = a/(a + b), \qquad (2.4.5)$$

and

$$NPV = Pr(D = 0|T = 0) = d/(c + d). \qquad (2.4.6)$$

Again, Eq. (2.4.5) is the conditional probability that the positive test predicts the patient being the diseased, namely, it represents the prognostic ability of the diseased for the positive test, whereas Eq. (2.4.6) is the conditional probability that the negative test predicts the patient being the nondiseased, or the prognostic ability of the nondiseased for the negative test.

5. By using Bayes' theorem, the predictive values of the PPV and NPV can be expressed in terms of Se, Sp and the prevalence of the disease $Pr(D = 1)$ (see Exercise 2.5-2) as follows:

$$PPV = \frac{Pr(D = 1) \times Se}{Pr(D = 1) \times Se + Pr(D = 0) \times \beta}, \qquad (2.4.7)$$

and

$$NPV = \frac{Pr(D = 0) \times Sp}{Pr(D = 0) \times Sp + Pr(D = 1) \times \alpha}. \qquad (2.4.8)$$

Vice versa, the sensitivity and specificity can be expressed in terms of the PPV, NPV and $Pr(T = 1)$ (see Exercise 2.5-3) as follows:

$$Se = \frac{PPV \times Pr(T = 1)}{PPV \times Pr(T = 1) + (1 - NPV) \times Pr(T = 0)}, \qquad (2.4.9)$$

and

$$Sp = \frac{NPV \times Pr(T = 0)}{NPV \times Pr(T = 0) + (1 - PPV) \times Pr(T = 1)}. \qquad (2.4.10)$$

6. In clinical practice the PPV/NPV is more useful than that of Se/Sp. In fact, the sensitivity/specificity is of limited relevance to practice because Se/Sp has no direct diagnostic interpretation. Many reports have demonstrated that Se/Sp are prone to vary across different populations owing to selection bias. Indeed, empirical evidences have shown that Se, Sp and the likelihood ratio vary not only across different populations, but also across different subgroups within particular populations.[11] For example, the sensitivity of the electrocardio graphic test was 0.65 for men and 0.3 for women, 0.61 for smokers and 0.52 for nonsmokers, and 0.39 for patients with one diseased vessel and 0.77 for patients with three diseased vessels, while the specificity was 0.89 for men and 0.97 for women. Therefore, in diagnostic studies the emphasis should be placed on clinical impact rather than on accuracy.[12]
7. Whether Se/Sp and/or PPV/NPV are constants depends on the causal assumptions: diagnostic, predictive and correlational.[4] Any claim that the sensitivity and specificity of testing one clinical population is the same as those in another clinical population must be empirically documented.

Example 2.4-1

Assume that the collected sample data are cross-classified into Table 2.4-2. Estimate the sensitivity/specificity and probabilities of false positive and false negative values of the given diagnostic test.

Solution

By using Eqs. (2.4.1) to (2.4.4), the estimates for the sensitivity/specificity and probabilities of false positives and false negatives of the given diagnostic test are obtained from Table 2.4-2 as

Table 2.4-2.   The Result of a Diagnostic Test for a Disease

Test Result (T)	Disease status (D)		Total
	Present (=1)	Absent (=0)	
Positive (= 1)	4	5	9
Negative (= 0)	1	90	91
Total	5	95	100

follows:

$$\hat{S}_e = \frac{4}{5} = 0.8, \quad \hat{S}_p = \frac{90}{95} = 0.947,$$

$$\hat{\alpha} = \frac{5}{95} = 0.053, \quad \text{and} \quad \hat{\beta} = \frac{1}{5} = 0.2.$$

Remarks

1. Since the data in Table 2.4-2 is the sample data, all we can do is to estimate the population parameters defined by Eqs. (2.4.1) and (2.4.2). Therefore, we add the hat to the population parameters (Se and Sp) to indicate that they are the sample estimates.
2. If only a subsample of those patients tested received eventual disease verification, there exists a verification bias in the estimation of the diagnostic accuracy. Adjustment for the verification bias is considered in Ref. 1.
3. A single test is never adequate for a physician to reach his/her final decision in clinical practice, because many variables (symptoms/signs) entering into each diagnosis are caused by the same underlying disease and hence are correlated. A multivariate analysis should be sought.[11]

Example 2.4-2

Six dichotomous questions were selected from a questionnaire form given to 230 patients with a clinical diagnosis of bronchial asthma, and a group of 517 randomly selected patients who were known to be free of asthma.[5] The specific set of questions tested were as follows:

	Yes	No
In the past year or two have you had:		

1. Shortness of breath that awakens you from sleep?

2. Shortness of breath with asthmatic (wheezing) breathing?

3. Coughing up of yellow or green sputum?

In the past year or two have you had a tight feeling or pain in your chest:

4. When angry or excited?

5. That awakens you at night?

6. That lasts more than five minutes?

Although there are $64(=2^6)$ possible combinations of answers to six questions, only 55 combinations occurred in this population sample. In order to determine the sensitivity and specificity for this screening test, we used the idea of a likelihood ratio to discriminate patients with bronchial asthma (D) from the nonasthma (N). For a set of symptoms (S) defined by the above six questions, let $p(S|D)$ and $p(S|N)$ denote the probability of a patient who has the set of symptoms between the asthma and nonasthma patients, respectively. Then the likelihood ratio is defined by

$$\lambda = p(S|D)/p(S|N). \qquad (1)$$

To calculate $p(S|D)$ and $p(S|N)$ in columns 2 and 3 of Table 2.4-3, we tally respectively the number of "yes" answers to each of the 55 combinations of six questions for asthma and nonasthma patients and calculate the relative frequencies to serve as the estimate for the true probabilities of $p(S|D)$ and $p(S|N)$. The details can be found in Table 2 in Ref. 5. Afterwards, we calculate the values of λ by using Eq. (1).

Then the values of λ is arranged in an increasing order as in column 1 of Table 2.4-3. Corresponding to each value of λ, the

Table 2.4-3.   The Values of the Likelihood Ratio (λ), Sensitivity (Se), Specificity (Sp), Probabilities of False-positives (α), and -negatives (β) for Screening the Asthma and Nonasthma Patients*

λ	p(S|D)	p(S|N)	Asthma Patients $\geq \lambda$		Nonasthma Patients $< \lambda$	
			Se	α	Sp	β
0.0	0	0.135	1.0	0.0	0.0	1.0
0.09	0.004	0.046	1.0	0.0	0.135	0.865
0.10	0.070	0.683	0.996	0.004	0.182	0.818
0.28	0.004	0.015	0.926	0.074	0.865	0.135
0.34	0.022	0.064	0.922	0.078	0.880	0.120
0.50	0.004	0.010	0.900	0.100	0.944	0.056
2.25	0.004	0.002	0.896	0.104	0.954	0.046
3.37	0.013	0.004	0.891	0.109	0.956	0.044
4.50	0.009	0.002	0.878	0.122	0.959	0.041
6.74	0.117	0.017	0.870	0.130	0.961	0.039
8.24	0.048	0.006	0.752	0.248	0.979	0.021
12.92	0.010	0.008	0.704	0.296	0.985	0.015
20.23	0.078	0.004	0.604	0.396	0.992	0.008
24.73	0.048	0.002	0.526	0.473	0.996	0.004
33.72	0.065	0.002	0.478	0.522	0.998	0.002
∞	0.413	0.0	0.413	0.587	1.0	0.0

*This table is adapted from Table 3 in Ref. 5.

sensitivity/specificity of α and β were calculated according to Eqs. (2.4.1-4) that were listed in columns 4 to 7 respectively of Table 2.4-3.

To determine the appropriate sensitivity and specificity for this screening test, we need to specify the acceptable level of α. For bronchial asthma, it is all right to choose the acceptable level of α to be as high as 0.10 (or 10%). After locating this value in column 5 in Table 2.4-3, we found Se = 0.90 (or 90%), Sp = 0.944 (or 94.4%), and $\beta = 0.056$ (or 5.6%) with corresponding $\lambda = 0.5$.

A scatter plot of (Se, Sp) is presented in Fig. 2.4-1. The inverse relationship between sensitivity and specificity is vividly seen in Fig. 2.4-1.

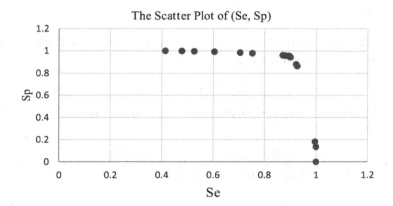

Figure 2.4-1. **The inverse relation between sensitivity and specificity**

Remarks

1. The six questions chosen here as the symptom for bronchial asthma neither represent the most diagnostic nor are in any aspect independent of one another. For sure, the determined sensitivity and specificity of the screening test will certainly be different for a different set of combinations of questions.
2. If we wish to detect bronchial asthma at a higher sensitivity, say $Se = 0.95$ (or 95%), this would result in a specificity of only 0.75 (or 75%) (estimated from Fig. 2.4-1). This implies that the probability of false positives is 0.25 (or 25%).

Example 2.4-3

A test for diabetes mellitus is evaluated in 100 subjects with known diabetes and in 100 normal control subjects with no evidence of the disease nor of any factors known to result in increased risk of the disease. It was found that the diabetic group yields 95% positive tests ($Se = 0.95$), whereas the normal group has only 5% positive tests ($Sp = 1 - 0.05 = 0.95$). What is the accuracy of a positive test in predicting diabetes in an unselected sample of 10,000 subjects, in which the actual prevalence of diabetes mellitus is 1%?

Solution

Let D denote the diasease of diabetes mellitus. Since the prevalence of diabetes mellitus is 1%,

$$\Pr(D = 1) = 0.01. \tag{1}$$

By substituting respectively Eq. (1), Se = 0.95 and Sp = 0.95 into Eq. (2.4.5),

$$PPV = \frac{0.01 \times 0.95}{0.01 \times 0.95 + 0.05 \times (1 - 0.01)} = \frac{0.0095}{0.059} = 0.1610 \cong 0.16. \tag{2}$$

Hence the probability that this patient with a positive has diabetes is only 0.16 (or 16%).

Remarks

1. By Eq. (2.4.6), the predicting probability of no diabetes with a negative test is

   $$NPV = \frac{(1 - 0.01) \times 0.95}{(1 - 0.01) \times 0.95 +).01 \times 0.05} = 0.999468 \cong 0.999.$$

   In fact, PPV increases with increasing diasease prevalence, but NPV is affected insignificantly.[13]

2. With the prevalence of the disease being fixed, the PPV depends chiefly on the specificity of the test, but it has a maximal value of 0.669 even at Se = Sp = 0.99. Sensitivity and specificity have relatively little effect on the NPV.

3. A warning is that despite the high efficiency of a diagnostic test in the preliminary evaluation in groups of known diseased and nondiseased subjects, one must be careful when applying the results to unselected groups because of the magnification of false positive errors by the relatively low prevalences of disease in the general population. The concepts of sensitivity and specificity are not adequate to predict test reliability under these circumstances. Rather, the PPV and NPV should be used in unselected populations because these two parameters take into account the actual prevalence of diseases in the general population.[13]

4. When the disease status of a patient is determined by the reference test rather than the true diagnosis, indices describing the proportional agreement between a reference and a screening test are called co-positivity and co-negativity, which are not identical with sensitivity and specificity.[2]

2.5 Exercises

1. Show that $Se = 1 - \alpha$ and $Sp = 1 - \beta$.
2. Show that Eqs. (2.4.7) and (2.4.8) hold.
3. Show that Eqs. (2.4.9) and (2.4.10) hold.
4. Several investigators carefully studied a group of men referred with chest pain. Following graded treadmill stress testing (the diagnostic test) and selective coronary arteriography (the gold standard), two tables were obtained (see Tables 2.4-4 and 2.4-5) for different disease prevalences.

   In both tables the CAS is defined as present whenever the stenosis of patients' arteriograms showed 75% or more. Make a comparison between their Se/Sp and PPV/NPV for the two tables.[9]
5. Let T be a screening test for the specific disease D, and $\pi = \Pr(D = 1)$ and $\tau = \Pr(T = 1)$ denote the disease prevalence and test prevalence, respectively. It can be shown[6] that

   (i) the estimate of π is given by

$$\hat{\pi} = \frac{\hat{\tau} - \alpha}{1 - \alpha - \beta},$$

(2.4.11)

Table 2.4-4. Postexercise Electrocardiogram (ECG) as a Predictor of Coronary Artery Stenosis (CAS) when the Disease is Present in Half the Men Tested

Test Result (ECG)	Disease Status (CAS)		Total
	Present ($= 1$)	Absent ($= 0$)	
Positive ($= 1$)	55	7	62
Negative ($= 0$)	49	84	133
Total	104	91	195

Table 2.4-5.   Postexercise Electrocardiogram (ECG) as a Predictor of Coronary Artery Stenosis (CAS) when the Disease is Present in One-sixth of the Men Tested

	Disease Status (CAS)		
Test Result (ECG)	Present (= 1)	Absent (= 0)	Total
Positive (= 1)	55	42	97
Negative (= 0)	49	478	527
Total	104	520	624

where α and β are given by Eqs. (2.4.3) and (2.4.4), respectively, $\hat{\tau}$ is the estimate of τ given by the proportion of number of persons with positive tests among a random sample of n tested persons.

(ii) the estimate of Eq. (2.4.5) is given by

$$P\hat{P}V = \frac{1-\beta}{1-\alpha-\beta}(1-\frac{\alpha}{\hat{\tau}}). \qquad (2.4.12)$$

(iii) when α and β are unknown but are estimated by $\hat{\alpha}$ and $\hat{\beta}$ based on the sample sizes of n_1 and n_2, respectively, from the diseased and nondiseased groups, the asymptotic sampling distribution of Eq. (2.4.12) is approximately normal with the mean PPV given by Eq. (2.4.5) and variance $\sigma^2(P\hat{P}V)$ given by

$$\sigma^2(P\hat{P}V) = \left\{ \frac{\alpha(1-\beta)}{\tau(1-\alpha-\beta)} \right\}^2 \frac{\tau(1-\tau)}{n\tau^2}$$
$$+ \left\{ \frac{\alpha\pi}{\tau(1-\alpha-\beta)} \right\}^2 \frac{\beta(1-\beta)}{n_1}$$
$$+ \left\{ \frac{(1-\beta)(1-\pi)}{\tau(1-\alpha-\beta)} \right\}^2 \frac{\alpha(1-\alpha)}{n_2}, \qquad (2.4.13)$$

as n, n_1 and n_2 increases indefinitely.

Remarks

1. Equation (2.4.11) can yield an estimate of the disease of the disease prevalence that does not lie between 0 and 1. To avoid such problems, one can define a truncated version $\dot{\pi}$ of $\hat{\pi}$ as

$$\dot{\pi} = \min[\max(\hat{\pi}, 0), 1]. \tag{2.4.14}$$

2. If α and β are known, the last two terms on the right side of Eq. (2.4.13) vanish because they reflect the variability of our estimate of the unknown true α and β of the screening test.
3. Application of Eqs. (2.4.11) to (2.4.14) to screen for AIDS and the lie detectors is given in Ref. 6.

References

1. Begg CB, Greenes RA. (1983) Assessment of diagnostic tests when disease verification is subject to selection bias, *Biometrics* **39**: 207–215.
2. Buck AA, Gart JJ. (1966) Comparing a screening test and a reference test in epidemiologic studies. *Am J Epidemiol* **83**: 586–592.
3. Carey RM, Reid RA, Ayers CR, *et al.* (1976) The Charlottesville Blood-Pressure Survey: Value of repeated blood-pressure measurements. *J Am Med Assoc* **236**: 847–851.
4. Choi BCK. (1997) Causal modeling to estimate sensitivity and specificity of a test when prevalence changes. *Epidemiology* **8**: 80–86.
5. Colleen MF, Rubin L, Neyman J, *et al.* (1964) Automated multiphasic screening and diagnosis. *Am J Public Health* **54**: 741–750.
6. Gastwirth JL. (1987) The statistical precision of medical screening procedures: Application to polygraph and AIDS antibodies test data. *Statist Sci* **2**: 213–222.
7. Guggenmoos-Holzmann I, van Houwelingen HC. (2000) The (in)validity of sensitivity. *Stat Med.* **19**: 1783–1792.
8. Hacking I. (1975) *The Emergence of Probability: A Philosophical Study of Early Ideads about Probability, Induction, and Statistical Inference.* Cambridge University Press, Cambridge, England.
9. Haynes RB. (1981) How to read clinical journals: II. To learn about a diagnostic test. *Canadian Med Assoc J* **124**: 703–710.
10. Lee T-S. (2015) *College Algebra: Historical Notes.* Applied Math Press, Lilburn, Georgia.

11. Moons KG, van Es GA, Deckers JW, *et al.* (1997) Limitations of sensitivity, specificity, likelihood ratio, and Bayes' theorem in assessing diagnostic probabilities: A clinical example. *Epidemiology* **8**: 12–17.
12. Moons KG, Harrell FE. (2003) Sensitivity and specificity should be de-emphasized in diagnostic accuracy studies. *Academic Radiology* **10**: 670–672.
13. Vecchio TJ. (1966) Predictive value of a single diagnostic test in unselected populations. *New Engl J Med* **274**: 1171–1173.

3 Classic Random Variables

In this chapter we are going to learn some classic random variables with their associated probability distributions. Oftentimes, these classic random variables are used to model real-world problems. As was pointed out in Chap. 1, a random variable is associated with a unique probability distribution. As a result, we sometimes describe a random variable without explicitly mentioning its probability distribution. Since all probability distributions are characterized by its parameters like the mean, variance, skewness and kurtosis, we will list them accordingly.

3.0 Preliminary

For a continuous randome variable (r.v.) X defined on $(-\infty, +\infty)$, its (cumulative) probability distribution is given by

$$F(x) = \int_{-\infty}^{x} f(s)ds, \tag{3.0.1}$$

where $f(s)$ is the probability density function (p.d.f.), while, for a discrete r.v. X defined on the set of nonnegative integers, its probability mass function is given by

$$p(x) = \sum_{s=0}^{x} \Pr(X = s). \tag{3.0.2}$$

All (population) parameters of a probability distribution are related to the following term.

Definition 3.0.1. The expected value of the nth power of a r.v. X is called the nth moment of X, that is,

$$M_n(X) \equiv E(X^n) = \begin{cases} \int_{-\infty}^{+\infty}(x^n \cdot f(x))dx, & \text{if } X \text{ is continuous;} \\ \sum(x^n \cdot \Pr(X = x)), & \text{if } X \text{ is discrete.} \end{cases}$$

(3.0.3)

Remarks

1. The symbol "E" in Eq. (3.0.3) refers to the expected value of a random variable.
2. The mean (μ_X) of X is nothing but the first moment of X, namely,

$$\mu_X = E(X). \tag{3.0.4}$$

3. The variance ($var_X \equiv \sigma_X^2$) of X is the second central moment of X, namely,

$$var_X \equiv \sigma_X^2 = E[(X - \mu_X)^2]. \tag{3.0.5}$$

4. The skewness (γ_X) of X is the third standardized central moment of X, namely,

$$\gamma_X = E\left[\left(\frac{X - \mu_X}{\sigma_X}\right)^3\right]. \tag{3.0.6}$$

5. Among these three parameters, the mean and the standard deviation are the most important one. They are used to transform any normal random variables into the standard (or unit) normal random variable. Also, they are used to set up the Chebyshev's inequality.

3.1   Discrete Random Variables

A.   *Bernoulli Distribution (X ~ BNOU(p))*

Let X be a Bernoulli random variable. Thus, its probability distribution is given by[1]

$$\Pr(X = x) = p^x q^{1-x}, \quad x = 0, 1, \quad q = 1 - p. \tag{3.1A.1}$$

It is easily shown (see Exercise 3.4-3) that

$$\mu_X = p \quad \text{and} \quad \sigma_X^2 = pq. \tag{3.1A.2}$$

Remarks

1. All cancer random variables in Example 1.3-1 can be modeled by the Bernoulli random variable with the value of p given by the corresponding $\Pr(X = 1)$. For example, if we let X = FB, then $p = 0.00122$.
2. If we create a new r.v. Y as the sum of n independent Bernoulli random variables, it leads to the Binomial random variable shown next (see Exercise 3.4-4).

B.   *Binomial Distribution (X ~ BIN(n, p))*

Let X be a binomial random variable. Thus, its probability distribution is given by[2]

$$\Pr(X = x) = \binom{n}{x} p^x q^{n-x}, \quad x = 0, 1, \ldots, n, \quad q = 1 - p. \tag{3.1B.1}$$

It is easily shown (see Exercise 3.4-4) that

$$\mu_X = np \quad \text{and} \quad \sigma_X^2 = npq. \tag{3.1B.2}$$

Remark

The value of p in the binomial distribution is exactly the same as that of the Bernoulli distribution. In fact, when n = 1, the binomial random variable reduces to the Bernoulli random variable.

C.　*Poisson Distribution (X ~ POI(λ))*

Let X be a Poisson random variable. Thus, its probability distribution is given by[2]

$$\Pr(X = x) = \frac{\lambda^x e^{-\lambda}}{x!}, \quad x = 0, 1, 2, \ldots \tag{3.1C.1}$$

It can be shown (see Exercise 3.4-5) that

$$\mu_X = \lambda \quad \text{and} \quad \sigma_X^2 = \lambda. \tag{3.1C.2}$$

Remarks

1. The Poisson distribution is very peculiar in the sense that its mean equals its variance. Hence, when using the sample data to estimate its variance, all we need to do is to set its sample mean as its sample variance.
2. It can be shown that a Poisson random variable is the limit of a binomial random variable when p is small and $np \to \lambda$ as $n \to +\infty$.

D.　*Hypergeometric Distribution*
   (X ~ HPY(N₁, N₂, n), where N = N₁ + N₂)

Let X be a random variable that out of n red marbles randomly drawn from an urn containing N_1 red and N_2 green marbles, it has x red ones. Then X is a hypergeometric random variable with its probability distribution given by[2]

$$\Pr(X = x) = \frac{\binom{N_1}{x}\binom{N_2}{n-x}}{\binom{N}{n}}, \tag{3.1D.1}$$

where $N = N_1 + N_2$.

It can be shown (see Exercise 3.4-6) that

$$\mu_X = \frac{nN_1}{N} \quad \text{and} \quad \sigma_X^2 = \frac{nN_1 N_2(N-n)}{N^2(N-1)}. \tag{3.1D.2}$$

Remarks

1. The classical application of the hypergeometric distribution is sampling without replacement.
2. The test based on the hypergeometric distribution is identical to the one-tailed version of Fisher's exact test in Sec. 11.1C.

3.2   Continuous Random Variables

A.   *Normal Distribution* ($X \sim N(\mu_X, \sigma_X^2)$)

Let X be a normal random variable. Thus, its probability density function is given by

$$f(x) = \frac{1}{\sigma_X \sqrt{2\pi}} \exp\left(-\frac{(x - \mu_X)^2}{2\sigma_X^2}\right), \quad -\infty < x < +\infty \qquad (3.2A.1)$$

It is easily shown that

$$\mu_X = E(X) \quad \text{and} \quad \sigma_X^2 = E([X - \mu_X]^2). \qquad (3.2A.2)$$

Remarks

1. It is a coincidence that Eq. (3.2A.2) is exactly the same as Eqs. (3.0.4) and (3.0.5).
2. All normal random variables can be transformed into a standard (or unit) normal random variable Z with $\mu_Z = 0$ and $\sigma_Z^2 = 1$ by letting

$$Z = \frac{X - \mu_X}{\sigma_X}. \qquad (3.2A.3)$$

Equation (3.2A.3) is also called the z-transformation.
3. An important implication of Eq. (3.2A.3) is that to calculate the probability of any normal random variable all we need is just a table of standard normal random variable. See Table A-1 in the appendix.
4. An interesting property of the family of normal random variables is that a linear combination of n independent normal

random variables is still a normal random variable (see Exercise 3.4-2).

5. A physical realization of a normal distribution is demonstrated by an ingenious design, called the Galton's Quincunx (see Ref. 6, pp. 275–281).

B. Exponential Distribution (X ~ EXP(ξ))

Let X be an exponential random variable. Thus, its probability density function is given by[3]

$$f(x) = \xi \exp(-\xi x), \quad \xi > 0, \quad -\infty < x < +\infty \tag{3.2B.1}$$

It is easily shown (see Exercise 3.4-6) that

$$\mu_X = \xi^{-1} \quad \text{and} \quad \sigma_X^2 = \xi^{-2} \tag{3.2B.2}$$

Remarks

1. The exponential random variable is very useful in modeling the lifetime distribution (see Chap. 12). If the hazard rate is constant, the corresponding survival distribution is an exponential random variable.
2. It is a particular case of a gamma distribution and has the key property of being memoryless.

C. Chi-squared Distribution (X ~ CHI(r) = χ_r^2)

Let X be a chi-squared random variable. Thus, its probability density function is given by[3]

$$f(x) = \frac{1}{\Gamma(r/2)\sqrt{2^r}} x^{\frac{r}{2}-1} \exp\left(-\frac{x}{2}\right), \quad 0 < x < +\infty. \tag{3.2C.1}$$

It can be shown that

$$\mu_X = r \quad \text{and} \quad \sigma_X^2 = 2r. \tag{3.2C.2}$$

Remarks

1. The chi-squared random variable arises as the result of the sum of r independent standard normal random variables squared, that is, $X = \sum_{j=1}^{r} Z_j^2$, where $\{Z_j\}$ are independently identically distributed (i.i.d.) standard normal random variables.
2. Unlike the normal distribution and exponential distribution, the chi-squared distribution is not as often applied in the direct modeling of natural phennmenon. Instead, it is primarily used in hypothesis testing, e.g., the chi-squared test for independence in contingency tables (see Chap. 11).

D. *Student t-Distribution* $\left(X \sim T_r = \dfrac{Z}{\sqrt{\chi_r^2/r}} \right)$

Let X be a t-random variable. Thus, its probability density function is given by[3]

$$f(x) = \frac{\Gamma((r+1)/2)}{\Gamma(r/2)\sqrt{r\pi}} \cdot \frac{1}{\left(1 + x^2/2\right)^{(r+1)/2}}, \quad -\infty < x < +\infty \qquad (3.2\text{D}.1)$$

where $r > 2$.

It can be shown that

$$\mu_X = 0 \quad \text{and} \quad \sigma_X^2 = \frac{r}{r-2}. \qquad (3.2\text{D}.2)$$

Remarks

1. The t-distribution is symmetric and bell-shaped, like the normal distribution, but has thicker tails, meaning that it is more prone to producing values that fall far from its mean.
2. The t-random variable arises as the small sample size test that will be covered in Chap. 5.

E. *F-distribution* $(X \sim F_{r_1, r_2})$

Let X be a F-random variable that is the ratio of sample variances of two independent random variables. Thus, its probability density function is given by[4]

$$f(x) = \frac{\Gamma((r_1 + r_2)/2)(r_1/r_2)^{n/2} x^{n/2-1}}{\Gamma(r_1/2)\Gamma(r_2/2)(1 + r_1 x/r_2)^{(r_1+r_2)/2}},$$ (3.2E.1)

where $\Gamma(u)$ is the Gamma function. It can be shown that

$$\mu_X = \frac{r_2}{r_2-2} \quad \text{and} \quad \sigma_X^2 = \frac{2r_2^2(r_1 + r_2 - 2)}{r_1(r_2 - 2)^2(r_2 - 4)}, \quad r_2 > 4. \quad (3.2E.2)$$

Remarks

1. It can be shown (see Ref. 4) that

$$X = \frac{\chi_{r_1}^2/r_1}{\chi_{r_2}^2/r_2}.$$ (3.2E.3)

2. F is not symmetric with respect to its arguments. In fact, it is easily shown by using Eq. (3.2E.3) that

$$F_{r_2,r_1} = F_{r_1,r_2}^{-1}.$$ (3.2E.4)

F. Bivariate Normal Distribution[5] ((X, Y) ~ BNOR($\mu_X, \sigma_X^2, \mu_Y, \sigma_Y^2, \rho_{XY}$))

Let (X, Y) be a bivariate normal random variable. Thus, its probability density function is given by

$$f(x, y) = \frac{1}{2\pi\sigma_X\sigma_Y\sqrt{1 - \rho_{XY}^2}}$$

$$\times \exp\left(\frac{\left(\frac{x-\mu_X}{\sigma_X}\right)^2 - 2\rho_{XY}\left(\frac{x-\mu_X}{\sigma_X}\right)\left(\frac{y-\mu_Y}{\sigma_Y}\right) + \left(\frac{y-\mu_Y}{\sigma_Y}\right)^2}{2(1 - \rho_{XY}^2)}\right),$$ (3.2F.1)

where ρ_{XY}, the population correlation coefficient between X and Y, is given by

$$\rho_{XY} \equiv \frac{cov_{XY}}{\sigma_X\sigma_Y} = \frac{E((X - \mu_X)(Y - \mu_Y))}{\sigma_X\sigma_Y}.$$ (3.2F.2)

It can be shown (see Ref. 1) that the conditional mean of Y given X is given by

$$E(Y \mid X) = \mu_Y + \rho_{XY} \cdot \frac{\sigma_Y}{\sigma_X}(X - \mu_X). \qquad (3.2\text{F.}3)$$

Remarks

1. The symbol cov_{XY} in the numerator of Eq. (3.2F.2) is called the covariance between X and Y.
2. Equation (3.2F.3) is a linear function of X. An extension of Eq. (3.2F.2) motivates the introduction of a linear regression model in Sec. 7.2.
3. The conditional mean of X given Y can be similarly defined.

3.3   Applications

In this section we will show how to apply classic random variables to model real-world problems.

Example 3.3-1

The percentage of female students in the Z-University is 40%. Ten students are randomly selected from the Z-University. Find the probability that at most two are females.

Solution

Let X be the number of females among ten randomly selected students. Then X is a binomial random variable with p = 0.4. By using Eq. (3.1B.1), the desired probability is given by

$$Pr(X \le 2) = \sum_{x=0}^{2} \binom{10}{x} 0.4^x 0.6^{10-x}$$

$$= \binom{10}{0} 0.4^0 0.6^{10-0} + \binom{10}{1} 0.4^1 0.6^{10-1} + \binom{10}{2} 0.4^2 0.6^{10-2}$$

$$= 0.6^{10} + 10 \times 0.4 \times 0.6^9 + 45 \times 0.4^2 \times 0.6^8 = 0.006046618$$

$$+ 0.040310784 + 0.120932352 = 0.167289754 \approx 0.17.$$

Thus, the probability that at most two are females is 0.17.

Example 3.3-2

The average number of phone calls per minute arriving at the hospital's emergency care unit is 4. Find the probability that no calls come in a given minute.

Solution

Let X denote the number of calls coming into the hospital's emergency care unit in any given minute. It is reasonable to assume that X is a Poisson random variable. Since the average number of calls per minute is 4, we thus have by Eq. (3.1C.2)

$$\lambda = \mu_X = 4. \tag{1}$$

By substituting Eq. (1) into Eq. (3.1C.1)

$$\Pr(X = 0) = \frac{4^0 e^{-4}}{0!} = e^{-4} = 0.018315639 \approx 0.02.$$

Thus the probability that no calls come in a given minute is 0.02.

Example 3.3-3

Patients arrive at a certain clinic on an average of 15 per hour. What is the probability that the clinic's physician must wait at least 10 minutes for the first patient?

Solution

Let X be the waiting time in minutes that the clinic's physician must wait for the first patient. Ordinarily, the waiting time is assumed to be an exponential r.v. Since patients arrive at an average of 15 per hour (or $\mu_X = 60/15 = 4$ per minute), the mean of X is given by Eq. (3.2B.2)

$$\xi = \mu_X^{-1} = 4^{-1} = 0.25. \tag{1}$$

Thus, we have by substituting Eq. (1) into Eqs. (3.0.1) and (3.2B.1)

$$\Pr(X \geq 10) = \int_{10}^{\infty} 4\exp(-0.25x)dx$$

$$= \exp(-2.5) = 0.0821 \approx 0.08.$$

Therefore, the probability that the clinic's physician must wait at least 10 minutes is merely 0.08.

Example 3.3-4

Consider the radioactive decay of Carbon-14 (C-14) atoms to Nitrogen-14 (N-14) with a mean time of 8267 years. Let X be the time in years that a C-14 atom takes to decay to N-14. Find the median time, x_{med}, of X.

Solution

It is reasonable to assume that X is an exponential r.v. Since the mean time of X is $\mu_X = 8267$, we have by Eq. (3.2B.2)

$$\xi = \mu_X^{-1} = 8267^{-1} = 0.000120963 \approx 0.000121. \tag{1}$$

To find the median time of X is equivalent to find x_{med} satisfying

$$\Pr(X \leq x_{med}) = 0.5.$$

By substituting Eq. (1) into Eqs. (3.0.1) and (3.2B.1),

$$\int_0^{x_{med}} 0.000121 e^{-0.000121x} dx = 0.5,$$

$$1 - e^{-0.000121 x_{med}} = 0.5. \tag{2}$$

By solving Eq. (2) for x_{med},

$$x_{med} = -8267 \times \ln 0.5 = 5730.2477 \approx 5730. \tag{3}$$

Thus, the median time of the radioactive decay of C-14 to N-14 is 5730 years.

Example 3.3-5

Let X be the birth weight of the newborn infants in the US, which is assumed to be a normal random variable with the mean birth weight $\mu_X = 3315$ and variance $\sigma_x^2 = 275{,}625$. What is the proportion of all newborn babies with the birth weight being greater than 3987 grams?

Solution

This is equivalent to finding the probability of $\Pr(X \geq 3987)$. In order to use Table A-1 in the appendix, we need to convert it into the standard normal random variable as follows:

$$\Pr(X \geq 3987) = \Pr\left(\frac{X - \mu_X}{\sigma_X} \geq \frac{3{,}987 - 3315}{\sqrt{275{,}625}}\right)$$

$$= \Pr\left(Z \geq \frac{672}{525}\right) = \Pr(Z \geq 1.28)$$

$$= 1 - \Pr(Z < 1.28) = 1 - 0.8997$$

$$= 0.1003 \approx 0.10 \tag{1}$$

From Eq. (1) the proportion is approximately 0.1 (or 10%).

Remark

To obtain the probability of $\Pr(Z < 1.28)$ in Eq. (1), first use the unit and tenths digits of 1.28, that is, to identify 1.2 in the first column of Table A-1 and then search along the line horizontally until the hundredths digit of 1.28, that is, to read the numerical value under the label of 0.08 in the first row, which is 0.8997.

3.4 Exercises

1. Let X and Y be two random variables, and c be a real number. Show that (i) $E(X + Y) = E(X) + E(Y)$, and (ii) $E(cX) = cE(X)$.

Remark

This implies that the expected value of a random variable is a linear operator.

2. Let $S_n = \sum_{i=1}^{n} c_i X_i$, where $\{X_i\}$ are mutually independent normal random variables and c_i are real constants, $i = 1, 2, \ldots, n$. Show that $\mu_{S_n} = \sum_{i=1}^{n} c_i \mu_{X_i}$ and $\sigma_{S_n}^2 = \sum_{i=1}^{n} c_i^2 \sigma_{X_i}^2$.

Remarks

The condition of mutually independence assures that the correlation between them is zero, namely, $\rho_{X_i X_j} = 0$.

3. Show that if $X \sim \text{BNOU}(p)$, then $\mu_X = p$ and $\sigma_X^2 = pq$.
4. Show that if $Y = \sum_{i=1}^{n} X_i$, where $\{X_i\}$ are independent BNOU(p), then $\mu_Y = np$ and $\sigma_Y^2 = npq$.
5. If $X \sim \text{POI}(\lambda)$, then $\mu_X = \sigma_X^2 = \lambda$.
6. If $X \sim \text{EXP}(\xi)$, then $\mu_X = \xi^{-1}$ and $\sigma_X^2 = \mu_X^2$.
7. Redo Example 3.3-5 when the variance of X is changed to $\sigma_X^2 = 330,625$. What is the proportion of all newborn babies with the birth weight being greater than 4,143 grams?

References

1. Hogg RV, Tanis EA. (1997) *Probability and Statistical Inference*, 5th ed. Prentice Hall Publishing Co., Upper Saddle River, NJ.
2. Johnson NL, Kemp AW, Kotz S. (2005) *Univariate Discrete Distributions*, 3rd ed. John Wiley & Sons, Inc., New York.
3. Johnson NL, Kotz S, Balakrisshnan N. (1994) *Continuous Univariate Distributions*, Vol. 1, 2nd ed. John Wiley & Sons, Inc., New York.
4. Johnson NL, Kotz S, Balakrisshnan N. (1995) *Continuous Univariate Distributions*, Vol. 2, 2nd ed. John Wiley & Sons, Inc., New York.
5. Kotz S, Balakrisshnan N, Johnson NL. (2000) *Continuous Multivariate Distributions*, Vol. 1, 2nd ed. John Wiley & Sons, Inc., New York.
6. Stigler, SM. (1986) *The History of Statistics: The Measurement of Uncertainty before 1900*. The Belknap Press of Harvard University Press, Cambridge, MA.

4 Inferential Statistics

4.0 A Preview on Significance Test and Hypothesis Testing

The formulation and philosophy of significance test and hypothesis testing was largely created during the period 1915–1933 by three persons: RA Fisher (1890–1962), J Neyman (1894–1981) and ES Pearson (1895–1980).[5]

Fisher was a great statistician and was regarded as the greatest theoretical statistician by his admirers. He was a contentious, polemical man. His life was filled with a sequence of scientific fights, often several at a time, at scientific meetings or in his papers.

Nevertheless, he made important contributions in many branches of modern statistics including the t-distribution, F-distribution, the distribution of the estimated correlation coefficient, randomization of the experiment, etc.[7] He rose as a new academic star by challenging K Pearson (1857–1936), the founding father of the school of biometrics, on issues concerning the method of parameter estimation, the correct way of counting degrees of freedom for contingency tables, and others. Later, his theory of significance test was challenged by the joint work on the theory of hypothesis testing by J Neyman and ES Pearson, the son of K Pearson.

During the period of 1926–1931, Neyman and Pearson (N–P) developed their theory of hypothesis testing in response to the inadequacy of Fisher's significance test (FST). In FST, Fisher mentioned neither the alternative hypothesis nor the power of the test. The reason was that Fisher just wanted to use the data as evidence to assess the degree of validity of the scientific (or null) hypothesis. His logic was that, just based on the available data, either something most improbable had happened or the (null) hypothesis was false. He was not concerned with the acceptance procedure for accepting or rejecting the null hypothesis. This led him to recourse to the tail area of the graph of the probability distribution by grouping outcomes as being more or less antagonistic to the given null hypothesis. This is what is known today as the so-called p-value of the observed evidence.

However, in their theory of hypothesis testing N–P identified an alternative hypothesis and recognized two types of error. Their approach focused on the power to detect alternative hypotheses and led to the identification of an optimal test criteria. It eventually served as the foundation for much later work in mathematical statistics. Based upon his work on hypothesis testing, Neyman formulated his theory on parameter estimation via applying the method of confidence intervals, which provided the interval estimates and has since prevailed over Fisher's point estimation by the method of maximum likelihood.

Remark

Despite basic philosophical differences, the two theories are complimentary rather than contradictory in their main practical aspects, and a unified approach is possible that combines the best features of both.[6]

4.1 Parameter Estimation

A. *Point Estimation*

A point estimator should possess a very desirable property of "unbiasedness" as defined in the following definition.

Definition 4.1.1. A point estimator $\hat{\theta}$ for the population parameter θ is said to be unbiased if the expected value of $\hat{\theta}$ equals θ, that is,

$$E(\hat{\theta}) = \theta. \tag{4.1.1}$$

Assume that the random sample data $\{x_i\}_{i=1}^n$ are collected with respect to the given continuous r.v. X. There are two methods for estimating the mean and variance of X.

(i) Method of Moments

By using Eq. (3.0.4), the estimator for the population mean and variance of X are given, respectively, by

$$\hat{\mu}_X = \bar{x} = n^{-1} \sum_{i=1}^n x_i, \tag{4.1.2}$$

and

$$\hat{\sigma}_X^2 = \frac{\sum_{i=1}^n (x_i - \bar{x})^2}{n}. \tag{4.1.3}$$

Remarks

1. Equation (4.1.2) is exactly the same as that of Eq. (1.4.1), while Eq. (4.1.3) is a little different from Eq. (1.4.9) for the ungrouped data.
2. It can be shown that the estimator $\hat{\mu}_X$ of Eq. (4.1.2) is an unbiased estimator for μ_X (see Exercise 4.4-1), but $\hat{\sigma}_X^2$ of Eq. (4.1.3) is not unbiased for σ_X^2. Rather, an unbiased estimator for σ_X^2 is given by Eq. (1.4.9).
3. The concept of unbiasedness for a point estimator is totally different from that of the unbiased sampling discussed in Sec. 1.2.

(ii) Method of Maximum Likelihood

First, we need to learn the notion of the likelihood function associated with collected random sample data.

Definition 4.1.2. The likelihood function of the random sample data $\{x_i\}_{i=1}^{n}$ is given by

$$L(\theta) = \prod_{i=1}^{n} f(x_i;\theta), \qquad (4.1.4)$$

where $f(x_i;\theta)$ is the p.d.f. of X. The maximum likelihood estimator (m.l.e.) of θ is obtained by finding the value of θ that maximizes the likelihood function $L(\theta)$, that is, solving

$$\frac{dL(\theta)}{d\theta} = 0, \qquad (4.1.5)$$

where $dL(\theta)/d\theta$ is the first derivative of $L(\theta)$.

Remarks

1. The m.l.e. may not exist because Eq. (4.1.5) has no solution. Also, the m.l.e. as a point estimator may not be unbiased.
2. An important result related to the sample mean is that the sample mean itself is a random variable whose limiting distribution is a normal random variable as shown in the following theorem.

Theorem 4.1.1. "Central Limit Theorem" *Assume that X is a continuous random variable with a finite mean μ_X and a finite variance $\sigma_X^2 > 0$. Then, as $n \to +\infty$,*

$$\frac{\bar{X} - \mu_{\bar{X}}}{\sigma_{\bar{X}}} \sim Z, \qquad (4.1.6)$$

where Z is a standard normal random variable, namely, $Z \sim N(0,1)$.

Remarks

1. Note that the sample mean $\bar{x}$ varies for different sets of sample data. The sample mean itself should be regarded as a random

variable. As a result, a new random variable corresponding to the sample mean $\bar{x}$ is defined by

$$\bar{X} = \frac{\sum_{i=1}^{n} X_i}{n}, \tag{4.1.7}$$

where $\{X_i\}, i = 1, \ldots, n$ are the independently identically distributed (i.i.d.) random variables as the original X, that is, $X_i \equiv X$.

2. It is easily shown (see Exercise 4.4-2) that

$$\mu_{\bar{X}} = \mu_X \quad \text{and} \quad \sigma_{\bar{X}}^2 = \frac{\sigma_X^2}{n}. \tag{4.1.8}$$

Thus, Eq. (4.1.6) is reduced to

$$\frac{\bar{X} - \mu_{\bar{X}}}{\sigma_{\bar{X}}} = \frac{\bar{X} - \mu_X}{\sigma_X / \sqrt{n}} \sim Z. \tag{4.1.9}$$

3. If the original X is required to be a normal random variable, Eq. (4.1.9) is always true without being required that $n \to +\infty$.
4. For practicality, the Central Limit Theorem is applicable whenever the sample size is no less than 30, namely, $n \geq 30$.

B. *Interval Estimation*

The interval estimator for the unknown population mean μ_X is given in the following theorem.

Theorem 4.1.2. *Assume that X is a continuous random variable with a finite mean μ_X and a finite variance $\sigma_{\bar{X}}^2 > 0$. Also, the sample data $\{x_i\}_{i=1}^n$ are randomly collected with respect to the given continuous r.v. X. Then, the $100 \times (1 - \alpha)\%(0 < \alpha < 1)$ confidence interval for the unknown μ_X is given by*

$$\bar{x} - z_{1-\frac{\alpha}{2}} \times \frac{\sigma_X}{\sqrt{n}} \leq \mu_X \leq \bar{x} + z_{1-\frac{\alpha}{2}} \times \frac{\sigma_X}{\sqrt{n}}, \tag{4.1.10}$$

where z_p denotes the $100 \times p^{th}$ percentile of the standard normal distribution, $0 < p < 1$.

Similarly, if $D = X - Y$, and the random sample data are collected with the respective sample size n and m for two independent continuous random variables (r.v.s) X and Y, the $100 \times (1 - \alpha)\%(0 < \alpha < 1)$ confidence interval for the unknown $\mu_X - \mu_Y$ is given by

$$\bar{x} - \bar{y} - z_{1-\frac{\alpha}{2}} \times \frac{\sigma_D}{\sqrt{n}} \leq \mu_X - \mu_Y \leq \bar{x} - \bar{y} + z_{1-\frac{\alpha}{2}} \times \frac{\sigma_D}{\sqrt{n}}, \qquad (4.1.11)$$

where σ_D is given by

$$\sigma_D \equiv \sigma_{X-Y} = \sqrt{\frac{\sigma_X^2}{n} + \frac{\sigma_Y^2}{m}}. \qquad (4.1.12)$$

Remarks

1. In Eqs. (4.1.10) to (4.1.12), the standard deviation σ_X or σ_Y can be substituted by their sample estimates s_X or s_Y, should they be unknown.
2. The proof of Theorem 4.1.2 is given in Exercise 4.4-3.
3. The confidence limit ratio (CLR) for μ_X is defined as

$$CLR = UCL/LCL, \qquad (4.1.13)$$

where UCL and LCL are the upper and lower confidence limit given in Eq. (4.1.10).

4.2 Hypothesis Testing

For any scientific investigation, an investigator often has an hypothesis in mind that he wishes to verify. This hypothesis is usually regarded as the alternative hypothesis. In contrast, the null hypothesis is the one that contradicts the alternative one. For a random variable X, the null and alternative hypotheses are mainly concerned with the unknown population parameter of X. Let θ denote such a parameter. At this moment to be concrete, let us imagine that θ is just the population mean of X.

Depending on the circumstance, there are three different ways of defining the null and alternative hypotheses as shown in the following definition.

Definition 4.2.1.

(i) A two-tailed hypothesis testing is a pair of null and alternative hypotheses H_0 and H_1 that are set up as follows:

$$H_0 : \theta = \theta_0 \text{ versus } H_1 : \theta \neq \theta_0, \qquad (4.2.1)$$

where θ_0 is a given number.

(ii) A right-tailed hypothesis testing is a pair of null and alternative hypotheses H_0 and H_1 that are set up as follows:

$$H_0 : \theta \leq \theta_0 \text{ versus } H_1 : \theta > \theta_0, \qquad (4.2.2)$$

(iii) A left-tailed hypothesis testing is a pair of null and alternative hypotheses H_0 and H_1 that are set up as follows:

$$H_0 : \theta \geq \theta_0 \text{ versus } H_1 : \theta < \theta_0, \qquad (4.2.3)$$

Remarks

1. Whether it is a two-tailed or one-tailed hypothesis testing depends on the form of the alternative hypothesis H_1. The form of H_0 remains the same for Equations (4.2.1) to (4.2.3).
2. Be aware that what we consider here are merely statistical hypotheses. There is a great difference between statistical hypotheses and scientific hypotheses. Statistical hypotheses only deal with mathematical properties of parameters in a distribution, while scientific hypotheses are trying to understand some natural phenomenon.[1] The final confidence a scientist can have in his scientific hypotheses is not dependent on statistical significance levels; it is ultimately determined by his ability to reject alternatives.

Table 4.2-1. **An acceptance-rejection decision chart**

		Decision	
		Accept	**Reject**
Status of H_0	**True**	correct	type I error
	False	type II error	correct

3. Before setting up the decision rule, we need to construct a testing statistics. For example, to test the hypothesis given by Eq. (4.2.1), a testing statistics is constructed by letting

$$z = \frac{\hat{\theta} - \theta_0}{\sigma_{\hat{\theta}}} = \frac{\hat{\theta} - \theta_0}{\sigma_X / \sqrt{n}}. \qquad (4.2.4)$$

Based upon the collected random sample data, we need to compute the value of Eq. (4.2.4) and make a decision whether to accept H_0.

Obviously, regardless of what decision we make, we unavoidably commit one of the two types — type I and type II — of errors. This can be illustrated in the following 2×2 table:

From Table 4.2-1 the type I and II errors are formally given in the above definition.

Definition 4.2.2. The type I error is an error in which a decision is made to reject H_0 when H_0 is true, while the type II error is an error in which a decision is made to accept H_0 when H_0 is false. Also, the (conditional) probabilities that commit type I and II errors are denoted, respectively, by α and β, that is,

$$\alpha = \Pr(\text{reject } H_0 | H_0 \text{ is true}), \qquad (4.2.5)$$

and

$$\beta = \Pr(\text{accept } H_0 | H_0 \text{ is false}). \qquad (4.2.6)$$

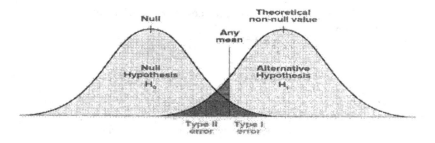

Fig. 4.2-1.   The figure of type I and type II errors.

Remarks

1. Between α and β, α has to be determined before seeing the data. Otherwise, an investigator is committing the sin of data peeking. Also, α is used in determining the critical region of the test.
2. The value of $1 - \alpha$ is the sensitivity of the test, whereas $1 - \beta$ is the specificity (or power) of the test.
3. For a fixed sample size n, the relationship between α and β is negatively correlated, that is, the value of β will increase if you intend to decrease the value of α, and vice versa. The only way to decrease the values of both α and β is by increasing the sample size (Fig. 4.2-1).

Definition 4.2.3.   The tail part of the probability distribution that forms the region in rejecting the null hypothesis is called the critical region of the test. The probability of committing a type I error α is called the size (or the significance level) of the test, while the probability of not committing a type II error is called the power of the test.

Remarks

1. The critical region is determined by the form of the alternative hypothesis H_1 as shown in the following definition.
2. The power of the test depends on the true unknown population parameter μ_X, that is a function of μ_X (see Example 4.3-2).

Decision Rule 4.2-1

For all the three tests below the significance level is α:

(i) A two-tailed test for Eq. (4.2.1) is to reject H_0 if the computed z of Eq. (4.2.4) is greater than $z_{1-\frac{\alpha}{2}}$ or less than $z_{\frac{\alpha}{2}}$. (4.2.7)

(ii) A right-tailed test for Eq. (4.2.2) is to reject H_0 if the computed z of Eq. (4.2.4) is greater than $z_{1-\alpha}$. (4.2.8)

(iii) A left-tailed test for Eq. (4.2.3) is to reject H_0 if the computed z of Eq. (4.2.4) is less than z_α. (4.2.9)

Remarks

1. If the original r.v. X is normal, the sampling distribution of Eq. (4.2.4) is also normal. Thus, the critical values in Eqs. (4.2.7) to (4.2.9) are the corresponding percentile of the standard normal distribution.
2. Otherwise, it depends on the sample size n. If $n \geq 30$, Eq. (4.2.4) is still approximately a normal r.v. However, if $n < 30$, Eq. (4.2.4) is a t-random variable with $n - 1$ degrees of freedom.
3. Once the null hypothesis H_0 is rejected, the test is said to be statistically significant at the level of α.

Another concept for assessing the degree of evidence for supporting the validity of the scientific hypothesis is called the p-value of the observed data as defined in the following definition.

Definition 4.2.4. The probability that under the assumption of no effect or difference the future observations are more extreme (equal to or greater) than the present observation, which is said to be the p-value of the present observation.

Remarks

1. The notion of the p-value introduced by RA Fisher in 1925 to evaluate the evidence of the data that support the null hypothesis is called the significance level.

2. Later, it was misused in the context of hypothesis testing by some people to compare the p-value of the testing statistics with the type I error. Once the p-value is less than the type I error, H_0 is rejected. Unfortunately, this common use of the p-value was misuse and abuse of that statistics. In fact, a pointedly criticism on the fallacy of using the p-value to evaluate the evidence of the collected data is given in Refs. 2 to 4.

3. A generalization of the p-value to become a bivariate function that defines the predictive evidence was proposed by Thompson.[8]

4.3 Examples

Example 4.3-1

Let X be a random variable to represent the forced expiratory volume per second for the population of all medical students in England. Suppose that the population mean of X is suspected to be greater than 3.8 before the sample data are collected. Let us assume that the sample data given in Example 1.4-1 are randomly collected.

Is our suspicion valid at the significance level of 0.05?

Solution

First, a pair of null and alternative hypotheses are set up as follows:

$$H_0 : \mu_X \le 3.8 \text{ versus } H_1 : \mu_X > 3.8. \tag{1}$$

By using Eq. (4.2.4) with $\bar{x} = 4.0607$ obtained in Example 1.4-2(a),

$$z = \frac{4.061 - 3.8}{2.033} = \frac{0.261}{2.033} = 0.12838 \approx 0.128. \tag{2}$$

Since the computed z of Eq. (2) is less than the critical value $z_{0.95} = 1.68$, our suspicion is invalid by DR 4.2-1.

Example 4.3-2

Let X denote SAT mathematics scores of students who attend a small liberal arts college. Assume that X is a normal random variable with an unknown mean, but with the variance 6400. We intend to test that $\mu_X < 540$. Suppose that a random sample of 36 students was selected from this college. Let the critical region for the sample average SAT Mathematics scores of these 36 students be chosen as $C = \{\bar{x} : \bar{x} \le 520\}$.

(a) Find the power function, $\Psi(\mu_X)$, for the test and sketch the graph of $\Psi(\mu_X)$.
(b) What is the value of significance level of this test?
(c) What is the value of $\Psi(510)$?
(d) Determine the sample size n such that the type I and II errors are given by $\alpha = 0.05$ and $\beta = 0.10$, respectively when $\mu_X = 500$.

Solution

(a) By the definition of the power function,

$$\Psi(\mu_X) = \Pr(\bar{X} \le 520; \mu_X) = \Pr\left(\frac{\bar{X} - \mu_X}{\sigma_{\bar{X}}} \le \frac{520 - \mu_X}{\sigma_{\bar{X}}}\right). \quad (1)$$

By substituting n = 36 into Eq. (4.1.8),

$$\sigma_{\bar{X}} = \frac{\sigma_X}{\sqrt{36}} = \frac{\sqrt{6400}}{6} = \frac{80}{6} = \frac{40}{3}. \quad (2)$$

By substituting Eq. (2) into Eq. (1),

$$\Psi(\mu_X) = \Pr\left(Z \le \frac{3(520 - \mu_X)}{40}\right) = \emptyset(z^*), \quad (3)$$

where $\emptyset(z)$ is the cumulative distribution of the standard normal random variable given by Eq. (3.2A.1), that is,

$$\emptyset(z) = \int_0^z \frac{1}{\sqrt{2\pi}} e^{-\frac{s^2}{2}} ds. \quad (4)$$

Table 4.3-1. The power function of Eq. (3) for different values of μ_X

μ_X	$z^* = \frac{3(520-\mu_X)}{40}$	$\emptyset(z^*)$
540	−1.5	0.0668
530	−0.75	0.2734
520	0	0.5
510	0.75	0.7734
500	1.5	0.9332
490	2.25	0.9778

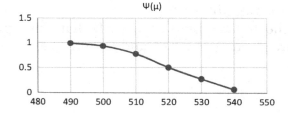

$\Psi(\mu)$

Fig. 4.3-1.   The graph of the power function of $\Psi(\mu_X)$.

By using the values of Table A-1 in the appendix, several values of $\Psi(\mu_X)$ of Eq. (3) are given in Table 4.3-1:

The graph of $\Psi(\mu_X)$ of Eq. (3) is given in Fig. 4.3-1.

(b) The significance level of this test is given by

$$\alpha = \Pr(\bar{X} \le 520 | \mu_X = 540) = \emptyset(-1.5) = 0.0668.$$

(c) By using Table 4.3-1, the value of $\Psi(510)$ is given by 0.7734.

(d) Consider the critical region to be of the form $\{\bar{X} \le c\}$. Since we want $\alpha = 0.05$ and $\beta = 0.10$ when $\mu_X = 500$, n has to be chosen to satisfy the following two equations:

$$0.05 = \Pr(\bar{X} \le c; \mu_X = 540) = \emptyset\left(\frac{\sqrt{n}(c - 540)}{80}\right), \qquad (5)$$

$$0.10 = \Pr(\bar{X} > c; \mu_X = 500) = 1 - \emptyset\left(\frac{\sqrt{n}(c - 500)}{80}\right). \qquad (6)$$

By finding the inverse value of $\emptyset(z^*)$ from Eqs. (5) and (6), we have

$$-1.645 = \frac{\sqrt{n}(c - 540)}{80}, \tag{7}$$

$$1.38 = \frac{\sqrt{n}(c - 500)}{80}. \tag{8}$$

By dividing Eq. (7) by Eq. (8),

$$-1.192 \approx \frac{c - 540}{c - 500} \implies c = \frac{540 + 1.192 \times 500}{2.192} = 518.25. \tag{9}$$

By substituting Eq. (9) into Eq. (8),

$$\sqrt{n} = \frac{80 \times 1.38}{18.25} = \frac{110.4}{18.25} = 6.049315 \approx 6.05. \tag{10}$$

By squaring Eq. (10),

$$n = 36.6025 \approx 37.$$

Therefore, the desired sample size is 37.

4.4   Exercises

1. Show that $\hat{\mu}_X$ of Eq. (4.1.2) is an unbiased estimator of μ_X, that is, $E(\hat{\mu}_X) = \mu_X$.
2. Show that Eq. (4.1.8) is valid, that is, $\mu_{\bar{X}} = \mu_X$ and $\sigma_{\bar{X}}^2 = \frac{\sigma_X^2}{n}$.
3. Prove that Theorem 4.2.1 is valid.
4. What is the difference between scientific and statistical hypothesis?
5. How to handle the importance between type I and type II errors in practical applications?

References

1. Bolles RC. (1962) The difference between statistical hypotheses and scienfitic hypotheses. *Psycho Reports* **11**: 639–645.
2. Goodman SN. (1992) A comment on replication, p-values, and evidence. *Stat Med* **11**: 875–879.
3. Goodman SN. (1993) p values, hypothesis tests, and likelihood: Implications for epidemiology of a neglected historical debate. *Am J Epidemiol* **137**: 485–496.
4. Goodman SN. (1999) Toward evidence-based medical statistics 1: The p-value fallacy. *Ann Intern Med* **130**: 995–1004.
5. Inman HF. (1994) Karl Pearson and R. A. Fisher on statistical test: A 1935 exchange from Nature. *Am Statis* **48**: 2–11.
6. Lehmann EL. (1993) The Fisher, Neyman–Pearson theories of testing hypotheses: One theory or two? *J Am Stat Assoc* **88**: 1242–1249.
7. Neyman J. (1967) R. A. Fisher (1890–1962): An appreciation. *Science* **156**: 1456–1460.
8. Thompson B. (2006) Critique of p-values. *Int Stat Rev* **74**: 1–14.

5 Inferences on Means and Variances

In contrast to Chap. 4, we are going to learn how to draw statistical inference when the sample size is small, that is, $n < 30$, and the true variance of the random variable is unknown.

5.1 The Mean of a Single Random Variable

When the true variance of the random variable (r.v.) X is unknown, we need to construct a new statistics for testing Eqs. (4.2.1) to (4.2.3) as follows:

$$t = \frac{\bar{x} - \mu_0}{s_X / \sqrt{n}}, \tag{5.1.1}$$

where s_X is the sample standard deviation given by Eq. (1.4.11). By employing the same argument on the sample mean, Eq. (5.1.1) is a new random variable. It can be shown that the sampling distribution of Eq. (5.1.1) is a t_{n-1}-distribution with $n-1$ degrees of freedom (see my remark under Definition 5.1.1.) The decision rules for the statistical test are defined in the following definition.

Decision Rule 5.1-1

For all the three tests below the significance level is α:

(i) A two-tailed test for Eq. (4.2.1) is to reject H_0 if the computed t of Eq. (5.1.1) is greater than $t_{n-1;1-\frac{\alpha}{2}}$ or less than $t_{n-1;\frac{\alpha}{2}}$. $$\tag{5.1.2}$$

(ii) A right-tailed test for Eq. (4.2.2) is to reject H_0 if the computed
    t of Eq. (5.1.1) is greater than $t_{n-1;1-\alpha}$.   (5.1.3)

(iii) A left-tailed test for Eq. (4.2.3) is to reject H_0 if the computed
     t of Eq. (5.1.1) is less than $t_{n-1;\alpha}$.   (5.1.4)

Remarks

1. It can be shown that the sampling distribution of the r.v. $(n-1)s_X^2/\sigma_X^2$ is a chi-squared distribution with $n-1$ degrees of freedom (see Sec. 5.3). This fact is used in proving that the sampling distribution of Eq. (5.1.1) is a t_{n-1}-distribution.
2. When the sample size n is large, Eqs. (5.1.2) to (5.1.4) are reduced to Eqs. (4.2.7) to (4.2.9).

Example 5.1-1

Let X be the serum uric acid levels of males. Assume that the population mean is $\mu_X = 5.4\,\text{mg}/(100 \cdot \text{ml})$, whereas the population variance is unknown. A random sample of 25 males was selected and the sample mean and standard deviation of the 25 measured uric acid levels were $\bar{x} = 5.7$ and $s_X = 1.2\,\text{mg}/(100 \cdot \text{ml})$. Is the sample mean significantly greater than the population mean at the level of significance 0.05?

Solution

To answer the question, we need to test the following hypotheses:

$$H_0 : \mu_X \leq 5.4 \quad \text{versus} \quad H_1 : \mu_X > 5.4. \tag{5.1.5}$$

First, we compute the testing statistics by using Eq. (5.1.1)

$$t = \frac{5.7 - 5.4}{1.2/\sqrt{25}} = \frac{0.3}{0.24} = 1.25. \tag{5.1.6}$$

Because the sample size is small, $n = 25 < 30$ and the population variance of X is unknown, we use Eq. (5.1.3) with $\alpha = 0.05$ to obtain the corresponding critical value $t_{24;0.95} = 1.71$. Since the computed value of Eq. (5.1.6) is less than the critical value, the observed sample mean is not significantly greater than the population mean.

5.2   The Means of Two Random Variables

In this section we are going to test whether the population means between two random variables are significantly different. It depends on whether these two random variables are independent or not. There are two different ways to test it.

Let X and Y be two continuous random variables. Three pairs of null and alternative hypothesis are thus set up as follows:

(i) $H_0: \mu_X = \mu_Y$ versus $H_1: \mu_X \neq \mu_Y$;   (5.2.1)
(ii) $H_0: \mu_X \leq \mu_Y$ versus $H_1: \mu_X > \mu_Y$;   (5.2.2)
(iii) $H_0: \mu_X \geq \mu_Y$ versus $H_1: \mu_X < \mu_Y$.   (5.2.3)

A.   *Independent Case*

First, assume that two samples of data, $\{x_i\}_{i=1}^n$ and $\{y_j\}_{j=1}^m$, are randomly collected from two independent random variables (r.v.s) X and Y in which $\sigma_X^2 = \sigma_y^2$. We then define the testing statistics as follows:

$$t = \frac{\bar{x} - \bar{y}}{\sqrt{\dfrac{(n-1)s_X^2 + (m-1)s_Y^2}{n+m-2}}}.$$ (5.2.4)

It can be shown that the sampling distribution of Eq. (5.2.4) is a t_{n+m-2}-distribution with $n + m - 2$ degrees of freedom. The decision rules of the statistical test are given in the following definition.

Decision Rule 5.2-1

For all the three tests below the significance level is α:

(i) A two-tailed test for Eq. (5.2.1) is to reject H_0 if the computed t of Eq. (5.2.4) is greater than $t_{n+m-2;1-\frac{\alpha}{2}}$ or less than $t_{n+m-2;\frac{\alpha}{2}}$.

$$(5.2.5)$$

(ii) A right-tailed test for Eq. (5.2.2) is to reject H_0 if the computed t of Eq. (5.2.4) is greater than $t_{n+m-2;1-\alpha}$. $\hspace{1cm}$ (5.2.6)

(iii) A left-tailed test for Eq. (5.2.3) is to reject H_0 if the computed t of Eq. (5.2.4) is less than $t_{n+m-2;\alpha}$. $\hspace{1cm}$ (5.2.7)

Remarks

1. The assumption of $\sigma_X^2 = \sigma_Y^2$ is required. Otherwise, we have difficulty in showing that the sampling distribution of Eq. (5.2.4) is a t_{n+m-2}-distribution. In the statistical literature this is the so-called Behrens–Fisher problem (see Ref. 3).
2. When both the sample sizes n and m are large, that is, n ≥ 30 and m ≥ 30, the t_{n+m-2}-distribution is reduced to the standard normal distribution Z. As a result, all the critical values in Eqs. (5.2.5) to (5.2.7) are replaced by that of the Z-distribution accordingly.

Example 5.2-1

From the finding that males are more variable than females on mathematics test scores, a professor in psychology, with his Ph.D. candidate student, wants to test a hypothsis that there might exist a phenomenon of gender-by-item-difficulty interaction such that easy items are easier for females than for males and hard items are harder for females than for males.[1] They conducted two studies. In Study 1 three forms of the minimum competency tests were derived from an item pool used in a pilot study. Item difficulty information obtained in the pilot study was used to create forms that were equally difficult. There were 68 items on each of the three forms. The data in Study 1 were gathered in 1995 from a representative sample of 10,321 8th-grade students

Table 5.2-1.   The Mean, Standard Deviation and Variance Ratio (Males/Females) for Study 1

| Test Package | Sex | Mean Package Scores | | | |
		Sample Size	Mean	SD	Variance Ratio
Form 1	Females	1,739	48.4	11.85	1.196
	Males	1,764	48.9	12.96	
Form 2	Females	1,734	47.8	12.67	1.221
	Males	1,725	47.9	14.00	
Form 3	Females	1,690	48.2	12.15	1.195
	Males	1,689	48.8	13.28	

from Minnesota. The mathematical tests used in each study were composed entirely of multiple-choice items. These tests were designed to assess competency in mathematical skills deemed essential for all high school graduates. Items emphasized application of mathematical concepts to real-life contexts. The data in Study 2 were gathered from a pilot project conducted in 1994 to develop the minimum competency mathematics tests used in Study 1. A representative sample of 5,332 9th-grade students participated in the study. Study 2 used six forms of the minimum competency mathematics achievement tests. Unlike Study 1, the forms in Study 2 varied in length; Forms 1 – 6 contained 40, 40, 41, 38, 39 and 40 items, respectively. Serial position was investigated as a potential confound by correlating it with item difficulties measured on the combined male-female samples for each form.

Mean, standard deviation and variance ratios (Males:Females) for all three forms in Study 1 are given in Table 5.2-1.

It is easily shown that the mean scores for males and females on all three forms were not significantly different at the level of 0.05 (see Exercise 5.5-1).

Remarks

1. The variance ratios of males to females are greater than one on all three forms, indicating that the spread of the males distribution is greater than that of females. It is found that there is a

greater percentage of males in the lowest score group and the three highest score groups, and there is a greater percentage of females in the middle score groups.[1]

2. In this study, item difficulty should receive more attention than it has to date. Future studies should examine whether the cognitive variables under study are confounded with difficulty such that difficulty offers an alternative explanation for any observed gender-by-difficulty interaction.[1]

B. *Dependent Case*

Let $D = X - Y$. Thus, $\mu_D = \mu_X - \mu_Y$. Then, we obtain the sample data of D from the collected sample data of X and Y, where $n = m$, that is, $d_i = x_i - y_i, i = 1, 2, \ldots, n$. Now, we wish to test the following three cases of null and alternative hypotheses:

(i) $H_0: \mu_D = 0$ versus $H_1: \mu_D \neq 0$; $\qquad\qquad$ (5.2.8)

(ii) $H_0: \mu_D \leq 0$ versus $H_1: \mu_D > 0$; $\qquad\qquad$ (5.2.9)

(iii) $H_0: \mu_D \geq 0$ versus $H_1: \mu_D < 0$. $\qquad\qquad$ (5.2.10)

Next, a testing statistics is constructed as follows:

$$t = \frac{\bar{d}}{s_D / \sqrt{n}}, \qquad\qquad (5.2.11)$$

here $\bar{d} = \sum_{i=1}^{n} d_i / n$ and $s_D^2 = \sum_{i=1}^{n} (d_i - \bar{d})^2 / (n - 1)$ are the sample mean and variance of the r.v. D.

The decision rules of the statistical test for Eqs. (5.2.8) to (5.2.10) are given in the following definition.

Decision Rule 5.2-2

For all the three tests below the significance level is α:

(i) A two-tailed test for Eq. (5.2.5) is to reject H_0 if the computed t of Eq. (5.2.11) is greater than $t_{n-1; 1-\frac{\alpha}{2}}$ or less than $t_{n-1; \frac{\alpha}{2}}$.

$$\qquad\qquad (5.2.12)$$

(ii) A right-tailed test for Eq. (5.2.6) is to reject H_0 if the computed
t of Eq. (5.2.11) is greater than $t_{n-1;1-\alpha}$.   (5.2.13)

(iii) A left-tailed test for Eq. (5.2.7) is to reject H_0 if the computed
t of Eq. (5.2.11) is less than $t_{n-1;\alpha}$.   (5.2.14)

Remarks

1. Equations (5.2.12) to (5.2.14) are almost the same as Eqs. (5.1.2)
   to (5.1.4) except that the computed t-values are defined differently.
2. The sample sizes for the dependent case are required to be the
   same, which is called the paired samples.

Example 5.2-2

The sleep pattern of 10 patients in the Michigan Asylum for insanity at Kalamazoo was measured without hypnotics (sleeping pills) and after treatment with hypnotics of (i) drug A (L-hyoscyamine hydrobromate), (ii) drug B (L-hyoscine Hydrobromate), or (iii) drug C (R-hyoscine hydrobromate). As a rule, a tablet was given on each alternate evening, and the duration of sleep and other features were noted and compared with patients to who no hypnotic was given.[4] Hyoscyamine was thus used on three occasions, and then racemic hyoscine, and then lavo-hyoscine. Then a tablet was given each evening for a week or more, the different alkaloids following each other in succession. The average number of hours of sleep of those with no use and use of the drug is tabulated in Table 5.2-2. Did the use of the drug gain additional hours of sleep for these ten patients at the significance level of 0.05?

Solution

Let X, Y and Z denote respectively the hours of sleep by the use of drugs A, B or C, and W for the no-use of any drug. Also, let

$$D_A = X - W, \quad D_B = Y - W, \quad \text{and} \quad D_C = Z - W.$$

Table 5.2-2. Additional Hours' Sleep Gained by the Use of Three Drugs

Patient	Controls (No Hypnotic)	Drug A	Drug B	Drug C
1	0.6	1.3	2.5	2.1
2	3.0	1.4	3.8	4.4
3	4.7	4.5	5.8	4.7
4	5.5	4.3	5.6	4.8
5	6.2	6.1	6.1	6.7
6	3.2	6.6	7.6	8.3
7	2.5	6.2	8.0	8.2
8	2.8	3.6	4.4	4.3
9	1.1	1.1	5.7	5.8
10	2.9	4.9	6.3	6.4

Thus, the paired sample data for the r.v.s D_A, D_B, D_C and their respective sample mean, standard deviation and t-value of Eq. (5.2.11) are obtained as given in Table 5.2-2.

Since $n = 10$ and $\alpha = 0.05$, the critical value of Eq. (5.2.13) is $t_{9;0.95} = 1.833$. From the computed t-value in the last row of Table 5.2-3, the use of drugs B and C gains additional hours of sleep for the ten patients significantly at the level of 0.05, but the use of drug A does not help the patients to gain more hours of sleep.

5.3   The Variance of a Single Random Variable

Consider a normal random variable X in which the population variance of X is unknown. Assume that the sample data of X, $\{x_i\}_{i=1}^n$ are randomly collected. We wish to test the following hypothesis cases:

(i) $H_0: \sigma_X^2 = \sigma_0^2$ versus $H_1: \sigma_X^2 = \sigma_0^2$; (5.3.1)

(ii) $H_0: \sigma_X^2 \le \sigma_0^2$ versus $H_1: \sigma_X^2 > \sigma_0^2$; (5.3.2)

(iii) $H_0: \sigma_X^2 \ge \sigma_0^2$ versus $H_1: \sigma_X^2 < \sigma_0^2$. (5.3.3)

Table 5.2-3. The Paired Sampled Data for the r.v.s D_A, D_B, and D_C

Patient	D_A	D_B	D_C
1	0.7	1.9	1.5
2	−1.6	0.8	1.4
3	−0.2	1.1	0.0
4	−1.2	0.1	−0.7
5	−0.1	−0.1	0.5
6	3.4	4.4	5.1
7	3.7	5.5	5.7
8	0.8	1.6	1.5
9	0.0	4.6	4.7
10	2.0	3.4	3.5
$\bar{d}$	0.75	2.33	2.32
s_D	1.79	2.0	2.27
t	1.33	3.68	3.24

The testing statistics is constructed as

$$\chi_2 = \frac{(n-1)s_X^2}{\sigma_0^2}, \tag{5.3.4}$$

where s_X^2 is the sample variance given by Eq. (1.4.11). It can be shown that the sampling distribution of χ of Eq. (5.3.4) is a chi-squared distribution with n − 1 degrees of freedom. The decision rules for testing Eqs. (5.3.1) to (5.3.3) are given in the following definition.

Decision Rule 5.3-1

For all the three tests below the significance level is α:

(i) A two-tailed test for Eq. (5.3.1) is to reject H_0 if the computed value χ of Eq. (5.3.4) is greater than $\chi^2_{n-1;1-\frac{\alpha}{2}}$ or less than $\chi^2_{n-1;\frac{\alpha}{2}}$; $\tag{5.3.5}$

(ii) A right-tailed test for Eq. (5.3.2) is to reject H_0 if the computed
    value χ of Eq. (5.3.4) is greater than $\chi^2_{n-1;1-\alpha}$ (5.3.6)
(iii) A left-tailed test for Eq. (5.3.3) is to reject H_0 if the computed
    value χ of Eq. (5.3.4) is less than $\chi^2_{n-1;\alpha}$.   (5.3.7)

Remarks

1. The requirement that X is a normal random variable is necessary; otherwise, the sampling distribution of Eq. (5.3.4) will not
   be a chi-squared distribution.
2. The probability tables of the chi-squared distribution is given
   in Table A-3 in the appendix.

Example 5.3-1

A psychology professor claimed that the variance of IQ scores
for college students is 100. Assume that the IQ scores of college
students is a normal r.v. X. To verify this claim, she decided to test
a pair of hypotheses as follows:

$$H_0 : \sigma^2_X = 100 \quad \text{versus} \quad H_1 : \sigma^2_X \neq 100. \qquad (5.3.8)$$

Suppose that the sample variance of the IQ scores calculated from
a random sample of 20 students is 147.8. Is the claim of this
professor valid at the significance level of 0.05?

Solution

To test Eq. (5.3.8), we use Eq. (5.3.4) to compute the value of the
testing statistics χ as follows:

$$\chi = (20 - 1) \times 147.8/100 = 13.3 \qquad (5.3.9)$$

The critical values for Eq. (5.3.8) are given by $\chi^2_{19,0.025} = 8.907$
and $\chi^2_{19,0.975} = 32.85$. Since the computed χ-value of Eq. (5.3.9) is
neither greater than 32.85 nor less than 8.907, H_0 is not rejected at
the significance level of 0.05. Hence the professor's claim is valid.

5.4   The Variances of Two Random Variables

Consider two independent normal r.v.s X and Y in which their variances σ_X^2 and σ_Y^2 are unknown. We wish to test the following three pair of hypotheses:

(i) $H_0 : \sigma_X^2 = \sigma_Y^2$ versus $H_1 : \sigma_X^2 \neq \sigma_Y^2;$ (5.4.1)

(ii) $H_0 : \sigma_X^2 \leq \sigma_Y^2$ versus $H_1 : \sigma_X^2 > \sigma_Y^2;$ (5.4.2)

(iii) $H_0 : \sigma_X^2 \geq \sigma_Y^2$ versus $H_1 : \sigma_X^2 < \sigma_Y^2.$ (5.4.3)

Assume that the sample data for X and Y are randomly collected as $\{x_i\}_{i=1}^n$ and $\{y_j\}_{j=1}^m$. Thus, the testing statistics for Eqs. (5.4.1) to (5.4.3) is constructed as follows:

$$\xi = \frac{s_X^2}{s_Y^2},$$ (5.4.4)

where s_X^2 and s_Y^2 denote the sample variance of X and Y, respectively. It can be shown that the sampling distribution of Eq. (5.4.4) is a $F_{n-1,m-1}$-distribution with the degrees of freedom $n-1$ and $m-1$. The decision rules for testing Eqs. (5.4.1) to (5.4.3) are given as follows.

Decision Rule 5.4-1

For all the three tests below the significance level is α:

(i)   A two-tailed test for Eq. (5.4.1) is to reject H_0 if the computed value ξ of Eq. (5.4.4) is greater than $F_{n-1,m-1;1-\frac{\alpha}{2}}$ or less than $F_{n-1,m-1;\frac{\alpha}{2}};$ (5.4.5)

(ii)   A right-tailed test for Eq. (5.4.2) is to reject H_0 if the computed value ξ of Eq. (5.4.4) is greater than $F_{n-1,m-1;1-\alpha};$ (5.4.6)

(iii)   A left-tailed test for Eq. (5.4.3) is to reject H_0 if the computed value ξ of Eq. (5.4.4) is less than $F_{n-1,m-1;\alpha}.$ (5.4.7)

Remarks

1. The derivation and sampling distribution of Eq. (5.4.4) is given in Ref. 2.
2. The degrees of freedom of $n-1$ and $m-1$ are associated respectively with the numerator and denominator of Eq. (5.4.4).

Example 5.4-1

A biologist who studies spiders believes that not only do female green lynx spiders (Y) tend to be longer than their male counterparts (X), but that their lengths seem to vary more too. Suppose that the data from a random sample of 30 male and 25 female spiders yield respectively, $\bar{x} = 5.92$, $s_X^2 = 0.44$, $\bar{y} = 8.15$ and $s_Y^2 = 1.41$. Is the biologist's latter belief true at the significance level of 0.05?

Solution

From the biologist's latter belief, we wish to test Eq. (5.4.3). The computed testing statistics is given by

$$\xi = \frac{0.44}{1.41} = 0.3120567 \approx 0.312. \tag{1}$$

Recall from Eq. (3.2E.4) that $F_{m-1,n-1} = \frac{1}{F_{n-1,m-1}}$. The critical value for Eq. (5.4.7) is given by

$$F_{29,24;0.05} = \frac{1}{F_{24,29;0.05}} = \frac{1}{1.89} = 0.5231. \tag{2}$$

Since the computed value of Eq. (1) is less than the critical value of Eq. (2), H_0 is rejected at the significance level of 0.05. Hence, the biologist's belief that the length of the female spiders is much varied is valid.

Remark

Since we are unable to get from the table in Ref. 2 the exact critical value for $F_{24,29;0.05}$, we use its closest approximation, that is, $F_{24,29;0.05} \cong F_{24,30;0.05}$.

5.5   Exercises

1. By using Table 5.2-1, show that there is no difference between the mean scores in the test of all three forms.

References

1. Bielinski J, Davison ML. (1998) Gender differences by item difficulty interactions in multiple-choice mathematical items. *Am Educ Res J* **35**: 455–476.
2. Hogg RV, Tanis EA. (1997) *Probability and Statistical Inference*, 5th ed. Prentice Hall Publishing Co., Upper Saddle River, NJ.
3. Kim SH, Cohen AS. (1998) On the Behrens–Fisher problem: A review. *J Educ Behav Statist* **23**: 356–377.
4. Student (1908) The probable error of a mean. *Biometrika* **6**: 1–25.

6 Inference on Proportions

In this chapter we are going to learn how to draw an inference on the unknown population proportion of a binomial random variable and a comparison on proportions of two binomial random variables.

6.1 The Proportion of a Single Binomial Random Variable

Consider a binomial random variable (r.v.) $X \sim \text{BIN}(n, p)$ with the unknown proportion p. We wish to test the following cases of hypotheses:

(i) $H_0: p = p_0$ versus $H_1: p \neq p_0$;   (6.1.1)

(ii) $H_0: p \leq p_0$ versus $H_1: p > p_0$;   (6.1.2)

(iii) $H_0: p \geq p_0$ versus $H_1: p < p_0$.   (6.1.3)

Assume that the sample data are collected, and let the total number of successes be k in n independent Bernoulli trials, where $n \geq 30$. The testing statistics for Eqs. (6.1.1) to (6.1.3) is constructed as follows:

$$z = \frac{k - np_0}{\sqrt{k(n-k)/n}}. \qquad (6.1.4)$$

It can be shown[1] that the sampling distribution of Eq. (6.1.4) is a normal random variable. The decision rules for testing Eqs. (6.1.1) to (6.1.3) are given as follows.

Decision Rule 6.1-1

For all the three tests below the significance level is α:

(i) A two-tailed test for Eq. (6.1.1) is to reject H_0 if the computed z of Eq. (6.1.4) is greater than $z_{1-\frac{\alpha}{2}}$ or less than $z_{\frac{\alpha}{2}}$.   (6.1.5)

(ii) A right-tailed test for Eq. (6.1.2) is to reject H_0 if the computed z of Eq. (6.1.4) is greater than $z_{1-\alpha}$.   (6.1.6)

(iii) A left-tailed test for Eq. (6.1.3) is to reject H_0 if the computed z of Eq. (6.1.4) is less than z_α.   (6.1.7)

Remarks

1. It can be shown[1] that the $100 \times (1 - \alpha)\%$ confidence interval is given by

$$\hat{p} - z_{1-\frac{\alpha}{2}}\sqrt{\hat{p}\hat{q}/n} \le p \le \hat{p} + Z_{1-\frac{\alpha}{2}}\sqrt{\hat{p}\hat{q}/n}, \qquad (6.1.8)$$

   where $\hat{p} = \frac{k}{n}$ is the point estimator for p and $\hat{q} = 1 - \hat{p}$.

2. If $n < 30$, all the critical values in Eqs. (6.1.5) to (6.1.7) are replaced by that of the corresponding t_{n-1}-distribution.

Example 6.1-1

A random survey of 1,324 Americans yielded 866 who favored the death penalty. Find the 95% confidence interval for the proportion of Americans who favor the death penalty.

Solution

Let p be the proportion of Americans who favored the death penalty. Since 866 out of the 1324 Americans favored the death penalty, a point estimator for the unknown p is given by

$$\hat{p} = \frac{866}{1324} = 0.65407855 \approx 0.654. \qquad (1)$$

It follows that

$$\hat{q} = 1 - \hat{p} = 1 - 0.654 = 0.346. \tag{2}$$

Since $1 - \alpha = 0.95$,

$$z_{1-\frac{\alpha}{2}} = z_{0.975} = 1.96. \tag{3}$$

By substituting Eqs. (1) to (3) into Eq. (6.1.8),

$$0.654 - 1.96 \times \sqrt{\frac{0.654 \times 0.346}{1324}} \leq p \leq 0.654 + 1.96$$

$$\times \sqrt{\frac{0.654 \times 0.346}{1324}}, \quad \text{or} \quad 0.63 \leq p \leq 0.68. \tag{4}$$

The 95% confidence interval for the true proportion p is given by
Eq. (4).

6.2   Proportions of Two Binomial Random Variables

Consider two independent Binomial r.v. $X \sim \text{BIN}(n, p_X)$ and $Y \sim \text{BIN}(m, p_Y)$, where both n and m are no less than 30, p_X and p_Y are unknown. We wish to test the following pairs of hypotheses:

(i) $H_0: p_X = p_Y$ versus $H_1: p_X \neq p_Y$;   (6.2.1)
(ii) $H_0: p_X \leq p_Y$ versus $H_1: p_X > p_Y$;   (6.2.2)
(iii) $H_0: p_X \geq p_Y$ versus $H_1: p_X < p_Y$.   (6.2.3)

Assume that the sample data are collected and the total number of successes in n and m independent Bernoulli trials for X and Y are given, by n_X and m_Y, respectively. The testing statistics for Eqs. (6.2.1) to (6.2.3) is constructed as follows if $\hat{p}_X > \hat{p}_Y$:

$$z = \frac{\hat{p}_X - \hat{p}_Y}{\sqrt{\hat{p}\hat{q}(n^{-1} + m^{-1})}}, \tag{6.2.4}$$

where $\hat{p}_X = \frac{n_X}{n}$, $\hat{p}_Y = \frac{m_Y}{m}$, $\hat{p} = \frac{n_X+m_Y}{n+m}$ and $\hat{q} = 1 - \hat{p}$. The decision rules for testing Eqs. (6.1.1) to (6.1.3) are given as follows.

Decision Rule 6.2-1

For all the three tests below the significance level is α:

(i) A two-tailed test for Eq. (6.2.1) is to reject H_0 if the computed z of Eq. (6.2.4) is greater than $z_{1-\frac{\alpha}{2}}$ or less than $z_{\frac{\alpha}{2}}$.   (6.2.5)

(ii) A right-tailed test for Eq. (6.2.2) is to reject H_0 if the computed z of Eq. (6.2.4) is greater than $z_{1-\alpha}$.   (6.2.6)

(iii) A left-tailed test for Eq. (6.2.3) is to reject H_0 if the computed z of Eq. (6.2.4) is less than z_α.   (6.2.7)

Remarks

1. It can be shown[1] that the $100 \times (1 - \alpha)\%$ confidence interval is given by

$$\hat{p}_X - \hat{p}_Y - z_{1-\frac{\alpha}{2}} \sqrt{\frac{\hat{p}\hat{q}}{n}} \le p \le \hat{p}_X - \hat{p}_Y + z_{1-\frac{\alpha}{2}} \sqrt{\frac{\hat{p}\hat{q}}{n}}. \qquad (6.2.8)$$

2. If $\hat{p}_Y > \hat{p}_X$, the numerator in Eq. (6.2.4) should be replaced by $\hat{p}_Y - \hat{p}_X$.

3. If $n < 30$, all the critical values in Eqs. (6.2.5) to (6.2.8) are replaced by that of the corresponding t_{n-1}-distribution.

Example 6.2-1

Let X and Y be two random variables that represent physicians with and without lung cancer (see Example 1.3-4), respectively. Assume that the sample data were randomly collected and cross-classified into Table 1.3-4. Is the smoker's mortality rate of physicians with lung cancer higher than that without it at the significance level of 0.05?

Solution

This is equivalent to testing Eq. (6.2.2). Since $\hat{p}_X = \frac{60}{63} = 0.952 > \hat{p}_Y = \frac{32}{43} = 0.744$, we use Eq. (6.2.4) to calculate the testing statistics z. First, we need to compute the pooled sample proportion from X and Y as follows:

$$\hat{p} = \frac{60 + 32}{63 + 43} = \frac{92}{106} = 0.8679245 \approx 0.868. \tag{1}$$

By using Eq. (6.2.4), we have

$$z = \frac{0.952 - 0.744}{\sqrt{0.868 \times 0.132 \times \left(\frac{1}{63} + \frac{1}{43}\right)}} = \frac{0.208}{0.066} = 3.1515 \approx 3.15. \tag{2}$$

Since the computed z-value of Eq. (2) is greater than the critical value for Eq. (6.2.6), $z_{0.95} = 1.645$, H_0 is rejected at the significance level of 0.05. Hence, the smoker's mortality rate for physicians with lung cancer is significantly higher than those without the disease.

6.3 Exercises

1. A random survey of 25 college seniors indicated that seven were planning to pursue a graduate degree. Find the 90% confidence interval for the proportion of all college seniors planning to pursue a graduate degree.
2. A national poll, based on interviews with 1200 voters in a presidential campaign, gave one candidate 52% of the vote. Find the 95% confidence interval for the proportion of voters supporting this candidate.
3. If 1244 out of a random sample of 5500 Amercians selected jogging, find the 95% confidence interval for the proportion of Americans who select jogging as one of their recreational activities.
4. The New England Journal of Medicine published a study in which 615 smokers (all who wanted to give up smoking) were randomly assigned either Zyban (an antidepressant) or a

placebo (a dummy pill) for six weeks. Of the 309 patients who received Zyban, 71 stopped smoking a year later. Of the 306 patients who received a placebo, 37 stopped smoking a year later. Test the hypothesis that taking an antidepressant drug helps smokers kick their habit at the level of significance 0.05.

References

1. Hogg RV, Tanis EA. (1997) *Probability and Statistical Inference*, 5th ed. Prentice Hall Publishing Co., Upper Saddle River, NJ.
2. McClave JT, Sinich T. (2000) *A First Course in Statistics*, 7th ed. Prentice Hall Publishing Co., Upper Saddle River, NJ.

7 Inference on Correlation and Regression

In this chapter we are going to learn mainly the subject of regression toward the mean (RTM), correlation, linear regression, and generalized linear regression models.

7.0 A Note on Regression toward the Mean

The notion of "regression toward the mean" comes from genetics and was introduced into statistics by Sir Francis Galton (1822–1911) during the late 19th century to describe a hereditary phenomenon.[10] He noted that although there was a tendency for tall parents to have tall children and for short parents to have short children, the distribution of height in a population did not change from generation to generation. In a very detailed paper he showed that this constancy could be explained by a tendency towards the mean height of children who had parents of a given height to regress or move toward the population average height.

Though Galton popularized the concept of regression, he mistook the RTM as an universal inheritance law. He failed to understand that RTM was a general statistical phenomenon. Just like the law of natural selection or the invisible hand in market economics, it is a consequence of natural phenomenon that simulates deliberate intervention. It is an inherent feature of change that is a statistical artifact. This phenomenon can be observed in many areas of society such as economy, politics, sports, and even in evolution.[25]

In fact, it can be shown that RTM will occur if any two correlated random variables has a less than perfect correlation. Let X and Y be the pre-test and post-test scores in a pre-test/post-test study. Assume that X and Y are distributed as bivariate normal distribution $(X, Y) \sim BN(\mu_X, \mu_Y, \sigma_X^2, \sigma_Y^2, \rho_{XY})$. Then it can be shown that the conditional mean of Y, given $X = x_0$, is given by

$$Y^* = E(Y|X = x_0) = \mu_Y + \rho_{XY} \cdot \frac{\sigma_Y}{\sigma_X} \cdot (x_0 - \mu_X), \qquad (7.0.1)$$

or expressed in terms of its standardized score

$$Z_{Y^*} = E(Z_Y|Z_{x_0}) = \rho_{XY^*} \times Z_{x_0}, \qquad (7.0.2)$$

where $Z_Y = \frac{Y - \mu_Y}{\sigma_Y}$ and $Z_{x_0} = \frac{x_0 - \mu_X}{\sigma_X}$. The effect due to RTM is then given by

$$\text{Effect-RTM} = Z_{Y^*} - Z_{x_0} = (\rho_{XY} - 1)Z_{x_0}. \qquad (7.0.3)$$

The key idea of RTM is simply expounded as scores that are extreme in standard deviation on one measure are not likely to be as extreme when measured on the other measure. Change is inevitable, but some components of scores hardly change at all. Consequently, there may be little or no RTM if selection is made on these components.

If statistical inference fails to account for the effect of RTM, this effect would cause a misleading conclusion, which is the "regression fallacy".[8] Here comes an interesting story to show you how a good researcher comes to absorb the new idea. After grasping the essential idea from a review on the book *The Triumph of Mediocrity in Business* written by his teacher H Hotelling,[12] M Friedman who is a 1976 Nobel Laureate in Economics introduced the concept to partition the income as the sum of two components — permanent and transitory — to avoid the trap of regression fallacy when studying the relation between incomes of the same individual in different years.[9]

If X and Y represent the first and second measurement without intervention of a characteristic of a human subject, thus

$\mu_X = \mu_Y \equiv \mu$ and $\sigma_X = \sigma_Y \equiv \sigma$. When $X > x_0$ is required in a screening program, the effect of RTM is given by[12]

$$\text{Effect-RTM} = E(X|X > x_0) - E(Y|X > x_0)$$

$$= (1 - \rho_{XY}) \cdot \sigma \cdot c_0, \qquad (7.0.4)$$

where $c_0 = \frac{\varphi(z_0)}{1 - \Phi(z_0)}$ and $z_0 = \frac{x_0 - \mu}{\sigma}$.

Remarks

1. Similar to Friedman's income theory, an individual's test score, regardless of an American SAT or a Chinese College Entrance Exam, has two components: permanent and stochastic. The permanent component that is more stable reveals the person's intrinsic capability, while the stochastic component that has much variation reflects the temporary luckiness. As a result, there exists the RTM effect related to his/her score. We are surely able to estimate this effect if the same person is examined for the second time.

2. More examples are involved with the RTM.[5] Here is listed an example from patients brought to the hospital's emergency care center.

Example 7.0-1. Calculation of the effect due to RTM

Patient charts were examined in the Grady Hospital Emergency Care Center.[23] Patients were excluded if their charts documented symptomatic hypertension when admitted to the hospital, received ED treatment with nitrates, β-agonists or antihypertensives, and having the following conditions: seizure within the preceding 24 hours, severe trauma, or evidence of severe distress. Of the remaining patients, blood pressures were measured on two occasions, 20 minutes to 4 hours apart.

Of 220 consecutive charts examined initially, 76 had two sets of vital signs and qualified for the all-patient sample. There was no difference in mean of initial diastolic blood pressure (DBP) between patients with and without a second set of vital signs. Another 195 consecutive patients with hypertensive

Table 7.0-1. **The mean and standard deviation of the first and second readings of the DBP**

DBP	All-patients	Patients with $DBP > 90$
Sample size	76	195
First reading mean	78.3	104.5
Second reading mean	74.6	92.9
Standard deviation	17.9	
Correlation coefficient	0.76	

(DBP > 90 mm Hg) on initial determination and two sets of vital signs were selected for the hypertensive-patient sample. The mean, standard deviation and correlation coefficients of DBP for the two groups are given in Table 7.0-1.

Calculate the effect due to RTM from Table 7.0-1.

Solution

Let X and Y be the first and second reading DBP scores of the all-patients. Assume that (X, Y) is a bivariate normal random variable with $\mu_X = \mu_Y \equiv \mu$ and $\sigma_X = \sigma_Y \equiv \sigma$. By using Eq. (7.0.4) with $\mu_X = 78.3, \sigma_X = 17.9, \rho_{XY} = 0.76$ and $x_0 = 90$, we first compute the standardized z-score

$$z_0 = \frac{90 - 78.3}{17.9} = 0.6536. \tag{1}$$

The effect due to RTM of Eq. (7.0.4) is given by

$$\text{Effect-RTM} = \frac{(1 - 0.76) \cdot \varphi(0.6536)}{1 - \Phi(0.6536)} = 6.83. \tag{2}$$

The observed difference in the first and second reading of DBP between the all-patients and patients with DBP > 90 is

$$(74.6 - 78.3) - (92.9 - 104.5) = 7.9. \tag{3}$$

Out of 7.9 in Eq. (3), 6.83 is due to the effect of RTM.

7.1 The Correlation Between X and Y

The population correlation for any bivariate random variables (r.v.s) (X, Y) is defined exactly the same as given by Eq. (3.2F.2), even without the assumption of normality. Assume that the sample data, $\{(x_i, y_i)\}_{i=1}^{n}$, are randomly collected. Thus, the point estimator for Eq. (3.2F.2) is given by

$$\hat{\rho}_{XY} \equiv \frac{c\hat{o}v_{XY}}{\hat{\sigma}_X \hat{\sigma}_Y} = \frac{\sum_{i=1}^{n}(x_i - \bar{x})(y_i - \bar{y})}{\sqrt{\sum_{i=1}^{n}(x_i - \bar{x})^2 \cdot \sum_{i=1}^{n}(y_i - \bar{y})^2}}. \qquad (7.1.1)$$

But Eq. (7.1.1) is not an unbiased estimator for ρ_{XY}. To find the sampling distribution of Eq. (7.1.1) when the population correlation coefficient is nonzero, we have to employ the Fisher's inverse-hyperbolic-tangent transformation defined by

$$\hat{\omega} = \tan h^{-1}(\hat{\rho}_{XY}) \equiv \frac{1}{2} \ln\left(\frac{1 + \hat{\rho}_{XY}}{1 - \hat{\rho}_{XY}}\right), \qquad (7.1.2)$$

where $\tanh^{-1}(x)$ is the inverse function of the hyperbolic tangent function, $\tanh(x) = (e^x - e^{-x})/(e^x + e^{-x})$. It can be shown[6] that

$$z_{\omega} = \frac{\hat{\omega} - \omega}{\sigma_{\hat{\omega}}} \sim N(0, 1), \qquad (7.1.3)$$

where $\omega = \tan h^{-1}(\rho_{XY})$, $\sigma_{\hat{\omega}}^2 = n - 3$ as $n \to \infty$. As a result, the interval estimator for ρ_{XY} is given in the following theorem (see Ref. 1, pp. 122–135).

Theorem 7.1.1

The $100(1 - \alpha)\%$ confidence interval for ρ_{XY} of Eq. (3.2F.2) is given by

$$\tanh\left(\hat{\omega} - \frac{z_{1-\frac{\alpha}{2}}}{\sqrt{n-3}}\right) \leq \rho_{XY} \leq \tanh\left(\hat{\omega} + \frac{z_{1-\frac{\alpha}{2}}}{\sqrt{n-3}}\right), \qquad (7.1.4)$$

where $\hat{\omega}$ is defined by Eq. (7.1.2)

Remarks

1. As is shown in Eq. (7.1.3), the asymptotic sampling distribution of Eq. (7.1.2) does not depend on the population correlation coefficient ρ_{XY}; it also tends to normality faster.
2. The sample size n is required to be greater than 3 as shown in Eq. (7.1.3).

   We wish to test the following three cases of hypotheses:

   (i) $H_0: \rho_{XY} = 0$ versus $H_1: \rho_{XY} \neq 0$;   (7.1.5)

   (ii) $H_0: \rho_{XY} \leq 0$ versus $H_1: \rho_{XY} > 0$;   (7.1.6)

   (iii) $H_0: \rho_{XY} \geq 0$ versus $H_1: \rho_{XY} < 0$.   (7.1.7)

   Equation (7.1.3) can also be used as the testing statistics for Eqs. (7.1.5) to (7.1.7).

   The decision rules for testing Eqs. (7.1.5) to (7.1.7) with the use of Eq. (7.1.3) are given as follows.

Decision Rule 7.1-1

For all the three tests below the significance level is α:

(i) A two-tailed test for Eq. (7.1.5) is to reject H_0 if the computed z_ω of Eq. (7.1.3) is greater than $z_{1-\frac{\alpha}{2}}$ or less than $z_{\frac{\alpha}{2}}$.   (7.1.8)

(ii) A right-tailed test for Eq. (7.1.6) is to reject H_0 if the computed z_ω of Eq. (7.1.3) is greater than $z_{1-\alpha}$.   (7.1.9)

(iii) A left-tailed test for Eq. (7.1.5) is to reject H_0 if the computed z_ω of Eq. (7.1.6) is less than z_α.   (7.1.10)

Remarks

1. Note that $\rho_{XY} = 0$ implies $\omega = 0$. If $\rho_{XY} = \rho_0 \neq 0$, instead of $\rho_{XY} = 0$, in Eqs. (7.1.5) to (7.1.7), then the value of ω in Eq. (7.1.3) is replaced accordingly by $\omega_0 = tanh^{-1}(\rho_0)$.
2. If $n < 30$, the critical value of the standard normal distribution is replaced by that of t_{n-3}-distribution.

Example 7.1-1

A sample of ten father and eldest son pairs was randomly selected and their heights were measured as given in Table 7.1-1.

Table 7.1-1.   The height data of 10 Father-son's pairs

Height of father in inches (X)	Height of son in inches (Y)
66	63
68	67
65	64
69	68
66	62
68	70
65	66
71	68
67	67
68	69

(a) Find the scatter plot for the sample data in Table 7.1-1.

(b) Find the 95% confidence interval for ρ_{XY}.

(c) Is the null hypothesis H_0 in a two-tailed hypothesis test of Eq. (7.1.3) true at the significance level of 0.5?

Solution

(a) The scatter plot is to plot the ten pairs of (x_i, y_i) in the Cartesian xy-plane (see Figure 7.1-1).

(b) Since $n = 10$ and $\alpha = 0.05$, the critical value $t_{n-3;1-\frac{\alpha}{2}}$ is given by

$$t_{7;0.975} = 2.365. \tag{1}$$

Next, we compute the point estimator $\hat{\rho}_{XY}$ of Eq. (7.1.1)

$$\hat{\rho}_{XY} = \frac{29.8}{5.6657 \times 7.8994} = 0.66626 \approx 0.6663. \tag{2}$$

By substituting Eq. (1) into Eq. (7.1.4), we have

$$\tanh^{-1}(0.6663) - \frac{2.365}{\sqrt{10-3}} \leq \tanh^{-1}(\rho_{XY})$$

$$\leq \tanh^{-1}(0.6663) + \frac{2.365}{\sqrt{10-3}},$$

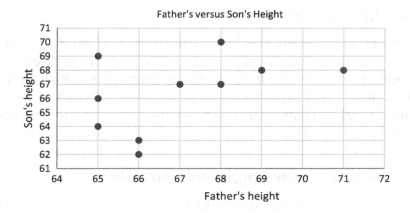

Fig. 7.1-1.   The scatter plot of the data in Table 7.1-1.

or

$$-0.09 \leq \rho_{XY} \leq 1.70. \qquad (3)$$

Equation (3) is the desired 95% confidence interval for ρ_{XY}.
(c) By substituting $n = 10$ and Eq. (2) into Eq. (7.1.4), we have
(d)

$$z_{\omega} = \frac{\tanh^{-1}(0.6663)}{\sqrt{10-3}} = \frac{0.8041}{2.6458} = 0.3039 \approx 0.3. \qquad (4)$$

Since Eq. (4) is less than Eq. (1), H_0 is not rejected at the significance level of 0.05, that is, the correlation coefficient between the father's and son's height is zero.

Remarks

1. Since the 95% confidence interval of Eq. (3) includes the number zero, this confirms the hypothesis testing result of Eq. (4).
2. That the correlation coefficient is zero does not imply that X and Y are independent.

7.2   Linear Regression

By observing that the conditional mean of Y of Eq. (7.0.3) is a linear function of X, FY Edgeworth (1845–1926) generalized it to a more general setting by relaxing the requirement that both X and Y follow a bivariate normal distribution. Thus, it frees us from a restricted confinement and opens a new era of regression modeling.

A.   *Simple Linear Regression Models*

Consider a new scenario in which the response variable Y is random and the explanatory variable X is non-random. We wish to find a linear relation between X and Y. Assume that the data set $\{x_i, y_i\}_{i=1}^{n}$ are collected in which only $\{y_i\}$ are subjected to errors, but $\{x_i\}$ are not. Thus, the relation between x and y is assumed to satisfy

$$y_i = a + bx_i + e_i, \qquad (7.2A.1)$$

where a and b are unknown regression coefficients, and $\{e_i\}$ denote the uncorrelated random errors with $E(e_i) = 0$, $\text{var}(e_i) = \sigma^2$ and $\text{cov}(e_j, e_k) = 0$ if $j \neq k$.

By using the least squares method, it can be shown[5] that the estimators for a and b are given, respectively, by

$$\hat{b} = \frac{\sum_{i=1}^{n}(x_i - \bar{x})(y_i - \bar{y})}{\sum_{i=1}^{n}(x_i - \bar{x})^2}, \qquad (7.2A.2)$$

and

$$\hat{a} = \bar{y} - \hat{b}\bar{x}. \qquad (7.2A.3)$$

Therefore, the desired prediction equation is given by

$$\hat{y} = \hat{a} + \hat{b}x. \qquad (7.2A.4)$$

Remarks

1. Although there seems to be a minor similarity between Eqs. (7.2A.2) and (7.1.1), there are no connections at all. In other words, Secs. 7.1 and 7.2 are intrinsically different.
2. The model given here is useful in the mathematical curve fitting.
3. When both variables are subjected to errors, the formula for the estimators of Eqs. (7.2A.2) and (7.2A.3) no longer applies; they become more complex.[5]

Since $\{y_i\}$ are subjected to errors, both the estimators of Eqs. (7.2A.2) to (7.2A.3) are random. Their standard errors are given in the following theorem.

Theorem 7.2A.1

The standard errors for Eqs. (7.2A.2) and (7.2A.3) and the covariance between $\hat{a}$ and $\hat{b}$ are given, respectively, by

$$se(\hat{b}) \equiv \sqrt{\operatorname{var}(\hat{b})} = \sqrt{\sigma^2 \left[\sum_{i=1}^{n} (x_i - \bar{x})^2 \right]^{-1}} ; \qquad (7.2A.5)$$

$$\operatorname{var}(\hat{a}) = \sigma^2 \left\{ n^{-1} + \bar{x}^2 \left[\sum_{i=1}^{n} (x_i - \bar{x})^2 \right]^{-1} \right\}; \qquad (7.2A.6)$$

and

$$\operatorname{cov}(\hat{a}, \hat{b}) = -\bar{x}\sigma^2 \left[\sum_{i=1}^{n} (x_i - \bar{x})^2 \right]^{-1} \qquad (7.2A.7)$$

Remarks

1. The proof is given in Ref. 29.
2. Equation (7.2A.7) implies that the estimators $\hat{a}$ and $\hat{b}$ are not independent; they are correlated.

3. In practical applications, the unknown σ^2 is replaced by its estimator given by

$$\hat{\sigma}^2 = \frac{\sum_{i=1}^{n} (y_i - \hat{y}_i)^2}{n-2}, \qquad (7.2A.8)$$

where $\hat{y}_i$ is given by Eq. (7.2A.4) at $x = x_i$.

We wish to test the following three pair of hypotheses:

(i) $H_0: b = 0$ versus $H_1 : b \neq 0$;   (7.2A.9)
(ii) $H_0: b \leq 0$ versus $H_1 : b > 0$;   (7.2A.10)
(iii) $H_0: b \geq 0$ versus $H_1 : b < 0$.   (7.2A.11)

If $n < 30$, the testing statistics is constructed as follows:

$$t = \frac{\hat{b}}{\sqrt{\widehat{var}(\hat{b})}}, \qquad (7.2A.12)$$

where $\widehat{var}(\hat{b})$ in Eq. (7.2A.12) is obtained by substituting Eq. (7.2A.8) for σ^2 in Eq. (7.2A.5). It can be shown that the sampling distribution of Eq. (7.2A.12) is a t_{n-2}-distribution with $n-2$ degrees of freedom if $n < 30$.

The decision rules for testing Eqs. (7.2A.9) to (7.2A11) are given in the following.

Decision Rule 7.2A-1

For all the three tests below the significance level is α:

(i)   A two-tailed test for Eq. (7.2A.9) is to reject H_0 if the computed t of Eq. (7.2A.12) is greater than $t_{n-2;1-\frac{\alpha}{2}}$ or less than $t_{n-2;\frac{\alpha}{2}}$;   (7.2A.13)
(ii) A right-tailed test for Eq. (7.2A.10) is to reject H_0 if the computed t of Eq. (7.2A.12) is greater than $t_{n-2;1-\alpha}$;   (7.2A.14)
(iii) A left-tailed test for Eq. (7.2A.11) is to reject H_0 if the computed t of Eq. (7.2A.12) is less than $t_{n-2;\alpha}$.   (7.2A.15)

Example 7.2A-1

By using the data in Example 7.1-1, find the linear regression model for the son's height in terms of the father's height.

Solution

Let X and Y denote the father's and the son's height, respectively. The linear regression model for Y in terms of X is given by Eq. (7.2A.1). By using Eqs. (7.2A.2) and (7.2A.3) the estimators for a and b are given by

$$\hat{b} = \frac{29.8}{31.2} = 0.9551 \approx 0.955, \tag{1}$$

and

$$\hat{a} = 67.2 - 0.955 * 66.4 = 2.1285 \approx 2.13. \tag{2}$$

By using Eqs. (1) and (2) the desired regression model is

$$\hat{y} = 2.13 + 0.955x.$$

Remark

Test of Eq. (7.2A.9) is given as Exercise 7.5-1.

B. *Multiple Linear Regression Models*

Linear regression models can be extended to multiple linear regression models in which we wish to investigate the relation between the random response variable Y and k non-random explanatory variables $X_1, X_2, \ldots, X_k$ on the interval scale. Assume that for $i = 1, 2, \ldots, n$ the collected data, $\{y_i, x_{1i}, \ldots, x_{ki}\}_{i=1}^{n}$, satisfy

$$y_i = b_0 + b_1 x_{1i} + \cdots + b_k x_{ki} + e_i, \tag{7.2B.1}$$

where $\{b_j\}, j = 0, 1, 2, \ldots, k$ are unknown regression coefficients, and $\{e_i\}$ denote the uncorrelated random errors with

$E(e_i) = 0, \text{var}(e_i) = \sigma^2$ and $\text{cov}(e_j, e_k) = 0$ if $j \neq k$. Equation (7.2B.1) is conveniently expressed in terms of the matrix notation:

$$\vec{y} = W\vec{b}, \qquad (7.2B.2)$$

where $\vec{y}$, W and $\vec{b}$ are respectively given by

$$\vec{y} = \begin{pmatrix} y_1 \\ y_2 \\ \vdots \\ y_n \end{pmatrix}, \quad W = \begin{bmatrix} 1 & x_{11} & \cdots & x_{k1} \\ 1 & x_{12} & \cdots & x_{k2} \\ \vdots & \vdots & \vdots & \vdots \\ 1 & x_{1n} & \cdots & x_{kn} \end{bmatrix}, \quad \text{and} \quad \vec{b} = \begin{pmatrix} b_0 \\ b_1 \\ \vdots \\ b_k \end{pmatrix}.$$

By using the least squares method, the estimators for the regression coefficients are given by

$$\hat{\vec{b}} = (W^T W)^{-1} W^T \vec{y}. \qquad (7.2B.3)$$

The prediction model is then given by

$$\hat{\vec{y}} = W\hat{\vec{b}}. \qquad (7.2B.4)$$

It can be shown[5] that the variance of the regression estimator of Eq. (7.2B.4) is given by

$$\text{var}(\hat{\vec{b}}) = \sigma^2 (W^T W)^{-1}. \qquad (7.2B.5)$$

If σ^2 is unknown, it can be estimated by

$$\hat{\sigma}^2 = (\vec{y} - W\hat{\vec{b}})^T (\vec{y} - W\hat{\vec{b}})/(n - k - 1). \qquad (7.2B.6)$$

Thus, in practical applications, Eq. (7.2B.5) is estimated by substituting Eq. (7.2B.6) for σ^2 in Eq. (7.2B.5) and given by

$$\hat{\text{var}}(\hat{\vec{b}}) = \hat{\sigma}^2 (W^T W)^{-1}. \qquad (7.2B.7)$$

Remarks

1. The numerator of the right side of Eq. (7.2B.6) is called the residual sum of squares in which the ith residual is given by $\hat{e}_i = y_i - \vec{w}_i^T \hat{\vec{b}}$, where $\vec{w}_i^T$ is the ith row of the coefficient matrix W in Eq. (7.2B.2).

2. A scatter plot of the ith residual against y_i is a useful tool to check whether the assumption of linearity between Y and X_1, $X_2, \ldots, X_k$ is valid. For details, see Ref. 29.
3. In order for the matrix $W^T W$ in Eq. (7.2B.3) to be nonsingular, the column vectors of the matrix W needs to be linearly independent. This assumption is not good enough. It could encounter another problem of multicollinearity.[5]

Example 7.2B-1

This example studies the incidence of post-operative wound infection and sepsis in 2903 patients from 12 hospitals.[17] Since various risk factors might combine in a multiplicative rather than an additive way on the risk φ of having sepsis due to wound infection, we need to take the following nonlinear transformation on φ to get the response variable Y

$$Y = \ln(\ln[1 - \varphi]^{-1}) = \sum_{k=1}^{K} X_k \cdot lnb_k, \tag{1}$$

whére ln is the logarithmic function with the natural base, $\{X_k\}$ are various risk factors, and $\{b_k\}, j = 0, 1, 2, \ldots, K$ are unknown regression coefficients. Five risk factors under consideration are: age, duration of operation, length of incision, insertion of drain, and whether appendectomy with abscess or peritonitis is used in an abdominal operation. They all are qualitative variables defined by the following dummy variables:

$X_1 = 1$ if age of the patient is ≥ 60 years, $= 0$ otherwise;
$X_2 = 1$ if the duration of operation of the patient is 31–60 minutes, $= 0$ otherwise;
$X_3 = 1$ if the duration of operation of the patient is over 60 minutes, $= 0$ otherwise;
$X_4 = 1$ if the incision is ≥ 6 in, $= 0$ otherwise;
$X_5 = 1$ if drain is inserted, $= 0$ otherwise;
$X_6 = 1$ if appendectomy with abscess or peritonitis is used in an abdominal operation, $= 0$ otherwise;
$X_7 = 1$ if the operation is appendix, $= 0$ otherwise;

$X_8 = 1$ if the operation is gall bladder, $= 0$ otherwise;
$X_9 = 1$ if the operation is any other, $= 0$ otherwise;
$X_{10} = 1$ if the operation is gastrectomy, $= 0$ otherwise;
$X_{11} = 1$ if the operation is thyroid, $= 0$ otherwise; and
$X_{12} = 1$ if the operation is thoracic, $= 0$ otherwise.

By applying Eq. (1) with the above X_k, $k = 1, 2, \ldots, 12$, the estimated regression equation is given by:[17]

$$
\ln\left(ln\left[1 - \varphi\right]^{-1} \right) = X_1 \cdot ln2.26 + X_2 \cdot ln2 + X_3 \cdot ln3.68
$$
$$
+ X_4 \cdot ln1.79 + X_5 \cdot ln2.05 + X_6 \cdot ln2.71
$$
$$
+ X_7 \cdot ln0.035 + X_8 \cdot ln0.033 + X_9 \cdot ln0.023
$$
$$
+ X_{10} \cdot ln0.012 + X_{11} \cdot ln0.007 + X_{12} \cdot ln0.009.
$$
$$
\tag{2}
$$

From Eq. (2), variables such as the age of the patient being over 60 years, duration of the operation exceeding 30 minutes, the incision being over 6 inches long and the insertion of a drain are found to be independently associated with a significantly increased risk of sepsis.

Remarks

1. The multiplicative form employed has the advantage that the predicted probabilities are confined within the range of 0–1.
2. The substantial differences associated with the operations performed in different hospitals are shown to be almost entiredly accounted for by differences in the operations performed in them.

7.3 Generalized Linear Regression

Through the use of the link function,[19] multiple linear regression models are extended to generalized linear regression models. Here we only consider two special models: Poisson and logistic regression models.

A. *Poisson Regression Model*

To model the rare disease, a Poisson regression model is useful to study the relation between the outcome variable and the risk factors.

Let Y be a Poisson random variable with the population parameter λ. Assume that the relationship between the logarithm of the expected value of Y and a set of explanatory variables $X_1, X_2, \ldots, X_k$ on the interval scale is linear, that is

$$\ln(E(y_i)) = b_0 + b_1 x_{i1} + \cdots + b_k x_{ik}, \tag{7.3A.1}$$

where $\ln = \log_e$, $\{y_i\}$, $i = 1, 2, \ldots$, n is the sample data randomly collected from Y, and $\{b_j\}$, $j = 0, 1, 2, \ldots, k$ are unknown regression coefficients.

The maximum likelihood method is used to estimate the unknown regression coefficients $\{b_j\}$, $j = 0, 1, 2, \ldots$, k. First, the likelihood function is the product of n probability distribution of Eq. (3.1C.1) for the sampled data $\{y_i\}$ as follows:

$$L(\vec{b}|\vec{y}; W) = \prod_{i=1}^{n} \frac{\exp(\vec{w}_i^T \vec{b}(y_i - \exp(\vec{w}_i^T \vec{b}))}{y_i!}, \tag{7.3A.2}$$

where $\vec{w}_i^T$ is the ith row of the coefficient matrix W in Eq. (7.2B.2). Note that it is very difficult to work with Eq. (7.3A.2). Since the maximum likelihood estimators of Eq. (7.3A.2) is the same as that of its log-likelihood is defined as follows:

$$\ell(\vec{b}) \equiv \ln L\left(\vec{b}|\vec{y}; W\right) = \sum_{i=1}^{n} \left\{ \vec{w}_i^T \vec{b}\left[y_i - \exp\left(\vec{w}_i^T \vec{b}\right)\right] - \ln\left(y_i!\right) \right\}.$$
$$\tag{7.3A.3}$$

To find the maximum likelihood estimator for $\vec{b}$, we differentiate Eq. (7.3A.3) with respect to $\vec{b}$ and set the resulting expression equal to zero, which are given by: for $j = 0, 1, 2, \ldots, k$

$$\frac{\partial \ell(\vec{b})}{\partial b_j} = \sum_{i=1}^{n} x_{ij}\left[y_i - \exp\left(\vec{w}_i^T \vec{b}\right)\right] = 0. \tag{7.3A.4}$$

Unfortunately, Eq. (7.3A.4) does not have a closed-form solution. Hence, it has to be solved by using the special statistical software packages.

Remarks

1. Many statistical software packages like SAS, BMDP and STATA can be used in practical applications.
2. The variance and covariance of the regression estimator $\hat{\vec{b}}$ can be obtained by taking the second partial derivative of Eq. (7.3A.3) with respect to $\vec{b}$.

Example 7.3A-1

This example applies the Poisson regression model to study the risk factors on the rate of bone and head cancers of female radium dial workers.[15] The study population was a cohort of 4337 females employed in the US radium-dial industry. Unaware of radium poisoning, dial painters tipped their brushes with their lips in order to provide a fine point for painting. As a result, dial painters were exposed to the intake of radium in their bodies. Several years after leaving the plant, former dial painters began developing a variety of mysterious medical problems; the most common symptoms experienced were teeth and jaw problems.

Because bone sarcomas and head carcinomas are rare cancers, the frequency count (Y) of bone sarcomas (or head carcinomas) was assumed to be a Poisson random varaiable with the probability distribution given by (see Sec. 3.3):

$$\Pr(Y = n) = \frac{\mu^n e^{-\mu}}{n!}, \quad n = 0, 1, 2, \ldots (\mu > 0) \tag{1}$$

where μ denotes the expected count number of bone (or head) tumors. A Poisson regression model with interaction terms was applied to model the expected frequency count of bone (or head) tumors as follows:

$$ln\mu = \alpha_0 + \ln(PYR) + \alpha_1 LDOSE + \alpha_2 AFE + \alpha_3 DOE$$
$$+ \alpha_4 TFE + \alpha_5 LDOSE \cdot AFE + \alpha_6 LDOSE$$
$$\cdot DOE + \alpha_7 LDOSE \cdot TFE, \tag{2}$$

where the explanatory variables are defined as follows:

> PYR = total exposure person years,
> LDOSE = the natural logarithm of the weighted
> systemic intake of radium,
> AFE = average age at 1st exposure,
> DOE = average duration of exposure,
> TFE = average time since 1st exposure.

After fitting Eq. (2) to the data, the final Poisson regression model for bone and head tumors are given respectively by

$$ln\mu = 4.8 - 1.2 LDOSE - 0.4 TFE + 0.051 LDOSE \cdot TFE,$$

and

$$ln\mu = -11.29 + 0.978 LDOSE. \tag{3}$$

For details see Ref. 15.

B. *Logistic Regression Model*

In some regression problems, the data of a response variable is dichotomous (quantal) or polychotomous. For such problems, normal errors do not correspond to a binary response. An important method that can be used in this situation is called the logistic regression.

Let Y be a binomial random variable with the total number of trials n and the population proportion of success p. Assume that the relationship between the expected value of Y and a set of explanatory variables $X_1, X_2, \ldots, X_K$ on the interval scale is linear logistic, that is,

$$\ln\left(\frac{p_i}{1-p_i}\right) = g(\vec{b}) \equiv b_0 + \sum_{k=1}^{K} b_k x_{ik}, \tag{7.3B.1}$$

where
$p_i = E(y_i|\vec{w}_i^T) = \exp(g(\vec{b}))[1 - \exp(g(\vec{b}))]^{-1}$, $\{y_i\}$, $i = 1,2,\ldots,n$ is a set of sample data randomly collected from the response variable Y, $\vec{w}_i^T$ is the ith row of the coefficient matrix W in Eq. (7.2B.2), $\{b_j\}$, $j = 0,1,2,\ldots,K$ are unknown regression coefficients and ln is the logarithmic function with the natural base, i.e., $\ln \equiv \log_e$.

The maximum likelihood method is used to estimate the unknown regression coefficients $\{b_j\}$, $j = 0,1,2,\ldots$, k. First, the likelihood function is the product of n probability distribution of Eq. (3.1B.1) for the sampled data $\{y_i\}$ as follows:

$$L(\vec{b}) = \prod_{i=1}^{n} p_i^{y_i} (1 - p_i)^{1-y_i}, \tag{7.3B.2}$$

where p_i is given by Eq. (7.2B.1). To find the maximum likelihood estimator for $\vec{b}$, we differentiate Eq. (7.3B.2) with respect to $\vec{b}$ and set the resulting expression equal to zero, which are given by

$$\sum_{i=1}^{n} \left[y_i - p_i(\vec{b}) \right] = 0, \tag{7.3B.3}$$

$$\sum_{i=1}^{n} x_{ik} \left[y_i - p_i(\vec{b}) \right] = 0, \quad k = 0,1,2,\ldots,K \tag{7.3B.4}$$

Unfortunately, Eqs. (7.3B.3) and (7.3B.4) do not have a closed-form solution. For a small project, an article contains a computer program for logistic regression to be used on an IBM PC.[20] However, for a large project in practical applications, the special statistical software packages such as the SAS must be used to solve it.

Remarks

1. The left side of Eq. (7.3B.1), the log of the odds is called the logit transformation. Incidentally, since the combinatorial quantity

in Eq. (3.2B.1) does not involve the unknown regression co-efficients $\vec{b}$, it is not included in the likelihood function of Eq. (7.3B.2).

2. The variance and covariance of the regression estimator $\hat{\vec{b}}$ can be obtained by taking the second partial derivative of Eq. (7.3B.2) with respect to $\vec{b}$.[11]

Example 7.3B-1

This example applies the logistic regression model of Eq. (7.3B.1) to analyze the effect of various risk factors on the risk of having coronary heart disease. To gather data on such associations, four large, prospective studies were established in the US between 1948 and 1957 in the order of initiation: Framingham, Los Angeles, Albany and Chicago studies. These studies followed samples from 1800 to 5000 men and women for up to 10 years.[27] The response variable is coronary heart disease, coded as $Y = 0$ if absent and $= 1$ if present, as determined by well-defined diagnostic criteria approximately 10 years from the date of the risk factor values for the given individual.

Various risk factors are defined as follows:

X_1 (Sex): $= 1$ if male, $= 2$ if female;

X_2 (Age): in years and hundredths;

X_3 (Height): in inches and hundredths;

X_4 (Systolic blood pressure): in mm.Hg;

X_5 (Diastolic blood pressure): in mm.Hg;

X_6 (Serum cholesterol): in mg. per ml;

X_7 (Electrocardiographic abnormality): $= 1$ if present, $= 0$ otherwise;

X_8 (Framingham relative weight): $=$ weight (lb) / median weight (lb) of sex-height group, as a percentage;

X_9   (Alcoholic consumption, oz/month):

Code	Oz. (men)	Oz. (women)
0	None	None
1	< 4	< 1
2	5–14	1–9
3	15–39	10–24
4	40–69	25–39
5	70–99	40–999
6	100–999	

By using the nine risk factors, the estimated regression coefficients $\{\hat{b}_k\}$ with the associated t-values $t_k = \hat{b}_k / s.d.(\hat{b}_k)$ are given in Table 7.3B-1.

From the t-values shown in Table 7.3B-1, almost all risk factors have a significant effect on the risk of coronary heart diasease, except X_5 (diastolic blood pressure) and X_9 (alcoholic consumption).

Table 7.3B-1*. The estimated regression coefficients and the values of testing statistics t_k

k	$\hat{b}_k$	t_k
0	−5.3695	—
1	−1.5883	−9.12
2	0.08095	10.15
3	−0.05279	−2.28
4	0.009116	2.50
5	0.005493	0.81
6	0.006631	5.41
7	0.8543	4.99
8	1.3586	3.77
9	−0.05873	−1.60

*This table was taken from Table 1b in Ref. 27. The sample size is n = 4671 after the removal of observations with missing values of one or more risk factors.

Remark

Incidentaly, an example applying the multiple logistic regression model to study the effect of PM_{10} on the health of residents living in the area of Hoopa Valley Indian Reservation is given in Ref. 16.

7.4 Discrimination/Classification

In the medical field, we are often confronted with the task of classifying a patient into one of two distinct populations on the basis of a number of data. Discrimination is a multivariate technique that deals with separating distinct sets of patients (or observations), while classification is concerned with allocating a new patient (or observation) to previously defined groups. As a result, the immediate goal of discrimination is to find "discriminants" whose numerical values are such that the collections are separated as much as possible. However, the emphasis of classification is to derive a rule that can be used to best assign patients to the labeled groups.

The technique of discrimination analysis between two groups was first suggested by Fisher (1936) to distinguish between two species of iris flowers — setosa and versicolor. This method yields the Fisher's linear discriminant function, which is known to be the best method in that it results in a minimal chance of misclassification, provided the observations follow a multinormal distribution with a common variance-covariance matrix for both populations.

Assume that there are J populations π_j, $j = 1, 2, \ldots, J$ and K predictor variables X_k, $k = 1, 2, \ldots, K$. A sample $\{x_{ik}^{(j)}\}$, $i = 1, 2, \ldots, n_j$, $k = 1, 2, \ldots, K$ of size n_j, $j = 1, 2, \ldots, J$ are randomly collected from the jth population π_j over K predictor factors, with the data matrix $A_{n_j \times K}^{(j)}$ given by the following table

In Table 7.4-1 the last row represents the sample average for each of the predictor factor X_k, namely,

$$\bar{x}_k^{(j)} = \sum_{i=1}^{n_j} x_{ik}^{(j)} \bigg/ n_j. \tag{7.4.1}$$

Table 7.4-1. The Data Matrix $A^{(j)}_{n_j \times K}$ for the jth Population π_j

	Predictor Factor		
$\mathbf{X_1}$	$\mathbf{X_2}$	$\cdots$	$\mathbf{X_K}$
$x^{(j)}_{11}$	$x^{(j)}_{12}$	$\cdots$	$x^{(j)}_{1K}$
$x^{(j)}_{21}$	$x^{(j)}_{22}$	$\cdots$	$x^{(j)}_{2K}$
$\vdots$	$\vdots$	$\vdots$	$\vdots$
$x^{(j)}_{n_j 1}$	$x^{(j)}_{n_j 2}$	$\vdots$	$x^{(j)}_{n_j K}$
$\bar{x}^{(j)}_1$	$\bar{x}^{(j)}_2$	$\vdots$	$\bar{x}^{(j)}_K$

Because K predictor variables X_k are not of equal importance, our goal is to find a composite variable Y that is a linear combination of K predictor variables X_k, with the optimal weights b_k of the form

$$Y = b_1 X_1 + b_2 X_2 + \cdots + b_K X_K = \vec{b}^T \vec{X} \qquad (7.4.2)$$

such that Y separates the J populations $\{\pi_j\}$, $j = 1, 2, \ldots, J$ as much as possible, where $\vec{X} = (X_1, X_2, \ldots, X_K)^T$ and $\vec{b} = (b_1, b_2, \ldots, b_K)^T$. By substituting the data in Table 7.4-1 into Eq. (7.4.2) for each j and taking the sample average,

$$\bar{y}^{(j)} = b_1 \bar{x}^{(j)}_1 + b_2 \bar{x}^{(j)}_2 + \cdots + b_K \bar{x}^{(j)}_K = \vec{b}^T \vec{\bar{x}}^{(j)}, \qquad (7.4.3)$$

where $\bar{y}^{(j)} = \sum_{i=1}^{n_j} y^{(j)}_i / n_j$, $y^{(j)}_i = \sum_{k=1}^{k} b_k x^{(j)}_{ik}$, $\vec{\bar{x}}^{(j)} = (\bar{x}^{(j)}_1, \bar{x}^{(j)}_2, \ldots, \bar{x}^{(j)}_k)^T$.

By finding the overall sample average of $\bar{y}^{(j)}$ given by Eq. (7.4.3),

$$\bar{\bar{y}} = \frac{\sum_{j=1}^{J} n_j \bar{y}^{(j)}}{\sum_{j=1}^{J} n_j} = \vec{b}^T \vec{\bar{\bar{x}}}, \qquad (7.4.4)$$

where $\vec{\bar{x}} = (\bar{x}_1, \bar{x}_2, \ldots, \bar{x}_K)^T$ and $\bar{x}_k$ is given by

$$\bar{x}_k = \sum_{j=1}^{J} \sum_{i=1}^{n_j} x_{ik}^{(j)} / \sum_{j=1}^{J} n_j. \tag{7.4.5}$$

According to the idea of Fisher,[7] the best discriminant function Y is obtained by maximizing the ratio of the sum of squares between-population variation over the sum of squares within-population variation, namely, finding the coefficients $\{b_k\}$ in Eq. (7.4.2) that solve the following maximization problem:

$$\text{Maximize}_{\{b_k\}} \frac{\sum_{j=1}^{J} [n_j(\bar{y}^{(j)} - \bar{y})]^2}{\sum_{j=1}^{J} \sum_{i=1}^{n_j} (y_i^{(j)} - \bar{y}^{(j)})^2} = \frac{\vec{b}^T B \vec{b}}{\vec{b}^T W \vec{b}}, \tag{7.4.6}$$

where the matrices B and W are given by

$$B = \sum_{j=1}^{J} n_j (\vec{\bar{x}}^{(j)} - \vec{\bar{x}})(\vec{\bar{x}}^{(j)} - \vec{\bar{x}})^T, \tag{7.4.7}$$

and

$$W = \sum_{j=1}^{J} \sum_{i=1}^{n_j} (\vec{x}_i^{(j)} - \vec{\bar{x}}^{(j)})(\vec{x}_i^{(j)} - \vec{\bar{x}}^{(j)})^T, \tag{7.4.8}$$

$$\vec{x}_i^{(j)} = (x_{i1}^{(j)}, x_{i2}^{(j)}, \ldots, x_{iK}^{(j)})^T.$$

Let $\hat{\lambda}_h, h \leq \min(J - 1, K)$, be the nonzero eigenvalues of the matrix $W^{-1}B$ and $\vec{e}_h$ the corresponding eigenvectors that are normalized so that $\|\vec{e}_h\|_S^2 \equiv \vec{e}_h^T S \vec{e}_h = 1$, where $S = W / (\sum_{j=1}^{J} n_j - J)$. It can be shown[11] that the coefficients $\{b_k\}$ that maximize Eq. (7.4.6) are given by

$$\hat{\vec{b}} = \vec{e}_h^* \equiv \vec{e}_h / \|\vec{e}_h\|_S, \tag{7.4.9}$$

where $\vec{e}_h$ is the eigenvector corresponding with the eigenvalue λ_h.

Remarks

1. In computing Eq. (7.4.8) we implicitly assume that J populations have a common variance-covariance matrix.
2. By substituting Eq. (7.4.9) into Eq. (7.4.3),

$$\bar{y}^{(j)} = \vec{e}_h^{*T} \vec{x}^{(j)} \qquad (7.4.10)$$

is called Fisher's h^{th} sample discriminant.
3. By adding the assumption of multinormal distribution on each of J populations with a common variance-covariance matrix, another form of Fisher's linear/quadratic discriminant function is given in Chap. 6 of Ref. 1.
4. When J = 2, it can be shown[4] that Fisher's linear discriminant function is a special case of the use of the likelihood ratio when the following three conditions are satisfied: (i) the two populations have multivariate normal distributions, (ii) they have common variance-covariance matrices, and (iii) sample estimates are substituted for unknown population parameters. Moreover, it also leads to minimal classification errors. However, if condition (ii) is not satisfied, it leads to a quadratic rather than a linear discriminant function.

If $\vec{x}_0 = (x_{01}, x_{02}, \ldots, x_{0K})^T$ is a new observation, a classification rule to assign $\vec{x}_0$ to the appropriate population is given as follows.

Decision Rule 7.4-1 (Classifying a new observation)

Suppose that only H eigenvalues of $W^{-1}B$, $\hat{\lambda}_h, h = 1, 2, \ldots, H$ are nonzero. Then allocate $\vec{x}_0$ to π_ℓ if the following inequality is satisfied:

For all $j \neq \ell$,

$$\sum_{i=1}^{H} \left[\hat{\vec{b}}_i^T \left(\vec{x}_0 - \vec{x}^{(\ell)} \right) \right]^2 \leq \sum_{i=1}^{H} \left[\hat{\vec{b}}_i^T \left(\vec{x}_0 - \vec{x}^{(j)} \right) \right]^2, \qquad (7.4.11)$$

where $\hat{\vec{b}}_i = \vec{e}_i, \vec{e}_i$ is defined by Eq. (7.4.9) and $\vec{x}^{(j)}$ is given by Eq. (7.4.3).

Remarks

1. Only the eigenvectors corresponding to the nonzero eigenvalues are used in computing Eq. (7.4.11).
2. When J = 2, Eq. (7.4.11) is reduced to a single critical discriminating value y^* so that $\vec{x}_0$ is assigned to population π_1 if $\hat{\vec{b}}^T (\vec{x}_0 - \vec{x}^{(1)}) < y^*$; it is assigned to π_2 otherwise.

Example 7.4-1

In discriminating the two populations of the Iris flower, setosa (π_1) and versicolor (π_2), four prognostic factors: Sepal length (X_1), Sepal width (X_2), Petal length (X_3) and Petal width (X_4) are used. Fifty measurements over X_k, k = 1, 2, 3, 4 were randomly collected from π_j, j = 1, 2 (see Table 7.4-2).[7]

Find Fisher's linear discriminant rule for π_j, j = 1, 2.

Solution

From Table 7.4-2, the sample sizes for π_j are $n_1 = n_2 = 50$. From the last row of Table 7.4-2,

$$\vec{x}^{(1)} = (5.006, 3.428, 1.462, 0.246)^T, \tag{1}$$

and

$$\vec{x}^{(1)} = (5.936, 2.77, 4.26, 1.326)^T.$$

By using Eq. (1),

$$\bar{\vec{x}} = \frac{1}{2}(\vec{x}^{(1)} + \vec{x}^{(2)}) = (5.471, 3.099, 2.861, 0.786)^T. \tag{2}$$

Table 7.4-2.   50 sample data of septal length, septal width, petal length, and petal width of two populations of iris flower

	π_1				π_2		
X_1	X_2	X_3	X_4	X_1	X_2	X_3	X_4
5.1	3.5	1.4	0.2	7	3.2	4.7	1.4
4.9	3	1.4	0.2	6.4	3.2	4.5	1.5
4.7	3.2	1.3	0.2	6.9	3.1	4.9	1.5
4.6	3.1	1.5	0.2	5.5	2.3	4	1.3
5	3.6	1.4	0.2	6.5	2.8	4.6	1.5
5.4	3.9	1.7	0.4	5.7	2.8	4.5	1.3
4.6	3.4	1.4	0.3	6.3	3.3	4.7	1.6
5	3.4	1.5	0.2	4.9	2.4	3.3	1
4.4	2.9	1.4	0.2	6.6	2.9	4.6	1.3
4.9	3.1	1.5	0.1	5.2	2.7	3.9	1.4
5.4	3.7	1.5	0.2	5	2	3.5	1
4.8	3.4	1.6	0.2	5.9	3	4.2	1.5
4.8	3	1.4	0.1	6	2.2	4	1
4.3	3	1.1	0.1	6.1	2.9	4.7	1.4
5.8	4	1.2	0.2	5.6	2.9	3.6	1.3
5.7	4.4	1.5	0.4	6.7	3.1	4.4	1.4
5.4	3.9	1.3	0.4	5.6	3	4.5	1.5
5.1	3.5	1.4	0.3	5.8	2.7	4.1	1
5.7	3.8	1.7	0.3	6.2	2.2	4.5	1.5
5.1	3.8	1.5	0.3	5.6	2.5	3.9	1.1
5.4	3.4	1.7	0.2	5.9	3.2	4.8	1.8
5.1	3.7	1.5	0.4	6.1	2.8	4	1.3
4.6	3.6	1	0.2	6.3	2.5	4.9	1.5
5.1	3.3	1.7	0.5	6.1	2.8	4.7	1.2
4.8	3.4	1.9	0.2	6.4	2.9	4.3	1.3
5	3	1.6	0.2	6.6	3	4.4	1.4
5	3.4	1.6	0.4	6.8	2.8	4.8	1.4
5.2	3.5	1.5	0.2	6.7	3	5	1.7
5.2	3.4	1.4	0.2	6	2.9	4.5	1.5
4.7	3.2	1.6	0.2	5.7	2.6	3.5	1
4.8	3.1	1.6	0.2	5.5	2.4	3.8	1.1
5.4	3.4	1.5	0.4	5.5	2.4	3.7	1

(*Continued*)

Table 7.4-2. (*Continued*)

	π_1				π_2		
X_1	X_2	X_3	X_4	X_1	X_2	X_3	X_4
5.2	4.1	1.5	0.1	5.8	2.7	3.9	1.2
5.5	4.2	1.4	0.2	6	2.7	5.1	1.6
4.9	3.1	1.5	0.2	5.4	3	4.5	1.5
5	3.2	1.2	0.2	6	3.4	4.5	1.6
5.5	3.5	1.3	0.2	6.7	3.1	4.7	1.5
4.9	3.6	1.4	0.1	6.3	2.3	4.4	1.3
4.4	3	1.3	0.2	5.6	3	4.1	1.3
5.1	3.4	1.5	0.2	5.5	2.5	4	1.3
5	3.5	1.3	0.3	5.5	2.6	4.4	1.2
4.5	2.3	1.3	0.3	6.1	3	4.6	1.4
4.4	3.2	1.3	0.2	5.8	2.6	4	1.2
5	3.5	1.6	0.6	5	2.3	3.3	1
5.1	3.8	1.9	0.4	5.6	2.7	4.2	1.3
4.8	3	1.4	0.3	5.7	3	4.2	1.2
5.1	3.8	1.6	0.2	5.7	2.9	4.2	1.3
4.6	3.2	1.4	0.2	6.2	2.9	4.3	1.3
5.3	3.7	1.5	0.2	5.1	2.5	3	1.1
5	3.3	1.4	0.2	5.7	2.8	4.1	1.3
5.006	3.428	1.462	0.246	5.936	2.77	4.26	1.326

Where the last row represents the sample average of X_k, k = 1,2,3,4 for the two populations π_j, j = 1,2.

By substituting Eqs. (1) and (2) into Eqs. (7.4.7) and (7.4.8),

$$B = \sum_{j=1}^{2} n_j (\vec{\bar{x}}^{(j)} - \vec{\bar{\bar{x}}})(\vec{\bar{x}}^{(j)} - \vec{\bar{\bar{x}}})^T$$

$$= \begin{bmatrix} 21.6225 & -15.2985 & 65.0535 & 25.11 \\ -15.2985 & 10.8241 & -46.0271 & -17.766 \\ 65.0535 & -46.0271 & 195.7201 & 75.546 \\ 25.11 & -17.766 & 75.546 & 29.16 \end{bmatrix}, \quad (3)$$

and

$$W = \sum_{j=1}^{2} \sum_{i=1}^{n_j} (\vec{x}_i^{(j)} - \vec{x}^{(j)})(\vec{x}_i^{(j)} - \vec{x}^{(j)})^T$$

$$= \begin{bmatrix} 19.14385 & 9.0356 & 9.7634 & 3.2394 \\ 9.0356 & 11.8658 & 4.6232 & 2.4746 \\ 9.7634 & 4.6232 & 12.2978 & 3.8794 \\ 3.2394 & 2.4746 & 3.8794 & 2.4604 \end{bmatrix}. \tag{4}$$

By using Eqs. (3) and (4),

$$W^{-1}B = \begin{bmatrix} -0.72422 & 0.512402 & -2.17888 & -0.84102 \\ -4.27588 & 3.025298 & -12.8644 & -4.96553 \\ 5.163892 & -3.65359 & 15.5361 & 5.996778 \\ 7.317634 & -5.17742 & 22.01585 & 8.497897 \end{bmatrix} \tag{5}$$

Since $J = 2$ and $K = 4$, Eq. (5) has only one nonzero eigenvalue. By applying the Mathematica's software "Eigenvalues", the nonzero eigenvalue is given by

$$\lambda_1 = 26.3351,$$

and the corresponding eigenvector is

$$\vec{e}_1 = (0.0728, 0.427, -0.5189, -0.7354)^T. \tag{6}$$

Since $S = W/(\sum_{j=1}^{J} n_j - J) = \frac{W}{50+50-2} = W/98$,

$$\|\vec{e}_1\|_S^2 = \vec{e}_1^T S \vec{e}_1 = 0.058679. \tag{7}$$

By dividing Eq. (6) by the square root of Eq. (7), the normalized eigenvector $\vec{e}_1^*$ is given by

$$\vec{e}_1^* = \frac{\vec{e}_1}{\|\vec{e}_1\|_S} \approx (0.3004, 1.7739, -2.1423, -3.0357)^T. \tag{8}$$

By substituting Eq. (8) into Eq. (7.4.10), Fisher's first sample discriminant for π_j is given by

$$Y = \vec{e}_1^{*T}\vec{X} = 0.3004X_1 + 1.7739X_2 - 2.1423X_3 - 3.0357X_4 \qquad (9)$$

Or equivalently, by making the largest optimal weight of X_2 in Eq. (9) to be one,

$$Y = 0.1693X_1 + X_2 - 1.2077X_3 - 1.7113X_4. \qquad (10)$$

Remark

All calcualations of Eqs. (3) to (5) were done on the Microsoft's EXCEL spreadsheets with the help of "MMULT" and "MINVERSE" for the matrix multiplication and the matrix inverse.

Example 7.4-2

Out of the 2571 patients discharged from Glen Lake Sanatorium from 1948 through 1953, 1534 patients were cases of uncomplicated adult type of pulmonary tuberculosis and could be adequately evaluated. Sufficient follow-up reports for periods ranging from 11 months to 6 years were obtained in 1259 of these patients.[21]

Approximately 1200 of these 1259 patients' records contained complete information for the following 13 predictor variables: (1) Sex (X_1), (2) State of disease on admission (X_2), (3) Unilateral or bilateral pulmonary lesions (X_3), (4) Age on admission (X_4), (5) Type of discharge (X_5), (6) Condition on discharge (X_6), (7) Bateriological findings on admission (X_7), (8) Bateriological findings on discharge (X_8), (9) Presence or absence of cavity on admission (X_9), (10) Presence or absence of cavity on discharge (X_{10}), (11) Length of hospitalization (X_{11}), (12) Regimens of chemotherapy (X_{12}), and (13) Type of treatment (X_{13}). The details of numerical coding for each variable are given in Ref. 22. Each case was designated as "relapsed" or "well" according to whether the patient did or did not suffer a relapse of pulmonary tuberculosis as of November 1954. There were 852 well cases and 348 relapsed cases.

The authors divided the entire sample (1200) into two sub-samples: the normative (900) and check (300) samples. The normative sample was used to compute the discriminant function, whereas the check sample was used for empirical validation of the computed function. In order that the two samples might be comparable in terms of relative frequency of "well" and "relapsed" cases as well as in the sex ratio, the 300 check-sample cases were done by the stratified (or quota) sampling scheme, and not by random sampling. Therefore, the 1200 cases were separated into four groups: (male, well), (male, relapsed), (female, well) and (female, relapsed), and one-fourth of each group was selected at random into the check sample. The result of the two subsamples is shown in Table 7.4-2a.

The sample means for the "well" (n_1 = 639), "relapsed" (n_2 = 261) and entire samples (n = 900) in the normative subsample are given in Table 7.4-2b.

Let the discriminant function Y be given by

$$Y = \sum_{k=1}^{13} b_k X_k, \tag{1}$$

where $\{X_k\}$ are defined in the second paragraph of this example. Since there are only two groups ("well" and "relapsed"), the authors applied the multiple regression technique to find the optimal weights $\{\hat{b}_k\}$ by adding a dummy variable "X_{14}" to Eq. (1) with $X_{14} = 1$ if a patient is well, and $X_{14} = 2$ if he is a relapsed. By

Table 7.4-2a. The data of normative and the check samples

	Normative Sample			Check Sample		
	Well (π_1)	Relapsed (π_2)	Row Total	Well (π_1)	Relapsed (π_2)	Row Total
Male	339	188	527	113	63	176
Female	300	73	373	100	24	124
Column Total	639	261	900	213	87	300

Table 7.4-2b. The sample mean of the well, relapsed, and entire sample in the normative subsample

	Normative Subsample		
k	$\bar{x}_k^{(1)}$ ("Well")	$\bar{x}_k^{(2)}$ ("Relapsed")	$\bar{\bar{x}}_k$ (Entire)
1	1.47	1.27	1.41
2	2.23	2.41	2.28
3	1.64	1.82	1.69
4	3.54	4.12	3.70
5	2.63	3.71	2.94
6	2.50	3.61	2.82
7	3.38	3.74	3.48
8	1.81	3.23	2.22
9	0.73	0.82	0.76
10	0.08	0.44	0.18
11	2.95	2.79	2.91
12	2.41	2.86	2.51
13	3.34	4.12	3.58

substituting the obtained optimal weights into Eq. (1),

$$\hat{Y} = -0.49X_1 - 0.04X_2 + 0.51X_3 + 0.06X_4 + 0.11X_5$$
$$+ 0.28X_6 + 0.06X_7 + 0.21X_8 - 0.48X_9 + X_{10}$$
$$+ 0.17X_{11} + 0.2X_{12} + 0.1X_{13} + 0.74, \tag{2}$$

where the constant term 0.74 was added merely to avoid having a negative value for any individual's discriminant function score, and also to make the mean of Y for the entire normative subsample equal to an integer.

By substituting the 2nd to the 4th column of Table 7.4-2b, respectively, for the values of $\bar{x}_k^{(1)}, \bar{x}_k^{(2)}$ and $\bar{\bar{x}}_k$ into Eq. (7.4.23),

$$\bar{y}^{(1)} = 3.5986 \approx 3.6,$$
$$\bar{y}^{(2)} = 5.023 \approx 5.0, \tag{3}$$
$$\bar{\bar{y}} = 3.9997 \approx 4.0.$$

Table 7.4-2c.   Outcome of Predictions for 300 Cases in the Check Sample

	Actual Status	
Prediction by Eq. (2)	Well	Relapsed
Well	163	30
Relapsed	50	57

Table 7.4-2c is adapted from Table 5 in Ref. 22.

Since there are only two groups ("well" and "relapsed"), the critical dividing point between these two groups is taken as equidistant in standard deviation from $\bar{y}^{(1)}$ and $\bar{y}^{(2)}$. By using Eq. (2), the critical discriminant score for dividing these two groups — "well" and "relapsed" — is given by finding the equal distance in standard deviations as 4.36.

A prediction of "well" or "relapsed" was made for each patient in the check sample, depending on whether his/her $\hat{Y}$ score of Eq. (2) was less than or greater than the critical score $\bar{y}^* = 4.36$. That the outcome thus predicted for each of the 300 cases in the check sample was then compared with the actual status of that patient as of November 1954 is given in Table 7.4-2c.

From Table 7.4-2c, 30 out of 87 who were actually relapsed would have received the misclassified forecast as being "well" and 50 out of 213 who were actually well were misclassified as being "relapsed". Hence, the overall empirical probability of misclassification is $(30 + 50)/300 = 0.267$, or 26.7%.

Remarks

1. The probability of misclassification (0.267) is not small. This is because some of the variables had the markedly skewed distributions, as evidenced by the fact that their standard deviations were of the same order of magnitude as the means. A possible way to reduce the probability of misclassification would be to introduce suitable transformations for these skewed variables.

2. Another way to reduce the misclassification is to look for additional and more significant factors to be used as predictor variables. One such factor is the socio-economic status of the patient.[22]

Example 7.4-3

Urinary steroid levels have been used for the prognosis of patients with advanced breast cancer. In the late 1950s women with advanced breast cancer received hypophysectomy or bilateral adrenalectomy with oophorectomy. Of the 11 hormone compounds determined from urine, only the 17-hydroxy-corticosteroid (17-OHCS: X_1) and the aetiocholanolone (X_2) levels might be of use in predicting the response to either operation. A linear discriminant function was determined as[3]

$$Y = 80 - 80X_1 + X_2. \qquad (1)$$

Values of Eq. (1) equal to zero are about equally likely to be found in successful and unsuccessful cases. Positive values of Eq. (1) are associated with a successful response to treatment, while negative values have no benefit.

Fifty-nine patients were randomly selected to be treated with either operation. On the basis of clinical findings, the results were graded into three groups (see Table 7.4-3):

(a) Remission: All visible and palpable lessions regressed;
(b) Intermediate: Cases in which the disease remained almost stationary or those in which regression was incompleted/shortlived; and
(c) Failure: The disease was apparently unaffected by treatment.

If the patients in the present series had actually been selected on the basis of their discriminants, 13 of the 25 treated by hypophysectomy would not have been treated in this way. Of the 13 rejected, 1 would have been denied remission of the disease, 1 could have had a marginal response, and the other 11 would

Table 7.4-3.   **The value of Eq. (1) for three groups after treatment of two operations**

Y of Eq. (1)	Treatment: (Adrenalectomy, Hypophysectomy)		
	Group: (a)	(b)	(c)
Positive (Y > 0)	(6, 7)	(1, 5)	(6, 0)
Negative (Y < 0)	(0, 1)	(11, 1)	(10, 11)

This table is adapted from Fig. 2 in Ref. 3.

have failed to respond. These figures indicate that 85%(= 11/13) of those rejected would have failed to respond to hypophysectomy.

Of the 12 patients who were selected for hypophesectomy, the remission rate was 60%(= 7/12), which was a substantial improvement over the original remission rate of 28%(= 7/25). Of the 13 patients who were selected for adrenalectomy, the remission rate would be 46%(= 6/13), which was not as effective as that for hypophysectomy.

Remarks

1. The linear discriminant function of Eq. (1) is valuable in indicating the probable response to hypophysectomy.
2. Other variables describing the clinical, surgical and natural histories of the patients are shown to have prognostic values. The reliability of a prognosis based on steroid levels is better for patients submitted for hypophysectomy than for adrenalectomy.[2]

7.5   Exercises

1. In Example 7.2A-1, test the hypothesis of Eq. (7.2A.9).
2. The basal rate (X) and total energy expenditure in 24 hours (Y) from a study of 9 obese women are given in Table 7.5-1.[24]
   By using Eq. (7.1.4), find the 95% confidence interval for the correlation coefficient ρ_{XY}.

Table 7.5-1. **The sample data of the basal rate (X) and total energy expenditure (Y) of 9 obese women**

Subject	X	Y
1	6.70	9.68
2	6.77	9.69
3	8.20	11.85
4	6.64	12.79
5	6.54	9.21
6	6.42	9.19
7	6.43	9.97
8	5.96	8.79
9	6.73	11.51

Table 7.5-2. **The data of mean arterial blood pressure (X) and the total glycosylated haemoglobin (Y) in the enalaparil group**

Subject	X	Y (%)
1	91	9.8
2	104	7.4
3	107	7.9
4	107	8.3
5	106	8.3
6	100	9.0
7	92	9.7
8	92	8.8
9	105	7.6
10	108	6.9

(a) Find the linear regression model for Y with respect to X.

(b) Find the 95% confidence interval for the slope of the regression line in (a).

3. The mean arterial blood pressure (X) and the total glycosylated haemoglobin (Y) of the enalaparil group are given in Table 7.5-2.[18]

(a) Find the linear regression model of Y with respect to X.

(b) Find the 95% confidence interval for the slope of the regression line in part (a).

References

1. Anderson TW. (2003) *An Introduction to Multivariate Statistical Analysis*, 3rd ed. Wiley, New York.
2. Armitage P, McPherson CK, Copas JC. (1969) Statistical studies of prognosis in advanced breast cancer. *J Chron Dis* **22**: 343–360.
3. Bulbrook RD, Greenwood FG, Hayward JL. (1960) Selection of breast cancer patients for adrenalectomy or hypophysectomy by determination of urinary 17-hydroxycorticosteroids and aetiocholanolone. *Lancet* **i**: 1154–1157.
4. Cornfield J. (1962) Discriminant functions. *Rev Int Stat Inst* **35**: 142–153.
5. Draper NR, Smith H. (1998) *Applied Regression Analysis*, 3rd ed. Wiley, New York.
6. Fisher RA. (1921) On the "probable error" of a coefficient of correlation deduced from a small sample. *Metron* **1**: 3–32.
7. Fisher RA. (1936) The use of multiple measurments in taxonomic problems. *Ann Eugen* **7**: 179–188.
8. Friedman M. (1992) Do old fallacies ever die? *J Econ Literature* **30**: 2129–2132.
9. Friedman M, Kuznets S. (1945) *Income from Independent Professional Practice*. National Bureau of Economic Research, New York.
10. Galton F. (1886) Regression towards mediocrity in hereditary statue. *J Anthropological Inst of Great Britain and Ireland* **15**: 246–263.
11. Hosmer DW, Lemeshow S. (2000) *Applied Logistic Regression*, 2nd ed. Wiley, New York.
12. Hotelling H. (1933) Review of the Triumph of Mediocrity in Business by Horace Secrist. *J Am Stat Assoc* **28**: 463–465.
13. James KE. (1973) Regression toward the mean in uncontrolled clinical studies. *Biometrics* **29**: 121–130.
14. Johnson RA, Wichern DW. (1998) *Applied Multivariate Statistical Analysis*, 4th ed. Prentice-Hall, Upper Saddle River, New Jersey.
15. Lee TS. (2012) A Poisson regression model with interaction for female radium dial workers. *J Mod Appl Stat Methods* **11**: 233–241.
16. Lee TS, Falter K, Meyer P, *et al.* (2009) Risk factors associated with clinic visits during the 1999 forest fires near the Hoopa Valley Indian Reservation. *Int J Environ Health Res* **19**: 315–327.
17. Lidwell, OM. (1961) Sepsis in surgical wounds: Multiple regression analysis applied to records of post-operative hospital sepsis. *J Hygiene* **59**: 259–270.
18. Marre M, Leblanc H, Suarez L, *et al.* (1987) Converting enzyme inhibition and kidney function in normotensive diabetic patients with persistent microalbuminuria. *British Med J* **294**: 1448–1452.

19. McCullagh P, Nelder JA. (1983) *Generalized Linear Models*. Chapman & Hall Ltd, London, UK.
20. McGee DL. (1986) Epidemiologic programs for computers and calculators: A program for logistic regression on the IBM PC. *Am J Epidemiol* **124**: 702–705.
21. Oyama, T. (1955) Factors influencing relapse in pulmonary tuberculosis: A statistical analysis of 1259 patients followed from eleven months to six years. *Am Rev Tuberc* **72**: 613–632.
22. Oyama, T, Tatsuoka, M. (1956) Prediction of relapse in pulmonary tuberculosis: An application of discriminant analysis. *Am Rev Tuberc* **73**: 472–484.
23. Pitts SR, Adams RP. (1998) Emergency department hypertension and regression to the mean. *Ann Emergency Med* **31**: 214–218.
24. Prentice AM, Black AE, Coward WA, *et al.* (1986) High levels of energy expenditure in obese women. *British Med J* **292**: 983–987.
25. Stigler SM. (1989) Francis Galton's account of the invention of correlation. *Statist Sci* **4**: 73–86.
26. Stigler SM. (1997) Regression toward the mean, historically considered. *Stat Methods Med Res* **6**: 103–114.
27. Truett J, Cornfield J, Kannel W. (1967) A multivariate analysis of the risk of coronary heart disease in Farmingham. *J Chron Dis* **20**: 511–524.
28. Walker SH, Duncan DB. (1967) Estimation of the probability as a function of several independent variables. *Biometrika* **54**: 167–179.
29. Weisberg S. (1985) *Applied Linear Regression*, 2nd ed. Wiley, New York.

8 Nonparametric Inference

8.0 A Preview

In previous chapters all the statistical tests depend on the parametric probability distributions, in particular, normal distribution. In this chapter we are going to learn the nonparametric statistical inference. The term "nonparametric" was originally suggested by J Wolfowitz.[7] It means that the populations under consideration could not be specified by a finite number of parameters.

Many textbook authors use the terms "nonparametric" and "distribution-free" interchangeably. Classical normal-theory tests depend on the actual sample data, whereas nonparametric tests depend on the sample data only through their ranks.

8.1 Order Statistics

Before defining the rank of the sample data, we first learn the notion of the order statistics.

Definition 8.1.1. Given that the sample data $\{x_i\}_{i=1}^n$ are randomly collected from the continuous random variable (r.v.) X, a set of the order statistics denoted by $\{x_{[j]}\}_{i=1}^n$ is obtained by arranging all the sample observations from the smallest to the largest according to their magnitudes, that is, they satisfy

$$x_{[1]} \leq x_{[2]} \leq \cdots \leq x_{[n]}. \tag{8.1.1}$$

The rank of the sample observation x_k is defined to be the subscript of its corresponding order statistic $x_{[l]}$, namely,

$$rank(x_k) \equiv rank(x_{[l]}) = l. \qquad (8.1.2)$$

Remarks

1. It can be shown that the order statistics $\{x_{[j]}\}_{j=1}^n$ partition the support of the r.v. X into $n + 1$ subintervals and each subinterval has the same expected value of the area under curve of the probability density function (p.d.f.) of X, that is, for $k = 1, 2, \ldots, n$

$$E[F(x_{[k+1]}) - F(x_{[k]})] = (n + 1)^{-1}, \qquad (8.1.3)$$

where $F(x)$ denotes the cumulative distribution of the r.v. X,

2. It can be shown[2] that the p.d.f. of the sampling distribution of the kth order statistics $x_{[k]}$ is given by:

$$g_k(x_{[k]}) = \frac{n!}{(k-1)!(n-k)!} [F(x_{[k]})]^{k-1} [1 - F(x_{[k]})]^{n-k} f(x_{[k]}),$$

$$(8.1.4)$$

where F and f denote the cumulative distribution function and the p.d.f. of the r.v. X.

3. In theory, all sample observations should be distinct for a continuous random variable since the probability that two observations equal to one another is zero. However, in practical applications, tied observations could occur. In this case, we simply assign their average rank to tied observations. See Example 8.2-1.

Example 8.1-1

Using the FEV1 data in Example 1.4-1, estimate the sample IQR by using the order statistics to first find the 1st and 3rd quartiles.

Solution

The 1st and 3rd quartiles are just the 25th and 75th percentiles. By using Eq. (8.1.3), the location of the 25th percentile lies at

$$(n+1) \times 0.25 = (57+1) \times 0.25 = 14.5. \tag{1}$$

Thus, we have by applying linear interpolation on Eq. (1)

$$x_{25\%} = x_{[14]} + 0.5 \times (x_{[15]} - x_{[14]})$$
$$= 3.54 + 0.5 \times (3.54 - 3.54) = 3.54.$$

Similarly, the location of the 75th percentile lies at:

$$(n+1) \times 0.75 = 58 \times 0.75 = 43.5. \tag{2}$$

Thus, we have by applying the linear interpolation on Eq. (2)

$$x_{75\%} = x_{[43]} + 0.5 \times (x_{[44]} - x_{[43]})$$
$$= 4.5 + 0.5 \times (4.56 - 4.5) = 4.53.$$

Hence, the sample estimator for the IQR is

$$I\hat{Q}R_X = x_{75\%} - x_{25\%} = 4.53 - 3.54 = 0.99.$$

Remarks

1. We read the order statistics $x_{[14]}, x_{[15]}, x_{[43]}$ and $x_{[44]}$ directly from Fig. 1.4-5.
2. The sample estimator for the IQR obtained here is more precise than that in Example 1.4-3.

Example 8.1-2

Let X be a uniform random variable on the open interval $(0, 1)$. Assume that the sample data of size five, $\{x_i\}_{i=1}^5$, are randomly collected on X. Find the probability that the order statistic $x_{[4]}$ lies between $\frac{1}{5}$ and $\frac{4}{5}$.

Solution

Since the p.d.f. of the uniform r.v. X is $f(x) = 1, 0 < x < 1$, its cumulative distribution is given by

$$F(x) = \int_0^x f(t)dt = \int_0^x 1 \cdot dt = t|_0^x = x - 0 = x. \qquad (1)$$

By applying Eqs. (8.1.4) and (1), the p.d.f. of $x_{[4]}$ is given by

$$g_4(x_{[4]}) = \frac{5!}{(4-1)!(5-4)!}[x_{[4]}]^{4-1}[1 - x_{[4]}]^{5-4} = 20x_{[4]}^3(1 - x_{[4]}). \qquad (2)$$

Thus, the probability that the order statistic $x_{[4]}$ lies between $\frac{1}{5}$ and $\frac{4}{5}$ is given by using Eq. (2)

$$\Pr\left(\frac{1}{5} < x_{[4]} < \frac{4}{5}\right) = \int_{\frac{1}{5}}^{\frac{4}{5}} g_4(t)dt = \int_{\frac{1}{5}}^{\frac{4}{5}} 20t^3(1-t)dt$$

$$= 20\int_{\frac{1}{5}}^{\frac{4}{5}} (t^3 - t^4)dt = 20\left[\frac{1}{4}t^4 - \frac{1}{5}t^5\right]_{\frac{1}{5}}^{\frac{4}{5}}$$

$$= 20\left\{\left[\frac{1}{4}\left(\frac{4}{5}\right)^4 - \frac{1}{5}\left(\frac{4}{5}\right)^5\right] - \left[\frac{1}{4}\left(\frac{1}{5}\right)^4 - \frac{1}{5}\left(\frac{1}{5}\right)^5\right]\right\}$$

$$= \frac{2283}{3125} = 0.73056 \approx 0.731.$$

Remarks

1. The order statistic $x_{[4]}$ is replaced by a dummy variable t in the above integration.
2. The readers need to know calculus in order to follow the above integration.

8.2 The Wilcoxon Signed-Rank Test

Now let us turn our attention to the hypothesis testing. We wish to test the following pairs of hypotheses:

(i) H_0: $med_X = m_0$ versus H_1: $med_X \neq m_0$,   (8.2.1)
(ii) H_0: $med_X \leq m_0$ versus H_1: $med_X > m_0$,   (8.2.2)
(iii) H_0: $med_X \geq m_0$ versus H_1: $med_X < m_0$,   (8.2.3)

where med_X is the median of the symmetric r.v. X.

Assume that the sample data of size n are randomly collected on X, $\{x_i\}_{i=1}^n$. Set $d_i = x_i - m_0$, i = 1,2,...,n. Let T^+ equal the sum of the rank of the positive differences. That is, let

$$T^+ = \text{sum of positive } T_i s, \tag{8.2.4}$$

where T_is are defined by

$$T_i = sign(d_i) \cdot rank(|d_i|), \tag{8.2.5}$$

and sign $(d_i) = +1, 0$, or -1 if $d_i > 0, = 0$, or < 0.

The testing statistic for Eqs. (8.2.1) to (8.2.3) is given by

$$z = \frac{T^+ - E(T^+|H_0)}{\sqrt{\text{var}(T^+|H_0)}}, \tag{8.2.6}$$

where $E(T^+|H_0)$ and $\text{var}(T^+|H_0)$ are given respectively by[2]

$$E(T^+|H_0) = n(n+1)/4, \tag{8.2.7}$$

$$\text{var}(T^+|H_0) = n(n+1)(2n+1)/24. \tag{8.2.8}$$

The decision rule for testing Eqs. (8.2.1) to (8.2.3) is given below.

Decision Rule 8.2-1

For all the three tests below the significance level is α:

(i) A two-tailed test for Eq. (8.2.1) is to reject H_0 if the computed z of Eq. (8.2.6) is greater than $z_{1-\frac{\alpha}{2}}$ or less than $z_{\frac{\alpha}{2}}$.   (8.2.9)

(ii) A right-tailed test for Eq. (8.2.2) is to reject H_0 if the computed z of Eq. (8.2.6) is greater than $z_{1-\alpha}$.   (8.2.10)

(iii) A left-tailed test for Eq. (8.2.3) is to reject H_0 if the computed z of Eq. (8.2.6) is less than z_α.   (8.2.11)

Remarks

1. By the Central Limit Theorem (Theorem 4.1.1), the testing statistic of Eq. (8.2.6) is a normal random variable as $n \to \infty$. When n < 30, the sampling distribution of Eq. (8.2.6) reduces to the t_n-distribution and the critical values of the z-distribution have to be accordingly replaced by that of the t_n-distribution.
2. When the symmetric assumption for the r.v. X does not hold, one of the two possible scenarios could occur: either H_0 is not true or the p.d.f. of the r.v. X is asymmetry if H_0 is rejected at the significance level α.
3. In addition to the Wilcoxon signed-rank test, there are other one-sample tests like the ordinary sign test and the Binomial test.[2]

Example 8.2-1

With the FEV1 data in Example 1.4-1, we wish to test

$$H_0: med_X = 4.1 \quad \text{versus} \quad H_1: med_X \neq 4.1. \tag{1}$$

Is the null hypothesis H_0 true at the significance level of 0.05?

Solution

By subtracting $m_0 = 4.1$ from the sample data of FEV1, we have $\{d_i\}_{i=1}^{57} = \{0.37, -1, 0.4, 0.8, -0.6, 0.04, 0.22, 0.7, -1, 0.58, 0.37, -0.53, -1.25, 1, 1, 1.1, 0.7, 1, 0.2, 0.6, -0.02, -0.62, 0.1, -0.4, 1.2, 0.61, 0, 0.2, -0.71, -0.41, 0.34, 0.9, 0.4, 0.1, 0.06, -0.4, -0.27, -0.2, 0.37, -0.8, 1.33, -0.68, -0.5, -0.9, 0.46, 0.68, -0.5, -0.14, -0.91, -1.25, -1.06, -0.3, -0.35, -0.05, -0.56, 0.04, -1.12, -0.56\}$.

Thus, by using Eq. (8.2.5), we have $\{T_i\}_{i=1}^{57} = \{19, -48.5, 22.5, 42.5, -33.5, 3.5, 13, 39.5, -48.5, 32, 19, -29, -55.5, 48.5, 52, 39.5, 48.5, 11, 33.5, -2, -36, 7.5, -22.5, 54, 35, 0, 11, -41, -25, 16, 44.5, 22.5, 7.5, 6, -22.5, -14, -11, 19, -42.5, 57, -37.5, -27.5, -44.5, 26, 37.5, -27.5, -9, -46, -55.5, -51, -15, -17, -5, -30.5, 3.5, -54, -30.5\}$.

From Eq. (8.2.4), we have

$$T^+ = 771. \tag{2}$$

After applying Eqs. (8.2.7) and (8.2.8), we have

$$E(T^+|H_0) = 57 \cdot (57 + 1)/4 = 826.5, \tag{3}$$

and

$$\sqrt{\text{var}(T^+|H_0)} = \sqrt{57(57 + 1)(2 \cdot 57 + 1)/24} = 125.862. \tag{4}$$

After substituting Eqs. (2) to (4) into Eq. (8.2.6), we have

$$z = \frac{771 - 826.5}{125.862} = -0.44096 \approx -0.441. \tag{5}$$

The z-value of Eq. (5) is neither greater than $z_{0.975} = 1.96$ nor less than $z_{0.025} = -1.96$ for $\alpha = 0.05$. By the decision rule of Eq. (8.2.9), H_0 is not rejected at the significance level of 0.05. In other words, the population median of the r.v. FEV1 indeed equals 4.1 at the significance level of 0.05.

Remarks

1. The value of m_0 chosen here is the same as the sample median obtained in Example 1.4-2.
2. Among the values of the magnitude of d_i, namely, $|d_i|$, there are several tied observations. As a result, their average rank are assigned to them as follows:

$$\text{rank}(\{0.04, 0.1, 0.2, 0.37, 0.4, 0.5, 0.56, 0.6,$$

$$0.68, 0.7, 0.8, 0.9, 1, 1.25\}$$

$$= \{3.5, 7.5, 11, 19, 22.5, 27.5, 30.5, 33.5, 37.5,$$

$$39.5, 42.5, 44.5, 48.5, 55.5\}.$$

3. All calculations were done on an EXCEL spreadsheet.

8.3 The Two-Sample Tests

Assume that the sample data, $\{x_i\}_{i=1}^n$ and $\{y_j\}_{j=1}^m$, are randomly collected on the two mutually independent continuous random variables (r.v.s) X and Y. We wish to test the following pairs of hypotheses:

(i) $H_0: F(t) = G(t)$ versus $H_1: F(t) \neq G(t)$,   (8.3.1)

(ii) $H_0: F(t) \leq G(t)$ versus $H_1: F(t) > G(t)$,   (8.3.2)

(iii) $H_0: F(t) \geq G(t)$ versus $H_1: F(t) < G(t)$,   (8.3.3)

where $F(x)$ and $G(y)$ denote the unknown cumulative distribution of X and Y, respectively. In this section we are going to learn two distribution-free tests available to test Eqs. (8.3.1) to (8.3.3).

A. *The Wilcoxon Rank-Sum Test*

Order the combined samples of X and Y from low to high, and assign a rank to each observation. If there are tied observations, assign the average of their ranks to them. Define a statistic W as follows:

$$W = \sum_{i=1}^n rank(x_i), \qquad (8.3A.1)$$

where rank (x_i) denote the rank of x_i in the combined samples of X and Y. It can be shown (see Ref. 5) that

$$E(W) = n(N+1)/2, \qquad (8.3A.2)$$

and

$$var(W) = nm(N+1)/12, \qquad (8.3A.3)$$

where $N = n + m$. The testing statistic for Eqs. (8.3.1) to (8.3.3) is given by

$$z_W = \frac{W - E(W)}{\sqrt{var(W)}} = \frac{W - n(N+1)/2}{\sqrt{nm(N+1)/12}}. \qquad (8.3A.4)$$

The decision rule for testing Eqs. (8.3.1) to (8.3.3) is given below.

Decision Rule 8.3A-1

For all the three tests below the significance level is α:

(i) A two-tailed test for Eq. (8.3.1) is to reject H_0 if the computed z_W of Eq. (8.3A.4) is greater than $z_{1-\frac{\alpha}{2}}$ or less than $z_{\frac{\alpha}{2}}$.

$$(8.3A.5)$$

(ii) A right-tailed test for Eq. (8.3.2) is to reject H_0 if the computed z_W of Eq. (8.3A.4) is greater than $z_{1-\alpha}$.   (8.3A.6)

(iii) A left-tailed test for Eq. (8.3.3) is to reject H_0 if the computed z_W of Eq. (8.3A.4) is less than z_{α}.   (8.3A.7)

Remarks

1. By the Central Limit Theorem (Theorem 4.1.1), the testing statistic of Eq. (8.3A.4) is a normal random variable as $n \rightarrow \infty$. When $n < 30$, the sampling distribution of Eq. (8.3A.4) reduces to the t_n-distribution and the critical values of the z-distribution has to be accordingly replaced by that of the t_n-distribution.

2. If the null hypothesis H_0 in Eq. (8.3.1) is true, then the equation of $med_X = med_Y$ surely holds. However, if $F(t) \neq G(t)$, it implies in many real situations that $Pr(X < Y)$ is no longer equal to $1/2$. As a result, Eqs. (8.3.1) to (8.3.3) can be replaced by:

   (i*) $H_0: Pr(X < Y) = 1/2$ versus $H_1: Pr(X < Y) \neq 1/2$,   (8.3.4)
   (ii*) $H_0: Pr(X < Y) \leq 1/2$ versus $H_1: Pr(X < Y) > 1/2$,   (8.3.5)
   (iii*) $H_0: Pr(rmX < Y) \geq 1/2$ versus $H_1: Pr(X < Y) < 1/2$.   (8.3.6)

B. *The Mann–Whitney (MW) Test*

Let U equal the sum of the number of y_j that are less than x_i for each x_i, that is,

$$U = \sum_{i=1}^{n} V_i,   (8.3B.1)$$

where V_i = the number of y_j that are less than x_i for each x_i in the combined sample. It can be shown[2] that

$$E(U) = \frac{1}{2} \cdot nm, \qquad (8.3B.2)$$

and

$$\text{var}(U) = \frac{1}{12} \cdot nm(N+1). \qquad (8.3B.3)$$

The testing statistic for Eqs. (8.3.4) to (8.3.6) is given by

$$z_{MW} = \frac{U - E(U)}{\sqrt{\text{var}(U)}} = \frac{U - nm/2}{\sqrt{nm(N+1)/12}}, \qquad (8.3B.4)$$

where $N = n + m$.

The decision rule for testing Eqs. (8.3.4) to (8.3.6) is given below.

Decision Rule 8.3B-1

For all the three tests below the significance level is α:

(i) A two-tailed test for Eq. (8.3.4) is to reject H_0 if the computed z_{MW} of Eq. (8.3B.4) is greater than $z_{1-\frac{\alpha}{2}}$ or less than $z_{\frac{\alpha}{2}}$.
$$(8.3B.5)$$

(ii) A right-tailed test for Eq. (8.3.5) is to reject H_0 if the computed z_{MW} of Eq. (8.3B.4) is greater than $z_{1-\alpha}$. $\qquad$ (8.3B.6)

(iii) A left-tailed test for Eq. (8.3.6) is to reject H_0 if the computed z_{MW} of Eq. (8.3B.4) is less than z_α. $\qquad$ (8.3B.7)

Remarks

1. By the Central Limit Theorem (Theorem 4.1.1), the testing statistic of Eq. (8.3B.4) is a normal random variable as $n \to \infty$. When $n < 30$, the sampling distribution of Eq. (8.3B.4) reduces to the t_n-distribution and the critical values of the Z-distribution has to be accordingly replaced by that of the t_n-distribution.
2. Equation (8.3B.1) is connected with Eq. (8.3A.1) by the relation of $U = W - n(n+1)/2$.
3. The Mann–Whitney test is unbiased and consistent (see Ref. 4).

Example 8.3-1

Let two r.v.s X and Y denote the length of remission (days) of endogenous versus neurotic depression patients. A sample of the data is randomly collected and given by $\{x_i\}_{i=1}^{12} = \{109, 214, 1818, 140, 179, 744, 105, 101, 105, 1547, 529, 140\}$ and $\{y_j\}_{j=1}^{12} = \{546, 844, 602, 87, 794, 643, 199, 91, 105, 479, 1296, 279\}$. By using the Wilcoxon rank-sum test and the Mann–Whitney test to test Eqs. (8.3.1) and (8.3.4), respectively.

Solution

We order the combined sample of $\{x_i\}_{i=1}^{12}$ and $\{y_j\}_{j=1}^{12}$ as follows:

$$\{87, 91, 101, 105, 105, 105, 109, 140, 140, 179, 199, 214, 279, 479,$$

$$529, 546, 602, 643, 744, 794, 844, 1296, 1547, 1818\}. \tag{1}$$

Assign the rank appropriately to each observation of Eq. (1), we have

$$\{1, 2, 3, 5, 5, 5, 7, 8.5, 8.5, 10, 11, 12, 13, 14, 15, 16, 17, 18, 19, 20,$$

$$21, 22, 23, 24\}. \tag{2}$$

By applying Eqs. (8.3A.1) and (8.3B.1) to Eq. (2), we have

$$W = 3 + 5 + 5 + 8.5 + 8.5 + 10 + 12 + 15 + 19 + 23 + 24 = 140, \tag{3}$$

and

$$U = 3 + 4 + 12 + 3 + 3 + 9 + 2 + 2 + 2 + 12 + 6 + 3 = 61. \tag{4}$$

By substituting $n = m = 12$, $N = 24$, and Eqs. (3) and (4) into Eqs. (8.3A.4) and (8.3B.4), we have

$$z_W = \frac{140 - 12 \times (24 + 1)/2}{\sqrt{12 \times 12 \times (24 + 1)/12}} = \frac{-10}{10\sqrt{3}} \approx -0.577, \tag{5}$$

and

$$z_{MW} = \frac{61 - 12 \cdot 12/2}{\sqrt{12 \cdot 12 \cdot (24 + 1)/12}} = -\frac{11}{10\sqrt{3}} \approx -0.635. \tag{6}$$

Since neither Eqs. (5) nor (6) is less than the critical value of $z_{0.025} = -1.96$, the null hypothesis H_0 is not rejected at the significance level of 0.05. In other words, the cumulative distributions of the endogenous versus neurotic depression patients are the same at the significance level of 0.05.

8.4 The Kolmogorov–Smirnov Test

A. *The One-sample Test*

Assume that the sample data of order statistics $\{x_{[j]}\}_{j=1}^{n}$ are randomly collected from a r.v. X with the unknown c.d.f. $F(x)$. We wish to test the following pair of hypotheses:

$$H_0 : F(x) = F_0(x) \text{ versus } H_1 : F(x) \neq F_0(x), \qquad (8.4A.1)$$

where $F_0(x)$ is the completely specified known function. Let the empirical distribution function (e.d.f.) of the r.v. X be defined by

$$S_n(x) = \begin{cases} 0, & \text{if} \quad x_{[j]} < x_{[1]} \\ \frac{j}{n}, & \text{if} \quad x_{[j]} \leq x < x_{[j+1]}. \\ 1, & \text{if} \quad x \geq x_{[n]} \end{cases} \qquad (8.4A.2)$$

It can be shown[5] that the mean and variance of $S_n(x)$ are

$$E(S_n(x)) = F(x), \qquad (8.4A.3)$$

and

$$\text{var}(S_n(x)) = F(x)(1 - F(x))/n. \qquad (8.4A.4)$$

In addition, $S_n(x)$ is a consistent estimator of $F(x)$. In other words, $S_n(x)$ converges in probability to $F(x)$.

The testing statistics for Eqs. (8.4A.1) are respectively given by

$$D_n = sup_x|S_n(x) - F_0(x)|, \qquad (8.4A.5)$$

where the supremum is taken over all x in the support of the r.v. X. It can be shown[3, 6] that if $F_0(x)$ is any continuous function, then for every $t \geq 0$,

$$\lim_{n\to\infty} \Pr(\sqrt{n}D_n \leq t) = KS(t). \qquad (8.4A.6)$$

where $KS(t)$, the Kolmogorov–Smirnov function, is given by

$$KS(t) = 1 - 2\sum_{i=1}^{\infty}(-1)^{i-1}e^{-2i^2t^2}.$$

The decision rule for testing Eq. (8.4A.1) is given below.

Decision Rule 8.4A-1

For the test below the significance level is α:

A two-tailed test for Eq. (8.4A.1) is to reject H_0 if the computed D_n of Eq. (8.4A.5) is greater than $d_{n;1-\alpha}$. $\qquad$ (8.4A.7)

Remarks

1. The $(1-\alpha)\%^{\text{th}}$ percentile $d_{n;1-\alpha}$ of Eq. (8.4A.7) is given in Table A-4 in the appendix.
2. To form the $100(1-\alpha)\%$ confidence band $[F_L(x), F_U(x)]$ for the true unknown distribution function F(x) based on a sample of size n, select a critical number $d_{n;1-\alpha}$ in Table A-4 such that

$$\Pr(D_n \geq d_{n;1-\alpha)}) = \alpha.$$

Then

$$1 - \alpha = \Pr[D_n \leq d_{n;1-\alpha}]$$
$$= \Pr[\text{Sup}_x |S_n(x) - F(x)| \leq d_{n;1-\alpha}]$$
$$= \Pr[S_n(x) - d_{n;1-\alpha} \leq F(x) \leq S_n(x) + d_{n;1-\alpha}].$$

As a result, let the lower band $F_L(x)$ and the upper band $F_U(x)$ be given respectively by

$$F_L(x) = \begin{cases} 0, S_n(x) - d_{n;1-\alpha} \leq 0 \\ S_n(x) - d_{n;1-\alpha}, S_n(x) - d_{n;1-\alpha} > 0 \end{cases} \qquad (8.4A.8)$$

and

$$F_U(x) = \begin{cases} S_n(x) + d_{n;1-\alpha}, S_n(x) + d_{n;1-\alpha} < 1 \\ 1, S_n(x) - d_{n;1-\alpha} \geq 1 \end{cases} \qquad (8.4A.9)$$

Example 8.4A-1

Given the following data: -0.6, -0.6, -0.53, -0.5, -0.47, -0.47, -0.42, -0.42, -0.37, -0.33, -0.32, -0.29, -0.26, -0.26, -0.24, -0.23, -0.23, -0.18, -0.18, -0.18, -0.18, -0.15, -0.14, -0.11, -0.08, -0.05, -0.005, 0.009, 0.02, 0.04, 0.04, 0.05, 0.07, 0.07, 0.12, 0.12, 0.13, 0.19, 0.2, 0.2, 0.2, 0.22, 0.22, 0.25, 0.31, 0.32, 0.32, 0.35, 0.36, 0.36, 0.41, 0.46, 0.51, 0.51, 0.56, 0.61, 0.67.

By using DR 8.4A-1, test at the significance level of 0.05 if the above data are generated from the standard normal distribution.

Solution

The sample size of the given data is n = 57. The empirical distribution function of Eq. (8.4A.4) is given by

$$S_{57}(x) = \frac{j}{57}, \quad \text{if } x_{[j]} \leq x < x_{[j+1]}. \qquad (1)$$

We wish to test

$$H_0 : F(x) = \Phi(x) \quad \text{versus} \quad H_1 : F(x) \neq \Phi(x), \qquad (2)$$

where $\Phi(x) = \frac{1}{\sqrt{2\pi}} \int_{-\infty}^{x} e^{-\frac{t^2}{2}} dt$. The testing statistics for Eq. (2) is

$$D_{57} = sup_x |S_{57}(x) - \Phi(x)|. \qquad (3)$$

Evaluating Eq. (3) over the given data point,

$$D_{57} = 0.2567 \approx 0.257. \qquad (4)$$

Because the value of the testing statistics D_{57} (Eq. 4) is greater than $d_{57;0.95} = 0.1767$, the null hypothsis H_0 in Eq. (2) is rejected at the level of 0.05.

B. *The Two-Sample Test*

Assume that the sample data of order statistics $\{x_{[i]}\}_{i=1}^{n}$ and $\{y_{[j]}\}_{j=1}^{m}$ are randomly collected from two mutually independent r.v.s X and Y with their unknown c.d.f.s $F(x)$ and $G(y)$. We wish to test the following pair of hypotheses:

$$H_0 : F(t) = G(t) \text{ versus } H_1 : F(t) \neq G(t), \qquad (8.4B.1)$$

Let the empirical distribution function (e.d.f.) of the r.v.s X and Y be defined respectively by

$$S_n(x) = \begin{cases} 0, & \text{if } x_{[i]} < x_{[1]} \\ \frac{i}{n}, & \text{if } x_{[i]} \leq x < x_{[i+1]}, \quad \text{for } i = 1,2,\dots n-1 \\ 1, & \text{if } x \geq x_{[n]} \end{cases} \qquad (8.4B.2)$$

and

$$T_m(x) = \begin{cases} 0, & \text{if } x_{[j]} < x_{[1]} \\ \frac{j}{m}, & \text{if } x_{[j]} \leq x < x_{j+1}, \quad \text{for } j = 1,2,\dots m-1 \\ 1, & \text{if } x \geq x_{[m]} \end{cases} \qquad (8.4B.3)$$

The testing statistics for Eq. (8.4B.1) are respectively given by

$$D_{n,m} = \sup_x |S_n(x) - T_m(x)|, \qquad (8.4B.4)$$

where the supremum is taken over all x in the joint support of the r.v.s X and Y. The limiting distribution of Eq. (8.4B.4) is given by[3,6]:

$$\lim_{n \to \infty} \Pr\left(\sqrt{\frac{nm}{n+m}} D_{n,m} \leq t\right) = KS(t), \qquad (8.4B.5)$$

where $KS(t)$ is given by Eq. (8.4A.6).

The decision rule for testing Eq. (8.4B.1) is given below.

Decision Rule 8.4B-1

For the test below the significance level is α:

A two-tailed test for Eq. (8.4B.1) is to reject H_0 if the computed $D_{n,m}$ of Eq. (8.4B.4) is greater than $d_{n,m;1-\alpha}$. $\qquad$ (8.4B.6)

Remarks

1. The Kolmogorov–Smirnov (K–S) two-sample test is an alternative to the MW test in Sec. 8.3B.
2. The MW test is more powerful when H_1 is the location shift. The K–S test has reasonable power against a range of alternative hypotheses.
3. For sufficiently large m and n, the critical value $d_{n,m;1-\alpha}$ in Eq. (8.4B.6) is given by

$$d_{n,m;1-\alpha} = c(\alpha)\sqrt{\frac{n+m}{nm}}, \qquad (8.4B.7)$$

where the value of $c(\alpha)$ = the inverse of the Kolmogorov–Smirnov distribution at α, is given below for the most common levels of α[8]:

α	0.1	0.05	0.025	0.01	0.005	0.001
$c(\alpha)$	1.073	1.224	1.358	1.517	1.628	1.858

Example 8.4B-1

By using the Kolmogorov–Smirnov two-sample test (DR 8.4B-1), determine at the level of significance 0.05 whether the following frequency data (Table 8.4B-1) for the age distributions of men and women are the same:

Table 8.4B-1.   The sample age distribution of men and women

Age	21–22	23–24	25–26	27–28	29–30	31–32	33–34	35–36	37–38	39–40
Men	4	11	5	7	0	5	9	13	20	6
Women	7	4	1	11	12	4	2	4	8	9

Table 8.4B-2.   The sampling distribution of X and Y

Age	$S_{80}(x)$	$T_{62}(x)$	$|S_{80}(x) - T_{62}(x)|$
21–22	$\dfrac{4}{80}$	$\dfrac{7}{62}$	0.0629
23–24	$\dfrac{15}{80}$	$\dfrac{11}{62}$	0.0101
25–26	$\dfrac{20}{80}$	$\dfrac{12}{62}$	0.0565
27–28	$\dfrac{27}{80}$	$\dfrac{23}{62}$	0.0335
29–30	$\dfrac{27}{80}$	$\dfrac{35}{62}$	0.2270
31–32	$\dfrac{32}{80}$	$\dfrac{39}{62}$	0.2290
33–34	$\dfrac{41}{80}$	$\dfrac{41}{62}$	0.1488
35–36	$\dfrac{54}{80}$	$\dfrac{45}{62}$	0.0508
37–38	$\dfrac{74}{80}$	$\dfrac{53}{62}$	0.0702
39–40	$\dfrac{80}{80}$	$\dfrac{62}{62}$	0.0

Solution

Let the r.v.s X and Y be the age distribution of men and women corresponding to the designate age range of 21 to 40. From Eqs. (8.4B-2) and (8.4B-3), the e.d.f. for X and Y corresponding to Table 8.4B-1 with n = 80 and m = 62 are calculated in Table 8.4B-2.

From the 4th column of Table 8.4B-2, we have

$$D_{80,62} = 0.229. \tag{1}$$

By using Eq. (8.4B.7) with $\alpha = 0.05$, n = 80 and m = 62,

$$d_{80,62;.95} = 1.224 \cdot \sqrt{\frac{80+62}{80 \cdot 62}} \approx 0.2071. \tag{2}$$

Since Eq. (1) is greater than Eq. (2), the null hypothesis is rejected at the significance level of 0.05, that is the age distributions between men and women are not the same.

8.5 Rank Correlation

Assume that the sample data of paired order statistics $\{x_{[i]}\}_{i=1}^{n}$ and $\{y_{[j]}\}_{j=1}^{n}$ are randomly collected from two r.v.s X and Y that have a continuous bivariate population. A nonparametric way to estimate the correlation between X and Y is via using the rank correlation. Thus, the Spearman rank correlation coefficient $\hat{\rho}_S$ is defined by

$$\hat{\rho}_S = 1 - 6[n(n^2 - 1)]^{-1} \cdot \sum_{i=1}^{n} d_i^2, \tag{8.5.1}$$

where $d_i = r_i - s_i, r_i = rank(x_i)$ and $s_i = rank(y_i), i = 1, \ldots, n$. It can be shown (see Exercise 8.6-2) that

$$E(\hat{\rho}_s) = 0 \quad \text{and} \quad var(\hat{\rho}_s) = (n-1)^{-1}. \tag{8.5.2}$$

Remarks

1. By substituting r_i and s_i respectively for x_i and y_i into Eq. (7.1.1) and then simplifying it, we obtain Eq. (8.5.1) (see Exercise 8.6-1).
2. Although Eq. (8.5.1) is obtained as shown in Exercise 8.6-1, it actually is an unbiased estimator for the grade correlation

coefficient of ρ_{FG} defined by[1]:

$$\rho_{FG} = \frac{\text{cov}(F(X), G(Y))}{\sqrt{\text{var}(F(x)) \cdot \text{var}(G(Y))}},$$ (8.5.3)

where F and G are the c.d.f. of X and Y.

We wish to test the three pairs of hypotheses:

(i) H_0: $\rho_{FG} = 0$ versus H_1: $\rho_{FG} \neq 0$,   (8.5.4)
(ii) H_0: $\rho_{FG} \leq 0$ versus H_1: $\rho_{FG} > 0$,   (8.5.5)
(iii) H_0: $\rho_{FG} \geq 0$ versus H_1: $\rho_{FG} < 0$,   (8.5.6)

Remark

Here X and Y are simply two random variables; they do not necessarily follow a bivariate normal distribution as we did in Sec. 7.1. Hence, correlation merely measures the association between X and Y.

The testing statistic for Eqs. (8.5.4) to (8.5.6) is given by

$$z_S = \frac{\hat{\rho}_S - E(\hat{\rho}_s)}{\sqrt{\text{var}(\hat{\rho}_S)}} = \sqrt{n-1}\hat{\rho}_S,$$ (8.5.7)

where $E(\hat{\rho}_S)$ and $\text{var}(\hat{\rho}_S)$ of Eq. (8.5.2) are used in Eq. (8.5.7).

The decision rule for testing Eqs. (8.5.4) to (8.5.6) is given below.

Decision Rule 8.5-1

For all the three tests below the significance level is α:

(i)   A two-tailed test for Eq. (8.5.4) is to reject H_0 if the computed z_S of Eq. (8.5.7) is greater than $z_{1-\frac{\alpha}{2}}$ or less than $z_{\frac{\alpha}{2}}$.   (8.5.8)

(ii) A right-tailed test for Eq. (8.5.5) is to reject H_0 if the computed z_S of Eq. (8.5.7) is greater than $z_{1-\alpha}$.   (8.5.9)

(iii) A left-tailed test for Eq. (8.5.6) is to reject H_0 if the computed z_S of Eq. (8.5.7) is less than z_{α}.   (8.5.10)

Remark

When the sample size is less than 30, the critical values in Eqs. (8.5.8) to (8.5.10) are replaced by that of the t_{n-2}-distribution accordingly.

Example 8.5-1

Using the sample data in Table 7.1-1, (a) find the Spearman rank correlation between the father's and son's height; and (b) test Eq. (8.5.3) at the significance level of 0.05.

Solution

(a) By ranking the sample data in Table 7.1-1, we have

Rank(x_i)	3.5	7	1.5	9	3.5	7	1.5	10	5	7
Rank(y_i)	2	5.5	3	7.5	1	10	4	7.5	5.5	9
d_i	1.5	1.5	−1.5	1.5	2.5	−3	−2.5	2.5	−0.5	−2

By using Eq. (8.5.1), we obtain

$$\rho_S = 1 - \frac{6 \cdot \sum_{i=1}^{10} d_i^2}{10(10^2 - 1)} = 1 - \frac{6 \cdot 41}{990} = 0.751515 \approx 0.75. \tag{1}$$

(b) By substituting Eq. (1) into Eq. (8.5.7), we have

$$z_S = 0.75 \cdot \sqrt{10 - 1} = 2.25. \tag{2}$$

Since Eq. (2) is less than the critical value $t_{8,0.975} = 2.365$, H_0 is not rejected at $\alpha = 0.05$. In other words, the father's and the son's height are not correlated.

8.6 Exercises

1. By substituting r_i and s_i respectively for x_i and y_i into Eq. (7.1.1) and then simplifying it, we obtain Eq. (8.5.1).
2. Show that Eq. (8.5.2) holds.

3. For independent weightings of a standard weight (in gram $\times 10^{-6}$) give the following discrepancies from the supposed true weight: $-1.2, 0.2, -0.6, 0.8, -1.0$. Are the discrepancies sampled from a standard normal r.v. Z?
4. Let the sample frequency data of two r.v.s X and Y be given in the following table:

Interval	50–53	54–57	58–61	62–65	66–69	70–73	74–77	78–81	82–85	86–89
X	3	2	1	1	3	1	0	1	1	1
Y	1	0	0	0	1	3	1	0	2	4

Do X and Y have the same cumulative probability distribution?

References

1. Conover WJ. (1971) *Practical Nonparametric Statistics*. John Wiley & Sons, Inc., New York.
2. Gibbons JD. (1971) *Nonparametric Statistical Inference*. McGraw-Hill Book Company, New York.
3. Kolmogorov A. (1933) Sulla determinazione empirica di una legge di distribuzione. *Giorn. Inst. Ital. Attuari* **4**: 83–91.
4. Lehmann EL, D'Abrera HJM. (1971) *Nonparametrics: Statistical Methods Based On Ranks*. Springer, New York.
5. Massey FJ. (1951) The distribution of the maximum deviation between two sample cumulative step functions. *Ann Math Stat* **22**: 125–128.
6. Smirnov NV. (1939) Estimate of deviation between empirical distribution functions in two independent samples (in Russian). *Bull Moscow Univ* **2**: 3–16.
7. Wolfowitz J. (1949) Non-parametric statistical inference. *Proc Berkeley Symp Math Statistics Prob*, p. 93.
8. https://en.wikipedia.org/wiki/Kolmogorov%2%80%93Smirnov_test.

9 Determination of Sample Size

In planning a scientific study, selecting the adequate sample size is vital to draw the meaningful statistical inference from sample to population. In this chapter we are going to learn how large the sample size should be in order to obtain a make-sense inference.

9.1 A Single Continuous Random Variable

A. *Estimation of the Mean*

Let X be a continuous random variable with the unknown mean μ_X. How large is the sample size (n) required to estimate μ_X with an accuracy of the $100(1 - \alpha)\%$ confidence interval within $\pm\delta$? Thus, from Eq. (4.1.10), δ is given by

$$\delta = z_{1-\frac{\alpha}{2}} \cdot \sigma_X / \sqrt{n}. \tag{9.1A.1}$$

Solving Eq. (9.1A.1) for n, we have

$$n = [(z_{1-\frac{\alpha}{2}} \cdot \sigma_X)/\delta]^2. \tag{9.1A.2}$$

Remarks

For fixed α and σ_X, n of Eq. (9.1A.2) is inversely proportional to the square of δ. Hence, the smaller the value of δ, the larger the sample size.

Table 9.1-1. Approximate Required Sample Size for Different δ

δ	0.05	0.1	0.2	0.3	0.4	0.5
n	984	246	62	28	16	10

Example 9.1A-1

Suppose that an estimate is desired of the average retail price of a new drug. A sample of retail pharmacy stores is planned to be selected. Based on a small pilot study, the standard deviation in price was estimated as 80 cents. How many pharmacy stores are required to be randomly selected so that the estimate is to be within δ cents of the true average price with 95% confidence?

Solution

Since the value of δ is not specified, we will calculate the sample sizes for a range of different values of δ as given in Table 9.1-1 by substituting $\sigma_X = 0.8, \alpha = 0.05$ and $z_{1-\frac{\alpha}{2}} = z_{0.975} = 1.96$ into Eq. (9.1A.2).

From Table 9.1-1, if the estimate for the average retail price of the tranquilizer is desired to be within 10 cents, 246 stores are required to be randomly selected.

Remarks

1. Table 9.1-1 confirms our remark below Eq. (9.1A.2).
2. For different values of α and σ_X, Table 9.1-1 is no longer applicable and we have to recalculate it (see Exercise 9.6-1).

B. *Hypothesis Testing on the Mean*

Suppose that we wish to test Eq. (4.2.1) in which $\theta \equiv \mu_X$ and $\theta_0 \equiv \mu_0$. How large is the sample size (n) required to estimate μ_X with an accuracy of the $100(1 - \alpha)\%$ confidence interval and the power of $1 - \beta$? Assume that the true unknown mean is μ_1. From Figure 4.2.1, the location of the x-coordinate (μ^*) of the intersection point between the probability curves for the null (H_0) and alternative (H_1) hypotheses can be expressed from the graph of H_0 and H_1, respectively, by

$$\mu^* = \mu_0 + z_{1-\frac{\alpha}{2}} \cdot \sigma_X / \sqrt{n}, \tag{9.1B.1}$$

and

$$\mu^* = \mu_1 + z_\beta \cdot \sigma_X / \sqrt{n}. \tag{9.1B.2}$$

By subtracting Eq. (9.1B.2) from Eq. (9.1B.1) and then solving for n, we thus have

$$n = \left[\frac{(z_{1-\frac{\alpha}{2}} - z_\beta) \cdot \sigma_X}{\mu_1 - \mu_0} \right]^2. \tag{9.1B.3}$$

Remarks

1. Since for fixed α and β, n of Eq. (9.1B.3) is inversely proportional to the square of $\mu_1 - \mu_0$, n is decreasing as the value of $\mu_1 - \mu_0$ is increasing as is shown in the next example.
2. If the testing hypothesis is of Eq. (4.2.2), then the critical value $z_{1-\frac{\alpha}{2}}$ in Eq. (9.1B.3) has to be replaced by $z_{1-\alpha}$.
3. If the testing hypothesis is of Eq. (4.2.3), then the critical values $z_{1-\frac{\alpha}{2}}$ and $-z_\beta$ in Eq. (9.1B.3) have to be replaced by $-z_\alpha$ and $z_{1-\beta}$, respectively.

Example 9.1B-1

A survey indicated that the average weight of men who are over 60 years with newly diagnosed heart disease was 220 lb. How large is a sample required to be tested at the 5% level of significance with a power of 90%, and would a change in average weight be detected with an estimated standard deviation of 25 lb?

Solution

Since a change in the average weight is not completely specified, we let $\eta = |\mu_1 - \mu_0|$. For a range of different values of η, we calculate the sample size by substituting $\sigma_X = 25, \alpha = 0.05$,

Table 9.1-2. **Approximate Sample Size for Different Values of** η

η	5	10	15	20	25	30
n	263	66	30	17	11	8

$1 - \beta = 0.9, z_{1-\frac{\alpha}{2}} = z_{0.975} = 1.96$ and $z_\beta = z_{0.1} = -1.28$ into Eq. (9.1B.3) as given in Table 9.1-2.

Hence, from Table 9.1-2, a sample of 263 men with their ages over 60 has to be randomly selected if the estimate for their average weight is to be within 5 lbs of the true average weight.

Remarks

1. Table 9.1-2 confirms our remark below Eq. (9.1B.3).
2. For different values of α and σ_X, Table 9.1-2 is no longer applicable and we have to recalculate it (see Exercise 9.6-2).

9.2 Two Independent Continuous Random Variables

A. *Estimation of Difference in Two Means*

When comparing the means of two independent continuous random variables X and Y with the unknown means μ_X, μ_Y and a common variance σ^2, how large should the minimum sample size be in order to detect the difference in either direction within an accuracy of $\delta > 0$ units in their means with $100(1 - \alpha)\%$ confidence? Assume that the sample size (n) is the same for both X and Y. Let $D = X - Y$. Then, $\bar{\mu}_D = \bar{x} - \bar{y}$ and $\text{var}(\bar{\mu}_D) = 2\sigma^2/n$. From Eq. (4.1.11) we have

$$\delta = z_{1-\frac{\alpha}{2}} \cdot \sqrt{\text{var}(\bar{\mu}_D)} = z_{1-\frac{\alpha}{2}} \cdot \sqrt{2\sigma^2/n}. \qquad (9.2A.1)$$

Solving Eq. (9.2A.1) for n, we thus have

$$n = 2z_{1-\frac{\alpha}{2}}^2 \cdot \sigma^2/\delta^2. \qquad (9.2A.2)$$

Remarks

For fixed α and σ, n of Eq. (9.2A.2) is inversely proportional to the square of δ. Hence, the smaller the value of δ, the larger the sample size.

Example 9.2A-1

Using Example 5.2-1, how large is the sample size required so that the difference in the number of hours of sleep in patients who are treated after treatment with hypnotics (drug A and drug B) can be detected with 90% confidence? Assume that the sleep hours of the two groups have a common variance of $\sigma^2 = 4$.

Solution

Since δ is not completely specified, we obtain the sample sizes for a range of different values of δ as given in Table 9.2-1, by substituting $\alpha = 0.1$, $z_{1-\frac{\alpha}{2}} = z_{0.95} = 1.65$ and $\sigma = 2$ into Eq. (9.2A.2).

Hence, from Table 9.2-1, a sample of 22 patients for each group has to be selected if the difference between their sleep is to be within 1 hour.

Remarks

1. Table 9.2-1 confirms our remark below Eq. (9.2A.2).
2. For different values of α and σ, Table 9.2-1 is no longer applicable and we have to recalculate it (see Exercise 9.6-3).

Table 9.2-1. Approximate Required Sample Size for Different δ

δ	0.5	1.0	1.5	2.0
n	88	22	10	6

B. *Hypothesis Testing*

Suppose that a study is designed to test Eq. (5.2.1). In terms of D, the original null and alternative hypotheses are reduced to Eq. (5.2.8). By following the similar derivation in Sec. 9.1B, the location of any mean (μ_D^*) can be expressed respectively from the graph of H_0 and H_1 by

$$\mu_D^* = 0 + z_{1-\frac{\alpha}{2}} \cdot \sqrt{\frac{2\sigma^2}{n}}, \qquad (9.2B.1)$$

and

$$\mu_D^* = \mu_D + z_\beta \cdot \sqrt{\frac{2\sigma^2}{n}}. \qquad (9.2B.2)$$

By subtracting Eq. (9.2B.2) from Eq. (9.2B.1) and then solving for n, the required sample size is thus given by

$$n = 2 \left[\frac{\sigma(z_{1-\frac{\alpha}{2}} - z_\beta)}{\mu_D} \right]^2. \qquad (9.2B.3)$$

Remarks

1. If the testing hypothesis is of Eq. (5.2.9), then the critical value $z_{1-\frac{\alpha}{2}}$ in Eq. (9.2B.3) has to be replaced by $z_{1-\alpha}$.
2. If the testing hypothesis is of Eq. (5.2.10), then the critical values $z_{1-\frac{\alpha}{2}}$ and $-Z_\beta$ in Eq. (9.2B.3) have to be replaced by $-z_\alpha$ and $z_{1-\beta}$, respectively.

Example 9.2B-1

A study is being planned to test whether a dietary supplement to pregnant women will increase the birthweight of babies. One group of women will receive the new supplement and the other group will receive the usual nutrition consultation. From a pilot study, the standard deviation in infant birthweight is estimated at 400 g and is assumed to be the same for both groups. The hypothesis of no difference is to be tested at the 5% level of significance.

It is desired to have 80% of power to detect an increase of 100 g. How large is the sample size required to detect such an increase?

Solution

By applying Eq. (9.2B.3) with $\sigma = 400$, $\mu_X - \mu_Y = 100$, $\alpha = 0.05$, $\beta = 0.2$, $z_{1-\frac{\alpha}{2}} = z_{0.975} = 1.96$ and $z_\beta = z_{0.2} = -0.84$, we have

$$n = 2 \cdot [400 \cdot (1.96 + 0.84)/100]^2 = 250.88 \approx 251.$$

Hence a sample of 251 women is required for each of the two groups.

9.3   A Single Binomial Random Variable

A.   *Estimation of the Unknown Proportion*

Let p be the population proportion of a binomial random variable (r.v.) X and δ be the distance in either direction from the true unknown p. How large is the sample size required to estimate the unknown p with an accuracy to be within δ? From Eq. (6.1.8), δ is given by

$$\delta = z_{1-\frac{\alpha}{2}} \sqrt{pq/n}, \tag{9.3A.1}$$

where $q = 1 - p$. Solving Eq. (9.3A.1) for n, we thus have

$$n = pq(z_{1-\frac{\alpha}{2}}/\delta)^2. \tag{9.3A.2}$$

Example 9.3A-1

A district medical officer seeks to estimate the proportion of children in the district receiving appropriate childhood vaccinations. Assuming a simple random sample from a community is to be selected, what is the minimum number of children required for the study if the resulting estimate is to fall within 10 percentage points of the true proportion with 95% confidence?

Solution

By applying Eq. (9.3A.2) with $\delta = 0.1$, $\alpha = 0.05$ and $p = 0.5$, we have

$$n = 0.5 \cdot 0.5 \cdot (1.96/0.1)^2 = 96.04 \approx 97.$$

Hence the minimum number of 97 children is required to be randomly selected.

Remarks

Since the product of $p \cdot q (= p - p^2)$ has the maximum at $p = 0.5$, the unknown value of p is conveniently set equal to the worst possible value of 0.5 in order to find the minimum number of children to be selected.

B. *Hypothesis Testing*

Under the same assumption in Sec. 9.3A, we wish to test Eq. (6.1.1). How large is the sample size (n) required to estimate p with an accuracy of the $100(1 - \alpha)\%$ confidence interval and the power of $1 - \beta$? Assume that the true unknown proportion is p_1. By following the derivation of Eq. (9.1B.3), we have

$$n = \frac{z_{1-\frac{\alpha}{2}} \cdot \sqrt{p_0 q_0} - z_\beta \sqrt{p_1 q_1}}{(p_1 - p_0)^2}. \qquad (9.3B.1)$$

Remarks

1. If the testing hypothesis is of Eq. (6.1.2), then the critical value $z_{1-\frac{\alpha}{2}}$ in Eq. (9.3B.1) has to be replaced by $z_{1-\alpha}$.
2. If the testing hypothesis is of Eq. (6.1.3), then the critical values $z_{1-\frac{\alpha}{2}}$ and $-z_\beta$ in Eq. (9.3B.1) have to be replaced by $-z_\alpha$ and $-z_{1-\beta}$.

Example 9.3B-1

Suppose that the success rate for surgical treatment of a particular heart condition is widely reported in the literature to be 0.65. A new medical treatment has been proposed that is alleged to offer equivalent treatment success. A hospital without the necessarily surgical facilities or staff has decided to use the new medical treatment on all new patients presenting with this condition. How many patients are required to test H_0: $p = 0.65$ versus $H_1 : p \neq 0.65$ at the significance level of $\alpha = 0.05$, if it is desired to have a 90% power of detecting a difference in proportion of success of 10 percentage points or greater?

Solution

We first consider the scenario that p_1 is greater than p_0 by 10%, namely, $p_1 = 0.75$. By applying Eq. (9.3B.1) with $\alpha = 0.05$ and $\beta = 0.1$, we have

$$n_1 = \frac{1.96 \cdot \sqrt{0.65 \cdot 0.35} + 1.28 \cdot \sqrt{0.75 \cdot 0.25}}{0.1^2} = 148.91 \approx 149.$$

We next consider the scenario that p_1 is less than p_0 by 10%, namely, $p_1 = 0.55$. By applying Eq. (9.3B.1) with $\alpha = 0.05$ and $\beta = 0.1$, we have

$$n_2 = \frac{1.96 \cdot \sqrt{0.65 \cdot 0.35} + 1.28 \cdot \sqrt{0.55 \cdot 0.45}}{0.1^2} = 157.17 \approx 158.$$

By taking the larger value between n_1 and n_2, it would require 158 patients to be studied using the new medical treatment.

9.4   Two Independent Binomial Random Variables

A.   *Estimating the Difference in Two Proportions*

Given that there are two independent binomial random variables (r.v.s) X and Y with unknown proportions p_X and p_Y. We wish to test H_0: $p_X = p_Y$ versus H_1: $p_X \neq p_Y$. Let $D = X - Y$. Thus, $p_D = p_X - p_Y$. Assume that the sample size required is the same for both X and Y. How large is the sample size (n) required to estimate p_D with an accuracy of δ in either direction at the $100(1 - \alpha)\%$

confidence level? The point estimator for p_D is given by $\hat{p}_D = \hat{p}_X - \hat{p}_Y$. In addition, we have $\text{var}(\hat{p}_D) = \text{var}(\hat{p}_X) + \text{var}(\hat{p}_Y) = (p_X q_X + p_Y q_Y)/n$. By letting half the length of $100(1 - \alpha)\%$ confidence interval for $p_D - \hat{p}_D$ equal to δ and solving for n, we have

$$n = z^2_{1-\frac{\alpha}{2}}(p_X q_X + p_Y q_Y)/\delta^2. \qquad (9.4A.1)$$

Remarks

1. Since both p_X and p_Y are unknown, we set them to equal the worst possible value, namely, $p_X = p_Y \equiv 0.5$.
2. If the alternative hypothesis is $H_1 : p_D > 0$, then the critical value $z_{1-\frac{\alpha}{2}}$ in Eq. (9.4A.1) has to be replaced by $z_{1-\alpha}$.
3. If the alternative hypothesis is $H_1 : p_D < 0$, then the critical values $z_{1-\frac{\alpha}{2}}$ in Eq. (9.4A.1) have to be replaced by $-z_\alpha$.

Example 9.4A-1

It is desired to estimate the risk difference in two industrial groups attributed to an environmental exposure to a certain toxicant. How large is the sample size required for the estimate to be within 5 percentage points of the true difference with 90% confidence, when no reasonable estimates of the exposure risk for either group are available?

Solution

By applying Eq. (9.4A.1) with $1 - \alpha = 0.9, \delta = 0.05$ and $p_X = p_Y \equiv 0.5$, we have

$$n = 1.65^2 \cdot (0.5 \cdot 0.5 + 0.5 \cdot 0.5)/0.05^2 = 544.5 \approx 545.$$

Hence, 545 subjects for each group are required in order for the estimated difference to be within 5 percentage points of the true exposure risk difference in two groups.

B.   *Hypothesis Testing in Difference of Two Proportions*

Under the assumption in Sec. 9.4A, the original null and alternative hypotheses can be expressed in term of D as $H_0 : p_D = 0$ versus $H_1 : p_D \neq 0$. How large is the sample size (n) required to estimate p_D with the $100(1 - \alpha)\%$ confidence and the power of $1 - \beta$? By following the derivation of Eq. (9.2B.3), we have

$$n = (z_{1-\frac{\alpha}{2}} - z_\beta)^2 (p_X q_X + p_Y q_Y)/p_D^2. \qquad (9.4B.1)$$

Remarks

1. For fixed α and β, n is inversely proportional to the square of p_D.
2. Since both p_X and p_Y are unknown, we set them to equal the worst possible value, namely, $p_X = p_Y \equiv 0.5$.
3. If the alternative hypothesis is $H_1 : p_D > 0$, then the critical value $z_{1-\frac{\alpha}{2}}$ in Eq. (9.4B.1) has to be replaced by $z_{1-\alpha}$.
4. If the alternative hypothesis is $H_1 : p_D < 0$, then the critical values $z_{1-\frac{\alpha}{2}}$ and $-z_\beta$ in Eq. (9.4B.1) have to be replaced by $-z_\alpha$ and $z_{1-\beta}$, respectively.

Example 9.4B-1

It is desired to estimate the risk difference in lung cancer between two groups — smokers and nonsmokers — of physicians How large should a sample of physicians be selected for each group with 90% confidence and a power of 80%, when no reasonable estimates of the risk of getting lung cancer are available?

Solution

Let p_X and p_Y be the risk of getting lung cancer for the two groups — smokers and nonsmokers — of physicians, respectively. Since no reasonable estimates for p_X and p_Y are available, we set

Table 9.4-1. **Approximate Required Sample Size for Different** p_D

p_D	0.1	0.2	0.3	0.4	0.5	0.6
n	311	78	35	20	13	9

both of them equal to 0.5. Also, as their desired difference p_D is not completely specified, the sample sizes for a range of different values of p_D are calculated as given in Table 9.4-1 by substituting $\alpha = 0.1$, $z_{1-\frac{\alpha}{2}} = z_{0.95} = 1.65$, $\beta = 0.2$, $z_\beta = z_{0.2} = -0.84$, and $p_X = p_Y = 0.5$ into Eq. (9.4B.1).

Hence, from Table 9.4-1, a sample of 78 physicians has to be randomly selected for each group, so that the risk difference p_D between these two groups is within 0.2 with 90% confidence and a power of 80%.

Remarks

1. Table 9.4-1 confirms our observation of our remark below Eq. (9.4B.1), that is, the smaller the value of p_D, the larger the sample size.
2. For different α and β, Table 9.4-1 needs to be recalculated accordingly (see Exercise 9.6-4).

9.5 Detecting the Correlation

A. *Estimating the Correlation*

Let ρ_{XY} be a correlation coefficient between two continuous r.v.s X and Y. How large is the sample size (n) required to estimate ρ_{XY} with an accuracy of δ in either direction at the $100(1 - \alpha)\%$ confidence level? By using Eq. (7.1.4), we have

$$\tanh^{-1}(\delta) = z_{1-\frac{\alpha}{2}}/\sqrt{n-3}. \qquad (9.5A.1)$$

Solving Eq. (9.5A.1) for n, we obtain

$$n = 3 + [z_{1-\frac{\alpha}{2}}/\tanh^{-1}(\delta)]^2. \qquad (9.5A.2)$$

Example 9.5A-1

Using the father and his eldest son in Example 7.1-1 as an example, how large is the sample size required so that an estimate of ρ_{XY} is with an accuracy of 0.2 in either direction of the true ρ_{XY} with 90% confidence?

Solution

By substituting $\delta = 0.2, \alpha = 0.1, z_{1-\frac{\alpha}{2}} = z_{0.95} = 1.65$ into Eq. (9.5A.2),

$$n = 3 + \left(\frac{1.65}{\tanh^{-1}(0.2)}\right)^2 = 3 + \left(\frac{1.65}{0.202733}\right)^2 = 69.24 \approx 70.$$

Hence, a random sample of 70 pairs of father/son's height is required so that the sample estimate of ρ_{XY} is within an accuracy of 0.2 in either direction from the true ρ_{XY} with 90% confidence.

B.   *Hypothesis Testing on the Correlation*

Under the same assumption of Sec. 9.5A, how large is the sample size (n) required to test Eq. (7.1.5) with the $100(1 - \alpha)\%$ confidence level and the power of $1 - \beta$? By following the derivation of Eq. (9.2B.3) with the use of Eq. (7.1.3), we have

$$n = 3 + [z_{1-\frac{\alpha}{2}} - z_\beta)/\tanh^{-1}(\rho_{XY})]^2. \qquad (9.5\text{B}.1)$$

Remarks

1. Since for fixed α and β, n of Eq. (9.5B.1) is inversely proportional to the square of $\omega = \tanh^{-1}(\rho_{XY})$ and ω is an increasing function of ρ_{XY}, n is decreasing as ρ_{XY} is increasing as shown in the next example.
2. If the hypotheses to be tested is of Eq. (7.1.6), then the critical value $z_{1-\frac{\alpha}{2}}$ in Eq. (9.4A.1) has to be replaced by $z_{1-\alpha}$.
3. If the hypothesis to be tested is of Eq. (7.1.7), then the critical value $z_{1-\frac{\alpha}{2}}$ in Eq. (9.4A.1) has to be replaced by $-z_\alpha$.
4. The value of $\tanh^{-1}(x)$ can be found by using the function "ATANH" in the EXCEL spreadsheet.

Table 9.5-1. **Approximate Sample Size Required to Detect a Correlation at 90% Confidence with a Power of 80%**

ρ_{XY}	0.01	0.05	0.1	0.3	0.5	0.7	0.9
n	62,000	2,479	619	68	24	12	6

Example 9.5B-1

Using the father and his eldest son in Example 7.1-1 as an example, how large is the sample size required so that a testing of Eq. (7.1.5) is with 90% confidence and a power of 80%?

Solution

For a range of the true ρ_{XY}, we obtain the approximate sample size in Table 9.5-1 by using $\alpha = 0.1$ and $\beta = 0.2$, and $z_{1-\frac{\alpha}{2}} = z_{0.95} = 1.65$ and $z_\beta = z_{0.2} = -0.84$ in Eq. (9.5B.1).

Remarks

1. Table 9.5-1 confirms the observation of our remark below Eq. (9.5B.1).
2. For different values of α and β, the required sample size is different from that given in Table 9.5-1 and has to be calculated again accordingly (see Exercise 9.6-5).

9.6 Exercises

1. Recalculate Table 9.1-1 with $\alpha = 0.1$ and $\sigma_X = 0.8$. What conclusion do you draw after comparing the new table with Table 9.1-1?
2. Recalculate Table 9.1-2 with $\alpha = 0.1, \beta = 0.2$ and $\sigma_X = 0.8$. What conclusion do you draw after comparing the new table with Table 9.1-2?
3. Recalculate Table 9.2-1 with $\alpha = 0.05$ and $\sigma = 3$. What conclusion do you draw after comparing the new table with Table 9.2-1?

4. Recalculate Table 9.4-1 with $\alpha = 0.05$ and $\beta = 0.1$. What conclusion do you draw after comparing the new table with Table 9.4-1?
5. Recalculate Table 9.5-1 with $\alpha = 0.05$ and $\beta = 0.1$. What conclusion do you draw after comparing the new table with Table 9.5-1?

References

1. Anderson TW. (2003) *An Introduction to Multivariate Statistical Analysis*, 3rd ed. Wiley, New York.
2. Lemeshow S, Hosmer Jr DW, Klar J, Lwanga SK. (1990) *Adequacy of Sample Size in Health Studies*. John Wiley & Sons, New York.

Chapter 10

Design of Observational/ Experimental Studies

In this chapter we are going to learn how to collect data for epidemiologic studies. Basically, there are two major categories of study designs — observational and experimental studies. The goal of analytic studies is to identify and evaluate causes or risk factors of diseases or health-related events. The difference between observational and experimental study designs is that no intervention is carried out in the former groups. In an observational study, the investigator does not intervene but merely "observes" and assesses the strength of the relationship between exposure and disease variable.

Cohort, cross-sectional, and case-control studies are collectively referred to as observational studies that are covered respectively in the first three sections of this chapter. Often these studies are the only practicable method of studying various problems, for example, studies of aetiology, instances where a randomized controlled trial might be unethical, or if the disease is rare. Cohort studies are used to evaluate incidence, differentiate cause and effect, and identify prognosis factors. Cross-sectional studies are used to determine prevalence. Case-control studies compare groups retrospectively. They seek to identify possible risk factors of the disease and are useful for studying rare diseases. They are often used to generate hypotheses that can be studied via prospective cohorts or other studies.

10.1 Cohort Studies

The term "cohort" is derived from the Latin word *cohors*. WH Frost (1880–1938), considered the father of modern epidemiology, was the first to use the word "cohort" in his 1935 publication assessing the age-specific mortality rates and tuberculosis.[5] Frost's personal life is rarely touched on, but one of the presumed reasons that he focused on tuberculosis was because he was diagnosed with incipient pulmonary tuberculosis when he was in his thirties. He had to spend several months in a sanatorium after being diagnosed. The modern-day definition of the word now means that a group of people with defined characteristics who are followed up to determine incidence, or mortality from, some specific disease, causes of death, or some other outcome.

Cohort studies are the best method for determining the incidence and natural history of diseases. The studies may be prospective or retrospective. For prospective studies a group of people is chosen who do not have the outcome of interest. The investigator then measures a variety of risk factors that might be relevant to the development of the condition. Over a period of time the people in the cohort are observed to see if they develop the outcome of interest. For retrospective cohort studies we use the data already collected for other purposes. The cohort is then followed up retrospectively. The methodology is the same except that the study is performed posthoc.

A Sketchy Guideline for Designing Cohort Studies

Step 1. Specify clearly the goal of the study.

Step 2. Select carefully a group of subjects who do not have the outcome of interest, yet each subject must have the potential to develop the outcome of interest.

Step 3. Observe over a period of time to see if any subject in the cohort develop the outcome of interest.

Step 4. Each variable must be accurately measured.

Step 5. Analyze the collected data at some fixed length of time.

Remarks

1. The use of cohort studies is mandatory if a randomized controlled clinical trial is unethical. For example, to study the effect of smoking cigarettes on lung cancer or cardiovascular heart disease we have to employ a cohort study because we cannot deliberately expose people to cigarette smoke.
2. As cohort studies measure potential causes before the outcome has occurred, the study can pinpoint these causes as having preceded the outcome. As a result, it avoids the cause-and-effect debate.
3. A single study can examine various outcome variables. For instance, a cohort study of smokers can simultaneously look at deaths from lung, cardiovascular, and cerebrovascular diseases.
4. A cohort study allows evaluation of the effect of each risk factor on the probability of developing the outcome of interest.
5. In prospective cohort studies the loss of follow-up events can significantly affect the calculation of incidence of the outcome. The rarer the outcome the more significant this effect.
6. When we compare two cohort studies, say, one has been exposed to the agent of interest and other has not, the effect of confounding could emerge because we are unable to control all other factors that might differ between the two cohorts. A confounding factor is independently associated with the variable of interest and the outcome of interest. The only way to eliminate all possibility of a confounding variable is by employing a prospective randomized controlled study.

Example 10.1-1

In Thailand, vascular diseases have been the leading cause of death since 1987. In 1998 there were over 54,000 deaths due to vascular causes. Between 1985 and 1997 the prevalence of heart disease in Thailand tripled, from 56 to 168 per 100,000 population. Cross-sectional studies have provided limited information about levels of vascular risk factors in different population groups within Thailand, but changes in risk factor levels with age and the association of established risk factors with mortality are not well-documented.[35]

Based upon our guidelines, a cohort study in the quoted article is decomposed into the following steps:

Step 1. The primary goal of the study is to depict 12-year changes in vascular risk factors of subjects in the cohort. A secondary aim is to determine the associations between levels of baseline risk factors and the risk of vascular death.

Step 2. All employees of the Electricity Generating Authority of Thailand (EGAT) whose ages were 35–54 years old were invited to take part in a survey of vascular risk factors. Of 7824 individuals who were potentially eligible for inclusion in the study in 1985, 3499 (2702 men and 797 women) volunteered to participate in the study. Volunteers completed a self-administered questionnaire, underwent a physical examination, provided fasting blood samples, and took an oral glucose tolerance test.

Step 3. Twelve years later, in 1997, efforts were made to re-contact all living participants by letter, telephone or personal contact. Over this period of time, 181 employees were uncontactable, 166 had died and 185 declined to participate. Only 2,967 living participants were re-surveyed using procedures similar to those employed at baseline. Information on the cause of death was sought for all subjects who had passed away. Consent and ethical approval were obtained.

Step 4. The data on sociodemographic variables, current and prior medical conditions, behaviors relating to vascular disease, and prescribed treatment were collected using a self-administered questionnaire. Blood pressure was measured after five minutes of rest, by using a calibrated mercury sphygmomanometer with systolic blood pressure (SBP) and diastolic blood pressure (DBP) recorded as the first and fifth Korotkoff sound, respectively. A single measurement had been made with participants in the supine position in 1985, while in 1997 two measurements were recorded using the seated position. On each occasion subjects were classified as hypertensive if their blood pressure was $\geq 140/90\,$mm Hg, or if they were taking prescribed blood pressure lowering therapy at that time.

Blood samples were obtained after a 12-hour overnight fast. Serum total cholesterol (STC), high density lipoprotein (HDL) cholesterol and triglycerides were measured using enzymatic assays. High total cholesterol (HTC) is defined as a total cholesterol level $\geq 6.2\,$mmol/L or current use of cholesterol lowering therapy. Blood glucose levels were measured using a glucose oxidase method on capillary blood samples in 1985 and on plasma samples in 1997. On each occasion oral glucose tolerance tests were performed by measuring blood glucose levels on fasting samples and on samples drawn 2 hours after ingestion of a 75 g glucose load. Diabetes was defined on the basis of any of the following measurements: (i) a prior clinical diagnosis, (ii) a fasting capillary glucose $\geq 6.1\,$mmol/L, (iii) a fasting plasma glucose $\geq 7.0\,$mmol/L or (iv) a 2-hour capillary or plasma glucose $\geq 11.1\,$mmol/L. Obesity was defined as the body mass index (BMI) $\geq 25\,$kg/m^2.

Step 5. Using the paired t-tests of Eq. (5.2.11) on mean of the SBP, DBP, serum total cholesterol, serum HDL, triglycerides and BMI levels in Table 10.1-1A all increased significantly for both sexes (all p-values < 0.001). Similarly, the proportion for each of the hypertension, HTC levels, diabetes and obesity in Table 10.1-1A rose markedly for both sexes (all p-values < 0.001).

By employing Cox's survival model the risk factors of age, SBP, DBP, diabetes and smoking were shown to be all positively and significantly associated with vascular mortality (all p-values <0.05), except for sex, BMI and total cholesterol, which have non-significant positive associations (see Table 10.1-1B). HDL cholesterol was significantly inversely associated with the vascular mortality (p-value $= 0.003$).

Remarks

1. The predominance of vascular causes of death in this cohort is consistent with the documented rise in the rates of vascular

Table 10.1-1A. Vascular Risk Factor Levels in 1985 and 1997 among 2967 Thai Men and Women[a]

	Male (n = 2252)		Female (n = 715)	
	1985	1997	1985	1997
Age (years)	42.8	54.8	41.4	53.4
BMI (kg/m^2)	23.2	24.7	22.7	24.8
SBP (mm Hg)	122	139	115	127
DBP (mm Hg)	76	84	71	77
STC	5.80	6.13	5.65	6.34
HDL cholesterol	1.18	1.33	1.36	1.48
Triglycerides	1.83	1.94	1.21	1.50
Hypertension (%)				
Diagnosed, on therapy	2.4	17.3	1.5	12.7
Undiagnosed	18.3	36.0	9.8	18.0
High Total Cholesterol				
Diagnosed, on therapy	0.0	13.8	0.1	14.5
Undiagnosed	34.0	37.2	26.2	43.7
Diabetes				
Diagnosed	1.3	11.5	0.7	8.2
Undiagnosed	4.8	5.9	3.6	4.1
Obesity (%)	25.5	43.2	20.7	40.9
Current smokers (%)	53.0	28.4	6.2	3.6

[a]This table is adapted from Table 1 in Ref. 35.

disease in Thailand, for which this study suggests deterioration in classical cardiovascular risk factors as an important case.
2. Because possible sources of bias may play a role, the absolute levels of risk factors and the absolute changes in risk factor levels over time are unlikely to be generalizable to the Thai nation as a whole.

Example 10.1-2

This is a continuation of Example 1.3-2 (The Framingham Heart Study). Here, factors related to the development and clinical manifestations of coronary heart disease (CHD) are studied in Ref. 6 of Chap. 1.

Table 10.1-1B.   Hazard Ratios (95% CI) for the Association of Risk Factors with Vascular Death Among 3318 Thais[a]

	Adjusted
Age (10 years)	2.7 (1.5–4.8)
Sex (male/female)	2.6 (0.6–11.1)
BMI (5 kg/m^2)	1.0 (0.6–1.6)
SBP (10 mm Hg)	1.3 (1.0–1.8)
DBP (5 mm Hg)	1.5 (1.1–1.9)
Total cholesterol (1.0 mmol/L)	1.0 (0.7–1.6)
HDL cholesterol (0.2 mmol/L)	0.7 (0.6–0.9)
Diabetes (yes/no)	3.3 (1.6–6.6)
Current smokers (yes/no)	2.2 (1.1–4.1)

[a]This table is adapted from Table 3 in Ref. 35.

Based on our guidelines, a cohort study is decomposed into the following steps:

Step 1. The goal of the study is to assess the factors that include blood pressure, serum cholesterol levels and certain electrocardiographic abnormalities on overt coronary heart disease.

Step 2. 5127 persons (2283 men and 2844 women) who were free of CHD were chosen as the study cohort. A 6-year longitudinal follow-up study from 1952 to 1958 was conducted.

Step 3. During the period of six years of follow-ups, clinical manifestations of CHD in both sexes were given, as seen in Table 10.1-2A.

There is clearly a difference in the predominant clinical manifestation of CHD in the sexes (see Table 10.1-2A). The CHD appearing in women was predominantly angina pectoris without being associated with myocardial infarction (68.9%). This is in contrast to men in whom angina pectoris, without associated myocardial infarction, constituted only 29.6% of CHD developing in the six years of observation. Among all cases of CHD, myocardial infarction with or without associated angina pectoris occurred

Table 10.1-2A. The six year follow-up of clinical manifestation of CHD in men and women

Clinical Manifestation	Number (%)	
	Men	Women
Total CHD	125 (100)	61 (100)
Definite MI* by history and ECG+	57 (45.6)	14 (23.0)
With AP#	32 (25.6)	7 (11.5)
Without AP	25 (20.0)	7 (11.5)
Definite MI by ECG only	7 (5.6)	2 (3.3)
Sudden death	24 (19.2)	3 (4.9)
With pre-existing MI	3 (2.4)	—
With pre-existing AP	6 (4.8)	—
Without pre-existing CHD	15 (12.0)	3 (4.9)
Definite AP	37 (29.6)	42 (68.9)

This table is adapted from Table 4 in Ref. 6 of Chap. 1.
*Myocardial infarction.
+Electrocardiogram.
#Angina pectoris.

as the manifestation of CHD almost twice as frequently in male coronary subjects.

Step 4. Higher mean cholesterol levels were demonstrated among subjects who developed CHD than in the population at risk (see Table 10.1-2B). This shows that there exists an association between serum cholesterol levels and the subsequent development of CHD. The risk associated with serum cholesterol was further analyzed in men in the age group of 40 to 59 years when the study began (see Table 10.1-2C). Separation of subjects in the population at risk into three categories according to increased levels of serum cholesterol are made at levels of 210 and 245 mg per 100 ml. An analysis of these groups reveals a gradient of risk of developing CHD with increasing levels of serum cholesterol, that is, those with serum cholesterols over 244 mg per 100 ml have more than three times the incidence of CHD, as do those with cholesterol levels less than 210 mg per 1000 ml (see Table 10.1-2C). Since no new CHD developed in women less than

Table 10.1-2B. **The mean serum cholesterol of new CHD in men and women**

Age at Entry	New CHD		Mean Serum Cholestrol: New CHD (Population at Risk)	
	Men	Women	Men	Women
30–34	5	—	257 (219)*	—
35–39	11	—	267 (222)*	—
40–44	14	3	259 (229)*	316 (222)*
45–49	14	14	250 (231)*	286 (240)*
50–54	27	13	245 (227)*	239 (250)
55–59	41	24	248 (229)*	260 (258)

This table is adapted from Table 5 in Ref. 6 of Chap. 1.
* Significantly elevated (at 5% level) compared with that of population at risk.

Table 10.1-2C. **The number of new and observed CHD rate in men and women**

Serum Cholesterol (mg/100 ml)	Number of New CHD (Population at Risk)		Observed (Expected) Incidence Rate (per 1000)	
	Men*	Women*	Men*	Women*
< 210	16 (454)	8 (445)	35.2 (69.4)#	18.0 (25.2)
210–244	29 (455)	16 (527)	63.7 (70.8)	30.4 (31.3)
> 245	51 (424)	30 (689)	120.3 (71.8)#	43.5 (38.7)

This table is adapted from Table 6 in Ref. 6 of Chap. 1.
* Aged 40–59.
# Significantly different (at 5% level) from the expected rate.

40 years of age, no analysis of the association of serum cholesterol level with the risks of CHD was possible. A significant elevation of mean serum cholesterol is evident for women, 40 to 49 years old, who developed CHD but not for women who were 50 to 59 years old (see Table 10.1-2B).

For men aged 35–39 or 55–59 and women aged 45–49 or 55–59 years on entry, blood pressure (systolic/diastolic) was significantly higher in the group who subsequently developed CHD than in

Table 10.1-2D. The mean SBP and DBP of new CHD in men and women

Age	Mean SBP[#]: New CHD (Population at Risk)		Mean DBP[+]: New CHD (Population at Risk)	
	Men	Women	Men	Women
30–34	128 (131)	—	83 (83)	—
35–39	144 (132)*	—	95 (85)*	—
40–44	133 (135)	125 (131)	90 (87)	81 (83)
45–49	144 (138)	158 (142)*	93 (88)*	97 (87)*
50–54	148 (140)*	171 (150)*	90 (89)	96 (90)
55–59	162 (145)*	178 (154)*	96 (88)*	100 (91)*

This table is adapted from Table 7A in Ref. 6 of Chap. 1.
[#] Systolic blood pressure.
[+] Diastolic blood pressure.
* Significantly elevated (at 5% level) compared with that of the population at risk.

Table 10.1-2E. The number and observed incidence rate of new CHD for men and women

Sex, Hypertensive Status, ECG Evidence of LVH[#]	Number of New CHD (Population at Risk)		Observed (Expected) Incidence Rate (per 1000)	
	Men*	Women*	Men*	Women*
Normotension	16 (454)	6 (704)	41.4 (68.8)	8.5 (26.5)
Borderline Hypertension	29 (455)	20 (647)	71.4 (68.6)	30.9 (35.0)
Definite Hypertension	51 (424)	31 (395)	123.7 (77.8)	78.5 (39.8)
Definite hypertension and ECG evidence				
No LVH	27 (265)	26 (357)	101.9 (75.8)	72.8 (40.0)
Possible LVH	3 (15)	1 (19)	200.0 (78.4)	52.6 (34.6)
Definite LVH	7 (19)	4 (19)	368.4 (105.1)	210.5 (42.2)

This table is adapted from Table 8 in Ref. 6 of Chap. 1.
[#] Left ventricular hypertrophy.
* Aged 40–59.

the whole population at risk (see Table 10.1-2D). In addition, hypertension associated with the electrocardiographic pattern of left ventricular hypertrophy was associated with a higher incidence of CHD than was hypertension alone (see Table 10.1-2E). In Table 10.1-2F the six-year incidence of CHD in persons who

Table 10.1-2F.   The number and observed incidence rate of new CHD for a combination of three symptoms in men and women aged 40–59

Sex, and Combinations of BP[#] SC[+] and ECG Evidence of LVH	Number of New CHD (Population at Risk)		Observed (Expected) Incidence Rate (per 1000)	
	Men[*]	Women[*]	Men[*]	Women[*]
Normal[$] on all three	29 (811)	15 (888)	35.8 (67.5)	16.9 (27.2)
Abnormal[$] on one only	43 (416)	24 (597)	103.4 (73.6)	40.2 (38.1)
Abnormal on two only	20 (98)	13 (162)	204.1 (81.4)	80.2 (42.1)
Abnormal on all three	4 (8)	2 (14)	500.0 (102.9)	142.9 (42.7)
Abnormal on two or three	24 (106)	15 (176)	226.4 (83.0)	85.2 (42.2)

This table is adapted from Table 11 in Ref. 6 of Chap. 1.
[#] Blood pressure.
[+] Serum cholesterol.
[*] Aged 40–59.
[$] Abnormal BP is defined as definite hypertension, abnormal SC is a reading of 260 mg/100 ml or higher, and abnormal LVH is a diagnosis of possible or definite LVH on the electrocardiogram. "Normal" means not abnormal; it includes normotension, borderline hypertension, SC less than 260 mg/100 ml, no LVH by ECG.

had various combinations of blood pressure, serum cholesterol and LVH by ECG is given. When only one of these character-istics was abnormal the risk in men almost tripled (103.4 per thousand) compared with normal characteristics on all three (35.8 per thousand). If two of these characteristics were abnormal, the six-year incidence climbs to 204.1 per thousand, approxi-mately doubling the rate had one of these characteristics been abnormal. In contrast, the incidence rates of risk associated with these characteristics are generally lower in women who were 40 to 59 years of age, 16.9 per thousand if all three characteristics were normal, rising to 40.2 per thousand when one characteristic was abnormal, and doubling to 80.2 per thousand when two abnormal characteristics were present. When two or more factors are abnormal, the incidence of 85.2 per thousand is noted.

Step 5. This study has confirmed the widely recognized influence of hypertension and hypercholestrolemia on the development of CHD. In addition, the electrocardiographic pattern of left ventric-ular hypertrophy is also shown to be associated with the increased risk of developing CHD. Although it is often stated that women tolerate hypertension better than men, the six-year incidence figures do not support this hypothesis. It appears that in assessing the contribution to risk of developing CHD of the three factors under consideration, hypertension represents a greater risk factor for women than men, whereas cholesterol contributes only slightly among women, but very significantly increasing the risk among men.

Remarks

1. There can be no doubt that the absence of these characteristics is advantageous since such persons demonstrate a relatively low risk of developing CHD.
2. Whether the correction of these abnormalities once they are discovered alter the risk of disease development remains to be demonstrated.

Example 10.1-3

Up to 1971, no cohort studies on physician mortality were ever performed,[39] although three cross-sectional studies on physician mortality in the US occurred in 1925, 1938–1942 and 1949–1951. Based upon our guidelines the cohort study is decomposed into the following steps:

Step 1. The mortality experience of graduates from the Harvard Medical School is first compared with that of the US white male population, then with that of the physician mortality provided in the three previous studies.

Step 2. All members of the nine classes who graduated from Harvard Medical School in the years 1923–1924, 1932–1934 and 1942–1944 were selected for the study. Incidentally, two classes that graduated in 1943 in an accelerated program were also included in this study.

Step 3. The dates of the births and deaths of all members of the nine classes who graduated from Harvard Medical School in the above years were obtained from records at the School's Alumni Office. All known deaths prior to 1 January 1970 were recorded.

Step 4. The appropriate comparison for the cohort members were made with a cohort "life" table for the US white males. Unfortunately, such a table does not exist. Hence, the authors used data closest in time from the stationary life table available in the US Vital Statistics Report. In order to compare the mortality experience of the chosen graduates with that of other physicians, age-specific mortality rates for physicians in the US in the years 1925, 1938–1942 and 1949–1951 were obtained from previously published studies. Using these rates, abridged life tables for physicians were calculated, according to the revised method described by the National Center for Health Statistics. Cohort physician life tables were then assembled and compared with the graduates.

Step 5. Cumulative mortality of graduates from the Harvard Medical School and their age distribution are given in Tables 10.1-3A and 10.1-3B, respectively. The figures of the white male population in Table 10.1-3A represent a weighted average with the weights proportional to the age distribution of Harvard graduates in Table 10.1-3B. The cumulative mortality of these three cohorts of medical school graduates is consistently less than that of comparable white males (see Table 10.1-3A).

In comparing the cumulative mortalities of the three groups of graduates with each other, each successive group has had fewer deaths at a comparable time after graduation than the group graduating in the preceding decade. The mean age at graduation has become steadily lower at 26.8, 26.1 and 24.8, respectively, and partially explains the improvement in mortality experience over these decades. However, the improved mortality experience of the graduates also reflects improvement in the mortality experience of the general white male population during this period. No differences existed between the improvement in mortality among groups of medical school graduates and that experienced by the general white male population.

Table 10.1-3A*. The mortality of three classes graduated from Harvard Medical School with a comparison with the general males in the US

Years after Graduation	Cumulative Mortality (%)					
	Classes 1923–24 N = 248	US White Males	Classes 1932–34 N = 399	US White Males	Classes 1942–44 N = 546	US White Males
5	2.0	2.6	0.8	1.9	0.6	1.2
10	4.4	4.8	2.5	3.4	1.1	2.2
15	6.9	7.5	4.0	5.4	1.7	3.5
20	8.1	10.3	5.8	7.7	2.4	5.3
25	9.7	14.4	8.0	11.2	4.9	8.2
30	14.9	19.5	12.0	16.2	—	—
35	23.4	26.8	17.8	23.3	—	—
40	29.0	36.1	—	—	—	—
45	40.7	47.6	—	—	—	—

*This table is taken from Table 1 in Ref. 39.

Table 10.1-3B*. The age distribution of three classes graduated from Harvard Medical School

Age at Graduation	Number		
	Classes		
	1923–24	1932–34	1942–44
20–24	32	37	161
25–29	186	342	370
30–34	28	17	14
35+	2	3	—

*This table is taken from Table 2 in Ref. 39.

Remarks

1. A study of the mortality experience of medical school graduates as compared with that of the US white male population was undertaken by using the cohort method for the first time.

2. In two of the three groups of medical school graduates, the medical specialist had a significantly higher mortality than the surgical specialists from about 15 to 25 years after graduation. Beyond 25 years after graduation, no difference was found.

10.2   Cross-sectional Studies

Cross-sectional studies are the best way to determine the prevalence and are useful at identifying association that can be rigorously studied using a cohort study or a randomized controlled study.

A Sketchy Guideline for Designing Cross Sectional Studies

Step 1. Formulate the research question and choose the sample population.
Step 2. Decide what variables are relevant to the research question.
Step 3. A method for contacting sample subjects must be devised and then implemented.
Step 4. Analyze the collected data.

Remarks

1. In general these kind of studies are quick and cheap.
2. Unlike cohort studies, it is difficult to differentiate cause and effect in cross-sectional studies.
3. Rarer conditions cannot efficiently be studied using cross-sectional studies because even in large samples there may be not a possible single occurrence with the outcome of interest.

Example 10.2-1

In the spring of 1981, the Centers for Disease Control and Prevention (CDC) received reports of the unexpected occurrence of Pneumocystis carinii pneumonia (PCP) and Kaposi's sarcoma

(KS) among young homosexual men in California and New York City. These illnesses were associated with an acquired cellular immunodeficiency of a type not previously described. This immune disorder and the accompanying illness became known as the acquired immune deficiency syndrome (AIDS). AIDS has been subsequently reported from other parts of the US and among heterosexual men and women.[18]

A national surveillance for these diseases was initiated by the CDC in June 1981. In terms of our guidelines on cross-sectional studies, it is expounded into the following steps:

Step 1. By February 1983, the CDC has received 1000 case reports. A hypothesis of a single-infectious-agent is to be examined to see if it could explain the AIDS epidemic.

Step 2. There are four disease groups: (i) KS but not PCP, (ii) PCP but not KS, (iii) KS and PCP, and (iv) neither KS nor PCP, but some other opportunistic infection. Five risk groups include: (i) homosexual or bisexual men, (ii) intravenous drug abusers, (iii) Haitians living in the US, (iv) patients with hemophilia, and (v) others. Decide if any association exists between disease groups and risk groups.

Step 3. AIDS surveillance has been both retrospective and current. Active retrospective surveillance methods include: (i) review of selected cancer tumor registries, (ii) contact with selected physicians in 18 major metropolitan areas, and (iii) review of requests received by the CDC's Parasitic Disease Drug Service for pentamidine isethionate. Current surveillance is predominantly passive in nature, through receipt of reports from individual physicians and local or state health departments.

Step 4. Mortality from AIDS has been high (see Table 10.2-1A). The overall crude mortality is 0.392, which is an underestimate of the true mortality rate because it does not consider most cases that have been diagnosed recently and have not been followed long enough to reasonably assess outcomes. To simplify data analysis, the 1000 cases were classified into a hierarchy of mutually exclusive risk groups (i) to (v) in step 2. Within this hierachial

Table 10.2-1A.   Mortality of AIDS by Disease Group[a]

Disease Group	No. of Cases	No. of Deaths	Mortality (%)
KS but not PCP	284	61	21.5
PCP but not KS	497	230	46.3
KS and PCP	83	40	48.2
Other	136	61	44.8
Total	1,000	392	39.2

[a]This table is taken from Table 2 in Ref. 18.

Table 10.2-1B.   Distribution of AIDS by Disease Group × Risk Group[a]

Risk Group	No. of Cases	Disease Group (%)			
		(i)	(ii)	(iii)	(iv)
(i)	727	36.0	43.7	11.1	9.1
(ii)	155	2.6	78.1	1.3	18.1
(iii)	50	4.0	38.0	0	58.0
(iv)	7	0	85.7	0	14.3
(v)	61	26.2	54.1	0	19.7
Total	1,000	28.4	49.7	8.3	13.6

[a]This table is taken from Table 4 in Ref. 18.

classification, risk group (i) was 44 times more likely to have KS (see Table 10.2-1B) in a comparison with risk groups (ii) to (iv). Only 3.8% of those patients belonging to risk groups (ii) to (iv) had KS, with or without PCP.

Remarks

1. Spontaneous return to normal immune function has not been reported in AIDS patients. Therefore, mortality is likely to remain high until a therapy to reverse the immune dysfunction of AIDS becomes available.
2. The spectrum of AIDS may not be limited to KS and opportunistic infection. The full range of illness associated with AIDS may not yet be known.

Example 10.2-2

Diabetes is a major risk factor for cardiovascular disease, and the prevalence is high and increasing in China. The China National Diabetes and Metabolic Disorder Study, a national cross-sectional study, was conducted from June 2007 through May 2008 as follow[40]:

Step 1. The goal of the study was to provide current and reliable data on the prevalence of diabetes and metabolic risk factors in the adult population in China. A total of 54,240 people whose ages were 20 years or older were selected and invited to participate in the study; 47,325 (18,976 men and 28,349 women) completed the study. After the exclusion of 538 persons whose demographic information were missing and 548 whose data on fasting or 2-hour plasma glucose levels were missing, 46,239 adults were included in the final analysis. Written informed consent was obtained from each participant before data collection.

Step 2. The 1999 World Health Organization diagnostic criteria were used to diagnose diabetes. Participants were instructed to maintain their usual physical activity and diet for at least three days before the oral glucose-tolerance test. Plasma glucose was measured with the use of a hexokinase enzymatic method, and serum cholesterol and triglyceride levels were assessed enzymatically with the use of commercially available reagents at the clinical biochemical laboratories in each province.

Step 3. A standard questionnaire was administered by trained staff to obtain information on demographic characteristics, personal and family medical history, and lifestyle risk factors. The interview included questions related to the diagnosis and treatment of diabetes, hypertension, dyslipidemia and cardiovascular events. "Cigarette smoking" was defined as having smoked at least 100 cigarettes in one's lifetime. "Alcohol drinking" was defined as the consumption of at least 30 g of alcohol for one year or more. "Regular leisure-time physical activity" was defined as

Table 10.2-2A. Characteristics of Study Participants According to Plasma Glucose Categories and Sex*

Characteristic	NGT	IIFG	IIGT	IFG+IGT	PUD	PDD
	\	\	Men (n = 18,419)			
Participants — No. (%)	13,426	686	1,691	395	1,327	894
	(73.3)	(3.2)	(11.0)	(1.9)	(6.5)	(4.1)
FPG (mg/dl)	87.3	114.9	93.1	116.2	135.7	158.6
OGT (mg/dl)	99.1	110.6	160.9	164.6	243.5	265.9
Age (yr)	42.5	48.5	50.2	50.2	52.1	55.8
FHD (%)	12.9	12.8	14.6	23.5	23.3	42.6
ELCH	25.3	19.2	18.7	22.6	16.8	16.4
CS (%)	57.5	56.8	58.6	60.1	59.4	50.5
CA (%)	44.3	41.7	39.5	51.6	40.5	35.2
RLPA (%)	33.3	31.6	36.2	39.2	30.3	49.7
BMI	23.6	24.5	24.8	26.6	25.8	25.2
WC (cm)	82.1	86.7	85.5	90.7	89.1	88.7
SBP (mm Hg)	121.0	127.4	129.2	132.1	133.2	132.0
HR (beats/min)	72.4	73.4	74.2	75.1	76.4	76.6
HDL (mg/dl)	48.5	47.1	48.9	45.6	48.1	44.5
LDL (mg/dl)	101.2	108.5	108.5	112.5	112.1	109.7
TGC (mg/dl)	141.7	176.5	169.5	204.3	198.6	172.4
Characteristic			**Women (n = 27,820)**			
Participants — No. (%)	20,867	783	2,880	562	1,581	1,147
	(76.4)	(2.2)	(10.9)	(1.7)	(5.2)	(3.5)
FPG (mg/dl)	86.9	114.7	93.7	115.5	135.3	165.2
OGT (mg/dl)	102.1	111.6	159.6	165.8	259.2	285.8
Age (yr)	42.1	46.6	51.9	53.9	54.8	59.3
FHD (%)	13.9	12.2	17.5	15.3	23.4	44.3
ELCH	20.3	11.1	9.6	11.0	6.3	4.6
CS (%)	3.0	2.3	4.4	3.7	4.6	4.2
CA (%)	4.1	4.3	3.8	4.0	4.7	3.4
RLPA (%)	30.9	22.9	34.6	30.9	35.5	49.2
BMI	22.9	24.2	25.8	25.9	24.8	24.6
WC (cm)	76.3	80.8	82.0	86.3	85.6	84.4
SBP (mm Hg)	116.4	123.6	128.6	134.2	134.9	136.1
HR (beats/min)	74.3	74.7	76.5	78.5	78.0	77.2

Table 10.2-2A. (*Continued*)

Characteristic	Women (n = 27,820)					
HDL-C (mg/dl)	52.4	51.4	52.0	50.6	51.4	51.4
LDL-C (mg/dl)	99.8	113.0	112.0	117.4	113.8	115.8
TG (mg/dl)	113.6	140.9	154.6	166.2	172.9	174.6

*This table is adapted from Table 1 in Ref. 40.

Note 1. Abbreviations: NGT = Normal Glucose Tolerance; IIFG = Isolated Impaired Fasting Glucose; IIGT = Isolated Impaired Glucose Tolerance; IFG+IGT = Combined Impaired Fasting Glucose and Impaired Glucose Tolerance; PUD = Previously Undiagnosed Diabetes; PDD = Previously Diagnosed Diabetes; FPG = Fasting Plasma Glucose; OGT = 2-hr plasma glucose in Oral Glucose-tolerance Test; FHD = Family History of Diabetes; ELCH = Education Level of College or Higher; CS = Cigarette Smoking; CA = Consumption of Alcohol; RLPA = Regular Leisure-time Physical Activity; BMI = Body Mass Index; WC = Waist Circumference; SBP = Systolic Blood Pressure; HR = Heart Rate; HDL-C = High Density Lipoprotein cholesterol; LDL-C = Low Density Lipoprotein cholesterol; TG = Triglycerides.

Note 2. All the data in the table are the sample mean.

participation in a moderate or vigorous activity for 30 minutes or more per day, at least 3 days a week.

Step 4. The prevalence of isolated impaired fasting glucose, isolated impaired glucose tolerance, combined isolated impaired fasting glucose and isolated impaired glucose tolerance, previously undiagnosed diabetes, and previously diagnosed diabetes were 3.2%, 11.0%, 1.9%, 6.5% and 4.1% among men and 2.2% 10.9%, 1.7%, 5.2% and 3.5% among women, respectively. The prevalence undiagnosed diabetes was 2.9% among men and 2.6% among women. The overall prevalences of total diabetes and prediabetes were 9.7% and 15.5%, respectively. Consequently, 92.4 million adults who are 20 years of age or older have diabetes, while 148.2 million adults have prediabetes, which is an important risk factor for the development of overt diabetes and cardiovascular disease. In the multinomial logit models, male sex, older age, a family history of diabetes, being overweight, obesity, central obesity, increased heart rate, elevated systolic blood pressure, elevated serum triglyceride level, educational level below college

Table 10.2-2B. **Multivariable-adjusted Odds Ratios for Diabetes and Prediabetes***

	Odds Ratio (*p*-value)	
Variable	Total Diabetes	Prediabetes
Sex/Male	1.26 (< 0.001)	1.06 (0.3)
Age (per 10-yr increment)	1.68 (< 0.001)	1.37 (< 0.001)
Family history of diabetes	3.14 (< 0.001)	1.32 (0.001)
Less than College Education	1.57 (< 0.001)	1.17 (0.02)
Overweight	1.43 (< 0.001)	1.42 (< 0.001)
Obesity	2.17 (< 0.001)	2.05 (< 0.001)
Central Obesity	1.39 (< 0.001)	1.22 (0.006)
Heart Rate (Per Increase of 10 beats/min)	1.29 (< 0.001)	1.15 (< 0.001)
Systolic Blood Pressure (Per Increase of 10 mm Hg)	1.17 (< 0.001)	1.12 (< 0.001)
Triglycerides (Per Increase of 50 mg/dl)	1.28 (< 0.001)	1.20 (< 0.001)
Urban Residence	1.22 (0.002)	0.90 (0.04)

*This table is adapted from Table 3 in Ref. 40.

and urban residence were all significantly associated with an increased risk of diabetes (see Table 10.2-2B).

Remarks

1. Population aging, urbanization, nutritional changes and a decreasing level of physical activity have probably contributed to the rapid increase in the diabetes burden in the Chinese population.
2. Dietary intake and work-related physical activity were not assessed in this study. Therefore, this study was not able to determine the association between these factors and the prevalence of diabetes.

10.3   Case-Control Studies

In contrast with cohort and cross-sectional studies, case-control studies are usually retrospective in nature. Retrospectively the investigator determines which individual was exposed to the agent, or treatment on people with the outcome of interest are matched with a control group who do not have the outcome of interest.

A Sketchy Guideline for Designing Case-control Studies

Step 1. Decide on the research questions that need to be answered.

Step 2. Formulate a hypothesis and then decide what will be measured and how.

Step 3. Specify the characteristic of the study group and decide how to construct a valid control group.

Step 4. Compare the exposure of the two groups for each variable.

Remarks

1. Case-control studies are not well suited for detecting weak association (odds ratio ≤ 1.5).[1]
2. Some problems encountered in the case-control study are low participation rates, differential misclassification and recall bias.[1]

Example 10.3-1

Alzheimer's disease is the major cause of dementia in the elderly, but little is known about the causative factors for this illness. Although some evidence suggests that the disease is related to a latent rival infection or the toxic effects of trace metals, genetic or environmental disorders, few epidemiologic studies have been carried out to confirm these hypotheses.

A case-control study was designed by Heyman *et al.*[19,20] as follows:

Step 1. To determine the possible contributing factors to the Alzheimer's disease.

Step 2. Previous genetic studies have reported an excess frequency of dementia, Down's syndrome, and hematological malignancies. Confirmation of the genetic findings was also sought in this study.

Step 3. Forty patients (12 men and 28 women) who had participated in a comprehensive clinical, genetic and epidemiological study of Alzheimer's disease at Duke University Medical Center served as a case group. The patients had a mean age of 60.8 years, ranging from 51 to 71 years of age. Because of the patients' mental impairment, information was uniformly collected from a close family member, usually the spouse, who served as a surrogate respondent. Through careful consideration of the possible information bias embedded in the patient's surrogate, we also collected information from each of the control's surrogate. Therefore, for each of the 40 patients, a matched control subject was selected by the telephone sampling technique of random-digit dialing and then an appropriate surrogate was selected from the same household. The kappa coefficient (κ) was calculated to measure the agreement between the control subjects and their surrogates to assess the validity of surrogate respondents for the various questionnaire items. The criteria for judging the degree of agreement is given as follows: the agreement is considerable if $\kappa > 0.6$; moderate if $0.4 \leq \kappa \leq 0.6$; poor if $\kappa < 0.4$.

A structured interview was used to collect information from each of the 40 patients and the 80 controls regarding selected illness, unusual dietary habits of lifestyle, occupational hazards, exposure to domesticated/wild animals, family history of dementia, mental retardation and leukemia.

Step 4. From Table 10.3-1A, approximately 48% (= 19/40) of the patients had education beyond high school, compared with 23% (= 18/80) of the controls. This difference is probably due to a selection bias in that the families of patients were likely to be well-educated. Indeed, the occupational histories of the patients indicated that there was a greater percentage of professionals among patients than among controls. There were no significant

Table 10.3-1A. Demographic Data[a]

Characteristic	Frequency	
	Patients	Controls
Education		
High school or less	10	30
High school graduation	11	32
Beyond high school	19	18
Marital status		
Never married	2	2
Married	31	64
Widowed	7	14
Residence since age 40		
City	17	55
Farm	4	14
Other	19	11

[a]This table is adapted from Table 1 in Ref. 20.

differences in marital status between patients and controls. However, residential history revealed that more patients (47.5% = 19/40) than controls (13.8% = 11/80) had lived in suburban areas. Both education and residence were potential confounders in comparing patients with controls. For this reason, educational and residential variables were used as covariates in the logistic regression analyses.

Information was also sought concerning the frequency of smoking and drinking in patients and controls. Approximately 31% of the subjects in each group had smoked a pack or more of cigarettes a day since the age of 40. The frequency of heavy coffee drinking (at least 4 cups a day) since the age of 40 was comparable between patients (33%) and controls (35%). Drinking beer was less common among patients (35%) than among controls (46%), as was drinking liquor among patients (38%) and controls (52%). However, the difference was not statistically significant.

A history of head injury was obtained more among patients than controls. Moreover, the odds ratio was significant. Yet, the kappa value (κ) of 0.42 indicated that the degree of agreement

Table 10.3-1B.   Frequency of Selected Illnesses and Accidents[a]

Prior Illnesses and Accidents	Patients	Controls (κ)	Odds Ratio
		Frequency	
Head injury	6	3 (0.42)	4.53[b]
Hypertension	6	30 (0.74)	0.31[b]
Myocardial infection	2	8 (0.93)	0.47
Diabetes	3	7 (0.88)	0.85
Stomach ulcer	3	8 (0.64)	0.73
Renal disease	9	16 (0.58)	1.16
Migraine/severe headache	8	28 (0.63)	0.46
Thyroid disease	7	5 (0.71)	3.18[b]
Influenza (World War I)	3	1 (0.33)	6.41
Shingles (herpes zoster)	5	3 (0.47)	3.67
Arthritis	16	29 (0.55)	1.17
Lung disease	3	7 (0.36)	0.85
Liver disease	1	1 (0.32)	2.03
Psychiatric disorders	6	6 (0.54)	2.18

[a]This table is adapted from Table 2 in Ref. 20.
[b]$p < 0.05$; With educational and residential variables as covariates, the odds ratio for head injury, hypertension and thyroid disease were 11.52, 0.19 and 6.87, respectively, each with $p < 0.05$.

between surrogate and control subjects was only moderate. The higher frequency of hypertension and prior myocardial infarction in control subjects was expected, because patients with severe hypertention or heart disease had been excluded from the study. Nevertheless, a significant higher frequency of prior thyroid disease was found in patients than in controls. There was no significant difference in chronic disease among patients and controls. Although severe influenza in World War I and shingles occurred more often in patients than controls, these findings were not significant (see Table 10.3-1B).

The use of medication for hypertensive/cardiac disorders was considerably more frequent in controls than in patients. This is compatible with the increased frequency of vascular diseases among the controls. For perhaps the same reason, the use of drugs

Table 10.3-1C. Frequency of Use of Selected Medications and Treatment Procedures[a]

	Frequency		
Treatment	**Patients**	**Controls (κ)**	**Odds Ratio**
Medications			
Analgesics	6	10 (0.85)	1.24
Antacids (with aluminum)	5	15 (0.84)	0.62
Diabetic medications	1	6 (0.93)	0.32
Estrogen replacement	6	6 (0.63)	2.18
Hypertensive/cardiac medications	5	28 (0.87)	0.27[b]
Thyroid medications	3	2 (0.79)	3.16
Other treatments and procedures			
Blood transfusion	2	17 (0.51)	0.20
Surgery with general anesthesia	34	72 (0.57)	0.63

[a]This table is adapted from Table 4 in Ref. 20.
[b]$p < 0.05$; With educational and residential variable as covariates, the odds ratio was 0.31 ($p = 0.06$).

for treating diabetes was more common in controls. Estrogen replacement therapy was found to be twice as frequent in patients than in controls, and a history of blood transfusion was found more frequently among controls than among patients, but both these differences were not significant (see Table 10.3-1C).

Dementia was significantly more frequent among the families of patients than among those of controls. It is not certain whether these relatives had Alzheimer's disease or some other type of dementia (see Table 10.3-1D).

Remarks

1. The present study failed to demonstrate any major premorbid demographic or clinical features that distinguished patients with Alzheimer's disease from their controls. However, there is an excess of prior thyroid disease among women with Alzheimer's disease. There was also an increased frequency of prior head trauma among patients with Alzheimer's disease.

Table 10.3-1D. Family History of Dementia, Mental Retardation and Leukemia[a]

Condition	Frequency		Odds Ratio
	Patients	Controls (κ)	
Dementiating illness	22	12 (0.33)	6.93[b]
Mental retardation (including Down's syndrome)	6	3 (0.56)	4.53[c]
Leukemia and hematological malignancies	4	8 (0.56)	1.0

[a]This table is adapted from Table 5 in Ref. 20.

[b] $p < 0.01$; With educational and residential variable as covariates, the odds ratio was 8.44 ($p < 0.01$).

[c] $p < 0.05$; With educational and residential variable as covariates, the odds ratio was 6.12 ($p < 0.05$).

2. The excess of relatives with dementia among family members of patients with Alzheimer's disease was confirmed in the authors' clinical study.[19]

Example 10.3-2

On 2 July 2002, Tropical Storm Chata'an hit Chuuk, one of the four states that comprise the Federated States of Micronesia. Almost 20 inches of rain fell on the islands within 24 hours. The US Geological Survey reported 265 landslides of various sizes and 12 of these landslides caused 43 deaths and injured at least 100 people.[33]

A case-control study was launched by the CDC:

Step 1. To identify the risk factors for mortality caused by landslides.

Step 2. To formulate strategies that can prevent future deaths in similar disasters.

Step 3. The case group consisted of people identified by Chuuk's Department of Health as having perished in the landslides in the 12 villages. The control group included individuals who survived after reportedly being in the path of a landslide. For each case subject, surrogate respondents were taken as relatives or neighbors who were familiar with the circumstances regarding the death of an individual. Surrogates were also sought for the control subjects if they were too young to answer questions for themselves. The authors interviewed 40 surrogates regarding the circumstances of the death(s) of either their relative(s), neighbor(s) or one or more of the 52 controls.

Although females accounted for a higher percentage (58% = 25/43) of the deaths, the risk of females dying during a landslide as compared with males was not statistically significant. Children under 15 years of age accounted for half (51% = 22/43) of the deaths and had a significantly higher (184% = (2.84 − 1) · 100%) risk of dying during a landslide when compared with people aged 15 years or older. Moreover, this association remains significant even after adjusting for gender or being inside a house or building. Being inside a house or building during the landslide was associated with a higher (74%) risk of mortality, but the association was not statistically significant. A majority of those who died were unaware (91% = 32/35) of the disaster and did not see or hear any signs warning them of danger (95% = 37/39). In addition, the risk of dying during the landslide was significantly associated with them being unaware of the disaster and not seeing or hearing any warning signs during the landslide (see Table 10.3-2A).

Of the 23 decedents who stayed in wood or concrete shelters or homes during the landslide, 17 (73% = 17/22) were located at the bottom of a slope or by the sea. Fifteen were found inside structures with concrete walls, and at least half (53% = 8/15) had taken refuge there instead of their own homes. For those staying inside a structure, the authors obtained complete information on 22 fatalities and 20 survivors regarding their locations during the landslide, and no significant association with the risk of becoming a fatality was found for either the location relative to the hill or the presence of concrete walls or roofs (see Table 10.3-2B).

By employing the conditional logistic regression and then stratifying first by island and then by village, being younger than

Table 10.3-2A. Crude Odds Ratio for Factors Associated with Mortality[a]

Factor	Deaths	Controls	Odds Ratio (95% CI)	*p*-value
Gender				
Male	18	29	0.57 (0.25–1.29)	0.18
Female	25	23	ref	
Age reported (yrs)				
< 15	22	14	2.84 (1.20–6.69)	0.02
≥ 15	21	38	ref	
adjusted gender[b]			3.00 (1.25–7.15)	0.01
adjusted location[b]			2.62 (1.07–6.40)	0.03
Location of person				
inside	23	22	1.74 (0.76–3.98)	0.19
outside	18	30	ref	
Awareness of landslides				
aware	3	16	0.21 (0.05–0.77)	0.02[c]
not aware	32	35	ref	
Natural warnings				
signs	2	25	0.06 (0.01–0.27)	< 0.0001[c]
no signs	37	27	ref	

[a]This table is adapted from Table 3 in Ref. 33.
[b]Cochran–Mantel–Haenszel statistics.
[c]Fisher's exact test.

15 years was a significant predictor for landslide mortality after being age adjusted by male gender (212%) and being inside (179%) for the former, and being age adjusted by male gender (231%) and being inside (179%) for the latter, when compared with people whose ages were over 15 years old (see Table 10.3-2C).

Table 10.3-2D indicated that the factors of being female and being inside were still associated with increased risk, but this increase was not statistically significant.

In this investigation deaths were most common among children. Children were clearly at a physical disadvantage during a natural disaster. Although women had a higher mortality rate, they had no increased risk of becoming a fatality during a landslide when compared with others in their control group. Because

Table 10.3-2B. Crude Odds Ratio for Factors for Those Inside a Structure[a]

Factor	Deaths	Controls	Odds Ratio (95% CI)	*p*-value
Position of house				
slope	5	4	1.18 (0.27–5.18)	1.00[b]
sea level	17	16	ref	
Walls				
concrete	15	13	1.15 (0.32–4.17)	0.83
tin, wood	7	7	ref	
Roof				
concrete	1	5	0.14 (0.02–1.35)	0.09[b]
tin, wood	21	15	ref	

[a]Thi table is adapted from Table 4 in Ref. 33.
[b]Fisher's exact test.

Table 10.3-2C. Odds Ratio for Age (Binary), Adjusted Individually to Other Potential Risk Factors after Controlling for Island and Village[a]

Age < 15 years	Odds Ratio (95% CI)	*p*-value	β
By island[b]			
age adjusted by male gender	3.12 (1.26–7.75)	0.01	1.14
age adjusted by being inside	2.79 (1.11–7.01)	0.03	1.03
age adjusted by awareness	2.52 (0.92–6.87)	0.07	0.92
age adjusted by natural signs	2.21 (0.81–6.05)	0.12	0.79
By village[b]			
age adjusted by male gender	3.31 (1.26–8.65)	0.02	1.20
age adjusted by being inside	2.79 (1.04–7.51)	0.04	1.03
age adjusted by awareness	2.91 (0.97–8.67)	0.06	1.07
age adjusted by natural signs	2.34 (0.80–6.85)	0.12	0.85

[a]This table is adapted from Table 5 in Ref. 33.
[b]Conditional logistic regression.

people were not aware that landslides were occurring, these findings suggest a need to improve the communication infrastructure and warning systems for emergency situations within or between islands.

Table 10.3-2D. Potential Predictors for 2002 Landslide-related Mortality after Controlling for Island and Village[a]

Parameters	Odds Ratio (95% CI)	*p*-value	β
By island			
children	2.91 (1.14–7.40)	0.03	1.07
female gender	1.63 (0.67–3.95)	0.28	0.49
being inside	1.34 (0.54–3.28)	0.53	0.29
By village			
children	2.95 (1.08–8.06)	0.04	1.08
female gender	1.53 (0.62–3.78)	0.36	0.42
being inside	1.44 (0.55–3.80)	0.46	0.37

[a]This table is adapted from Table 6 in Ref. 33.

Remarks

1. The nonrandomized recruiting of controls, the use of proxies for decedents, and the self-reported nature of exposure in the survey make it potentially susceptible to selection and misclassification bias.
2. The issue on how to test the assumption of non-differential misclassification was studied in Ref. 25.

10.4   Clinical Trial Studies

In his talk presented to the faculty and staff of the Department of Preventive Medicine, Harvard Medical School,[21] AB Hill (1897–1991) shared his experience gained while working as a statistician on several clinical trials conducted by the British Medical Council. First, he expressed his dismay on the most frequent criticism concerning the statistical approach in medicine that human beings are too variable to allow the contrasts inherent in a controlled trial of remedy. Nevertheless, the use of random allocation of patients to the treatment/control groups is capable of alleviating this concern. Of course, due to the play of chance, this random allocation might not provide groups that are sufficiently alike because of the heterogeneity among patients' individual characteristics. But this issue can be taken care of by using the stratifying technique to divide the heterogeneous group of patients into more homogeneous subgroups.

A case in point was the joint drug trial (cortisone and ACFH versus salicylates) that treated patients with rheumatic fever in a number of centers in the United Kingdom, US and Canada. It was noted that rheumatic fever runs a different course in young children and in adolescents. Therefore, patients with rheumatic fever were subdivided by age into two age groups: those under 16 years and those over 16 years. There were six subgroups. Apart from age, the course of disease in relation to treatment, particularly a concern about any possible permanent damage to the heart, may be influenced by the speed by which treatment is instituted after the onset of the attack. Within each of the two age groups, three divisions were divided by the duration of time that had elapsed between the onset of attack and the start of treatment. Every patient who was eligible for entry into the trial was first allocated to one of the six subgroups. He was then allocated a specific treatment, by means of random orders set up for each subgroup, and, separately, for each center taking part in the trial. Hill admitted that no method of random allocation can absolutely ensure the equality of the groups in all these aspects. Nevertheless, the purpose of randomization can safeguard against selection bias, as insurance, in the long run against accidental bias and as the sinew of statistical tests.[17]

Clinical trials used in the pharmaceutical industry to develop new drugs are roughly divided into four phases. A phase I study is the initial assessment of a new drug in humans; it takes place using healthy volunteers and is designed to investigate the drug toxicity on the determination of the maximally tolerated dose. Details on the choice of initial dose, dose escalation schemes, number of subjects at each dose level, volunteer selection and clinical pharmacology studies of the drug can be found in Geller.[15] Phase II studies take place in patients with diseases of interest and are designed to give firm evidence of a clinical effect of possible benefit, to detect common adverse reactions and to establish appropriate therapeutic dose ranges. Phase III studies constitute the full clinical trial program to complete a submission to a regulatory authority. Bioavailability in the final formulation in patients, the size of the beneficial effect, and appropriate dose regimes must all be established. Safety must be confirmed and a range of information must be collected on concomitant use with other medications and use in the whole range of disease states of interest. After marketing permission has been obtained, phase IV studies are conducted to answer the long-term efficacy concerning the confirmation of clinical benefits in large population during normal use, the incidence of rare adverse reactions, and the relative efficacy compared with other medications.

A Sketchy Guideline for Writing the Protocol for a Clinical Trial[1]

Step 1. It needs to provide a brief rationale and background for the study.

Step 2. It needs to clearly state the specific objective of the investigation.

Step 3. It should include a clear concise statement of the design to be used. Is it to involve the random allocation of patients to treatment? If not, document the reason why randomization is not necessary. If a study were to test the efficacy of a drug, the modes of administration need to be clearly outlined. The number of patients planned to be included in each treatment regimen must be specified.

Step 4. The patient's definition has to be completely defined, that is, the inclusion/exclusion criteria must be clear and specific.

Step 5. The treatment must be carefully outlined. Whether the treatment is a surgical procedure or the administration of a drug, it is imperative that all patients are uniformly treated, according to the random assignment for each patient.

Step 6. All aspects of the methodology must be explicitly and specifically defined. In particular, the methods must assure, measure and document the quality of the data collected. Incidentally, the data forms need to be included.

Step 7. The response variables of interest and the end points to be reached must be clearly identified for all participants. Provisions must be made for observing and recording side effects.

Step 8. With every study involving human subjects, it is essential to obtain informed consent. The forms for obtaining such consent and the anticipated approaches to patients in obtaining such consent needs to be fully spelled out in appendices.

Remarks

1. Before a trial is undertaken, the investigator has to decide what clinically significant difference he is interested in detecting and consult a statistician to determine the sample size needed to demonstrate such a difference if it exists within the generally acceptable error limits ($\alpha = 0.05$ and $\beta = 0.10$). Alternatively, should the investigator know roughly the expected sample size, a statistician can help to find the probability where such a difference is likely to be found if it exists (power of the test) and the probability that the real difference of other magnitudes will be found (beta error).[13]
2. Because of inadequate reporting, it fueled the development of the original CONSORT (Consolidated Standards of Reporting Trials). Although the 25 items in the checklist in the CONSORT statement does not include recommendations for designing, conducting and analyzing trials, CONSORT can still help researchers in designing their trials.[34]

Example 10.4-1

Since the natural course of pulmonary tuberculosis is so variable and unpredictable, the evidence of improvement or cure following the use of a new drug in a few cases cannot be accepted as proof of the effect of that drug. A new drug, streptomycin, was discovered in 1944, the clinical results of using it in treating pulmonary tuberculosis were encouraging but inconclusive. Because the history of chemotherapeutic trials in tuberculosis is filled with errors due to empirical evaluation of drugs, it had become obvious that conclusions regarding the clinical effect of a new drug in tuberculosis could be considered valid only if based on adequately controlled clinical trials. In 1946 no controlled trial of streptomycin had been undertaken in the US.

After receiving the limited amount of streptomycin generously supplied by the US, the Medical Research Council in Britain decided in September 1946 to use a small amount of the streptomycin for research purposes. They carefully planned a clinical trial to investigate the effect of streptomycin in pulmonary tuberculosis.[29] Historically, this was hailed as the first truly "randomized controlled" clinical trial.

The first accepted patient was admitted to the centers in January 1947. By September 1947, 109 patients had been accepted and no more were admitted to this trial. Two patients died within the preliminary observation week; they were excluded from the analysis. Of the remaining 107 patients 55 were allocated to the streptomycin group and 52 to the control group.

Determination of whether a patient would be treated by streptomycin and bed-rest (S case) or by bed-rest alone (C case) was made by reference to a statistical series based on random sampling numbers drawn up for each gender at each center; the details of the series were unknown to any of the investigators or to the coordinator and were contained in a set of sealed envelopes, each bearing only the name of the hospital and its number. After the panel accepted a patient, and before admitting this patient to the streptomycin center, the appropriate numbered envelop was opened at the central office; the card inside told if the patient was to be a S or a C case, and this information was then given to the medical officer of the center.

Table 10.4-1A. Data on Admission for Patients in the S and C Groups*

	S Group	C Group
Sample size	55	52
Gender		
Male	22	21
Female	33	31
General condition		
Good	8	8
Fair	17	20
Poor	30	24
Maximal evening temperature in 1st week		
98–98.9°F	3	4
99–99.9°F	13	12
100–100.9°F	15	17
101°+F	24	19
Sedimentation rate		
0–10	0	0
11–20	3	2
21–50	16	20
51+	36	29
X-ray classification (large/multiple cavities)		
Yes	32	30
No	23	22
Segmental atelectasis		
Yes	19	19
No	36	33

*This table is adapted from Table I in Ref. 29.

At the end of six months 7% of the S patients and 27% of the C patients had died. Considerable radiological improvement was noted in 51% of the S cases and 8% of the C cases (see Table 10.4-1B). The main difference between the S and C series was among the patients who were clinically acutely ill on admission (see Table 10.4-1A). More S patients than C patients showed clinical improvement but the difference between the two series was smaller than in respect of radiological changes. Results of tests

Table 10.4-1B. Assessment of Radiological Appearance at Six Months as Compared with that at Admission*

Radiological Assessment	S Group	C Group
Considerable improvement	28 (51%)	4 (8%)
Moderate/slight improvement	10 (18%)	13 (25%)
No material change	2 (4%)	3 (6%)
Moderate/slight deterioration	5 (9%)	12 (23%)
Considerable deterioration	6 (11%)	6 (11%)
Deaths	4 (7%)	14 (27%)
Total	55 (100%)	52 (100%)

*This table is adapted from Table II in Ref. 29.

for streptomycin sensitivity of infecting strains are given for 41 cases. In 35 cases tests revealed in-vitro resistence from 32 to over 8000 times than that of the original strain. In most cases streptomycin resistence emerged in the second month of treatment. It seemed that streptomycin resistence was responsible for much of the deterioration seen in S cases after the first treatment.

Remarks

1. The discovery of streptomycin can be found in Ref. 37.
2. While working in the Brompton hospital in 1935, N Oswald[30] recalled that about four-fifths of the inpatients had tuberculosis. Many of them were young women. Unfortunately, there were no effective drugs available in treating tuberculosis. The physicians at the hospital had little help to offer beyond rest, fresh air, good food and sympathy. Not until the mid-1940s were several anti-tuberculosis drugs discovered. Although various forms of collapse therapy were applied with confidence, their overall value was not proven because a well-designed clinical trial was lacking. Had this controlled clinical on using the streptomycin as a new drug not happened, effective treatment on tuberculosis would have been delayed several years.

Example 10.4-2

Among currently available therapeutic agents the adrenal corticosteroids produces the highest rate of remission induction. However, these remissions are relatively short. Moreover, they are usually not prolonged significantly by maintenance corticosteroid therapy. The Acute Leukemia Group B was therefore proposed a model for the evaluation of new and more effective therapeutic agents. The drug 6-mercaptopurine was selected as an agent to test such an experimental design in acute leukemia.[14]

The entire experimental design was divided into three phases: (i) remission induction (phase 1), (ii) remission maintenance (phase 2), and (iii) 6-MP therapy (phase 3). In phase 1, corticosteroid therapy was continued until complete bone marrow remission was achieved or a maximum of 28 days had passed (A-1). Prednisone was selected as the corticosteroid used in this phase. Patients who failed to show marrow improvement after 28 days were grouped as NRS patients. They were then given 6-MP as their next course of therapy for remission induction (phase 3). Patients with marrow remission (A-1) before 28 days or marrow remission (A-1 or A-2) on the 28th day were assigned randomly (double-blind) to 6-MP therapy or a placebo for the remission maintenance of the study (phase 2). This part of the study employed a sequential design so that the study could be stopped as soon as one treatment showed superior results to the other.

A full dosage of 6-MP (3mg/Kg/day) was used for maintenance therapy unless it was a toxicity modified dose. At this time, an envelope was opened and those patients who received the placebo maintenance treatment were now to receive the 6-MP therapy instead. Those who had originally received the 6-MP maintenance went on for the study.

Because corticosteroids are primarily active against acute lymphocytic leukemia during childhood years, the study was confined to patients under the age of 20 years. All suitable patients with proven acute leukemia when admitted to the participating

Table 10.4-2A. **Patients Classified by Response in Phase 1 (Randomization Category) and Best Response in Phases 1 and 2**[a]

Response in Phase 1		Best Response in Phases 1 and 2	
Randomization		CR	PR
A-1 marrow			
6-MP	24	24	0
placebo	24	23	1
A-2 marrow			
6-MP	9	5	4
placebo	5	3	2
No response	30	—	—
All patients	92	55 (60%)	7 (8%)

[a]This table is adapted from Table 2 in Ref. 14.

institution and had received no chemotherapy prior to admission were entered into the study.

The first patient was entered in April 1959 and the last one in April 1960. A total of 97 patients with acute leukemia were entered into the study by the 11 participating institutions. Of these patients, 92 were considered acceptable for analysis.

Of the 92 patients, 62 improved to complete or partial remission marrow after 28 days of corticosteroid therapy while 30 had no response. Among the 30 patients in the NRS group, 10 were dead before phase 3. With phase 1's corticosteroid therapy, 60% of patients went into complete remission (CR) and 8% into partial remission (PR) (see Table 10.4-2A).

The relative frequency of remissions in the age group of 15–19 years old was significantly lower than the younger age groups. Those with myelocytic leukemia had a significantly lower relative frequency of remission than patients classified "lymphocytic" or "unclassified". The difference among the categories in the onset of symptoms to diagnosis is not significant. For patients classified by the initial white blood count, there is evidence that the response rate decreased significant linearly with increasing white blood count. Similarly, there is evidence of a linear trend in the response rate of the initial platelet count; the higher the platelet count, the higher the probability of responding to steroids. For patients classified according to initial platelet count and number of blasts, those with a platelet count below 30,000 and a blast count above 5000 had a significant response rate of only 25%, as compared to others who had a response rate of about 77% (see Table 10.4-2B).

A comparison is made between patients who received 6-MP and who received a placebo in phase 2 with respect to a number of factors known to be associated with therapy and survival. There are no important differences between them. However, there is a marked difference in their remission curves. For patients who were maintained on 6-MP the median length of complete remission was 33 weeks, while for those on the placebo, the median length was only 9 weeks. Moreover, after 10 weeks of therapy, all patients receiving the 6-MP were still in remission, whereas only 40% of the patients who received the placebo were still in remission. For the patients in partial remission, the number was too small (only seven) to make any definite comparison between them.

Nevertheless, the number of patients in remission having greater than the median remission time with respect to age, type of leukemia, the duration of symptoms to diagnosis, white blood count, platelet count, platelet and number of blasts is given in Table 10.4-2C. There is evidence that remission are longer for patients with longer duration of symptoms to diagnosis and those with low initial white blood counts. The chi-squared test showed that the trend was significantly linear in each case. Yet, no evidence shows that the length of remission is related to age, type of leukemia, initial platelet count or number of blasts.

Remarks

1. Although corticosteroids therapy can induce remissions in almost 80% of patients under 15 years of age with acute lymphocytic leukemia, the prognosis for patients who fail to respond

Table 10.4-2B.   Response to Steroids for Patients Classified by Initial Status[a]

Initial Status	No. of Patients	No. of Patients in CR and PR (%)
Age (yrs.)		
0–4	44	30 (68)
5–9	25	19 (76)
10–14	4	11 (79)
15–19	9	2 (22)
Type		
lymphocytic	72	54 (75)
myelocytic	13	3 (23)
unclassified	7	5 (71)
Symptoms to diagnosis (wks.)		
0–1	13	8 (62)
2–3	28	18 (64)
4–5	25	15 (60)
6–7	13	11 (85)
8 and over	13	11 (85)
Starting WBC		
Below 5000	27	22 (81)
5000–9999	23	18 (78)
10,000–19,999	9	6 (67)
20,000–49,999	17	9 (52)
50,000 and over	16	8 (50)
Starting platelet count		
under 25,000	30	17 (57)
25,000–49,999	33	22 (67)
50,000–99,999	14	11 (79)
100,000 and over	13	12 (92)
Platelet No. of blasts		
Under 30,000		
under 5000	17	13 (76)
5000 and over	16	4 (25)
30,000 and over		
under 5000	38	30 (78)
5000 and over	9	6 (67)

[a]This table is adapted from Table 3 in Ref. 14.

Table 10.4-2C. Effects of Initial Status on Duration of Remission in Phase 2[a]

Initial Status		No. of Patients	No. of Patients Remitting Greater than Median Remission Time[b] (%)
Age (years)			
0–4		28	16 (57)
5–9		18	10 (56)
10–14		11	3 (27)
15–19		2	1 (50)
Type			
lymphocytic		52	26 (50)
myelocytic		2	1 (50)
unclassified		5	4 (80)
Symptoms to diagnosis (wks.)			
0–3		23	8 (35)
4–7		25	13 (52)
8 and over		11	9 (82)
Starting WBC			
Below 5000		21	14 (67)
5000–19,999		24	14 (58)
20,000 and over		14	2 (14)
Starting platelet count			
under 25,000		15	6 (40)
25,000–99,999		32	19 (59)
100,000 and over		11	5 (45)
Platelet	No. of blasts		
Under 30,000			
	under 5000	13	6 (46)
	5000 and over	4	1 (25)
30,000 and over			
	under 5000	27	17 (63)
	5000 and over	6	1 (17)

[a] This table is adapted from Table 6 in Ref. 14.

[b] Median remission time (complete and partial) for 6-MP and placebo patients are given by 29 weeks and 8, respectively.

is poor (33% mortality in 4 weeks). The observation that 6-MP therapy may prolong remissions in patients in whom it would fail to induce remissions suggests that the activity of remission-induction and -maintenance are not identical.

2. Chemotherapeutic agents differ markedly in these two activities. Perhaps some agents are almost inactive in remission induction, but could prove useful for remission maintenance. Clinical study of these two separate parameters of antileukemic activity may provide data for more precise correlation with preclinical anti-tumor screening systems.

10.5   Types of Bias

Unlike its colloquial use as "prejudice" or "unfairness", bias, in the context of research methodology, refers to the presence of systematic error in a study. In practice, this means that an estimate of association from the study population differs systematically from the true association in the target population of the study. Bias is intrinsically different from random (sampling) error. Systematic error does not diminish as the sample size of the study population increases, whereas random error does. Consequently, statistical significance does not reflect the presence or absence of bias.[16]

In observational studies four basic experimental principles including (i) verification of quality and accuracy in raw data, (ii) avoidance of major biases in comparison, (iii) vigilance in checking methodological errors, and (iv) maintenance of a careful distinction between research data that generate hypotheses and the new data needed to test these hypotheses are often overlooked. This is the reason why case-control/cohort studies lead to contradictory results.[11]

Horwitz and Feinstein[22] found that conflicts were noted in conclusions either among case-control studies or between case-control and cohort studies of the same topic. A total of 17 topics consisted of 95 investigated studies, of which 85 were of case-control type and 10 were cohorts. The 17 topics include the etiologic relationship of myocardial infarction to coffee-drinking and aspirin, and of various neoplastic diseases to reserpine, estrogens, coffee-drinking, herpesvirus, oral contraceptives, appendectomy, tonsillectomy, early age of menarche and tuberculosis.

The 12 methodologic standards that would enhance scientific quality in research were selected to evaluate the 85 case-control studies for the fulfillment of these standards. The standards include (i) predetermined method of patient selection, (ii) specification of the causal agent, (iii) unbiased data collection, (iv) anamnestic equivalence, (v–vi) avoidance of constrained selection for cases and controls, (vii) equal diagnostic examination, (viii) equal prehospital surveillance, (ix–x) equal demographic and clinical susceptibility, (xi) avoidance of protopathic bias, and (xii) avoidance of Berkson's bias. These standards were commonly violated in the 85 reviewed investigations.

Based on stages of research, Sackett[32] cataloged 56 biases into seven categories: (i) reading-up on the field, 5 items, (ii) specifying and selecting the study sample, 22 items, (iii) executing the experimental manoeuver for exposure, 5 items, (iv) measuring exposures and outcomes, 13 items, (v) analyzing the data, 5 items, (vi) interpreting the analysis, 6 items, and (vii) publishing the result, none. Delgado-Rodriguez and Llorda[6] collected 72 biases to subsume them into four classes: (i) selection bias, 35 items, (ii) information bias, 30 items, (iii) confounding bias, 3 items, and (iv) bias in clinical trials, 4 items. In addition, Vineis and McMichael[36] proposed a categorization of bias in molecular epidemiologic studies into four classes: (i) selection bias, (ii) information bias, (iii) intra-individual variation, and (iv) confounding.

A randomized controlled trial (RCT) is less susceptible to bias than other study designs for assessing therapeutic interventions. However, a study that is randomized does not mean that it is unbiased. There are at least seven important potential sources of bias in RCTs: (i) poor allocation concealment, (ii) imbalance in baseline prognostic variables, (iii) unblinding and no blinding, (iv) missing data, (v) lack of intention to treat analysis, (vi) count death as a good outcome, and (vii) competing interest. For a detailed discussion, see Refs. 26 and 27.

Here I select some of them for a detailed discussion. Example 10.5-1 considers Berkson's bias, while Example 10.5-2 studies the exclusion, susceptibility, or protopathic bias.

Example 10.5-1

(a) In 1946, J Berkson[3] published a paper in which he presented a theory that distinct hospitalized disease rates in hospital-based studies could possibly cause the spurious association between the case and control diseases in the target population. Such a phenomenon has become known as "Berkson's fallacy" or "Berkson's bias".

Let me recite what Berkson did in his paper. There was a prevailing expression that cholecystitis is a causal risk factor for diabetes. Berkson examined the patients' hospital records and chose non-diabetic patients as the control group to obtain the following 2×2 table:

Table 10.5-1A[a].   The hospital sample data of diabetes and not diabetes

	Diabetes	Not Diabetes
Cholecystitis	28	1,326
Not Cholecystitis	548	39,036

[a]This table is adapted from Table 2 in Ref. 3.

The odds ratio for Table 10.5-1A is

$$\hat{\theta}^{(A)}_{2 \times 2} = \frac{28 \cdot 39,036}{548 \cdot 1,326} = 1.504 \approx 1.5.$$

An objection that might be brought against Table 10.5-1A is that some of the "not diabetes" group might contain a variety of diagnoses, some of which may themselves be correlated with cholecystitis; hence the controls may be considered "no good". To meet this objection, he did not use all the nondiabetic patients, but took as the control group the diagnosis of "refractive errors" patients that could not reasonably be thought of to be correlated with cholecystitis. A new 2×2 table was obtained as Table 10.5-1B.

Table 10.5-1B[a]. **The hospital sample data of diabetes and refractive errors**

	Diabetes	Refractive Errors
Cholecystitis	28	68
Not Cholecystitis	548	2,606

[a]This table is adapted from Table 3 in Ref. 3.

The odds ratio for Table Table 10.5-1B is

$$\hat{\theta}^{(B)}_{2\times2} = \frac{28\cdot2,606}{68\cdot548} = 1.958 \approx 1.96.$$

It is easily shown that both the odds ratio estimates of $\hat{\theta}^{(A)}_{2\times2}$ and $\hat{\theta}^{(B)}_{2\times2}$ are statistically significant (see Exercise 10.6-3). After seeing this empirical evidence, Berkson asked himself a question: "Can this "statistical" result from the empirical data in Tables 10.5-1A and 10.5-1B permit a conclusion as to whether cholecystitis is "biologically" correlated with diabetes?"

Berkson then built a theoretical model to answer this question. He considered a hypothetical example in which, in a (source) population of 10 million people, the occurrence of three diseases — cholecystitis (C), diabetes (D) and refractive errors (R) — were assumed to be independently distributed, that is, the occurrence of one disease in a person does not affect the likelihood of that person also having one of the other diseases. The prevalence of cholecystitis, diabetes and refractive errors was assumed to be given by 3%, 1% and 10%, respectively. In terms of the Venn diagram, the calculated result from the target population is given in Fig. 10.5-1. After assembling the fourfold table with the "not diabetes" or "refractive errors" chosen as the control group from Fig. 10.5-1, the calculated odds ratio values for both tables were shown to be one in the source population (see Table 5 in Ref. 3).

On the other hand, if we let S_C, S_D and S_R denote the probability of selecting people from the source population for cholecystitis, diabetes and refractive errors, respectively, into the study

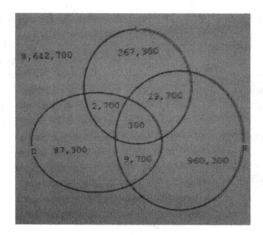

Figure 10.5-1. The hypothetical data of the source population of 10 million (By the way, a figure with a better resolution is attached separately).

Table 10.5-1C. $(S_C = S_D = S_R = 0.05)^a$

	Diabetes	Refractive Errors
Cholecystitis	306	2896
Not Cholecystitis	5311	48,015

^{a}This table is adapted from Table 7 in Ref. 3.

(hospitalized) population and assume that the mechanism of hospitalization for each disease operates independently. If all three selection rates are small and equal to 0.05, a 2 × 2 table for the expected number of patients in the study population is given by Table 10.5-1D.

The odds ratio for Table 10.5-1C is

$$\hat{\theta}_{2\times2}^{(C)} = \frac{306 \cdot 48{,}015}{2{,}896 \cdot 5{,}311} = 0.955 \approx 0.96.$$

When all three selection rates are unequal, say, $S_C = 0.15$, $S_D = 0.05$ and $S_R = 0.2$, a 2 × 2 table for the expected number of patients in the hospital sample is given by Table 10.5-1D.

Table 10.5-1D. $(S_C = 0.15, S_D = 0.05, S_R = 0.2)^a$

	Diabetes	Refractive Errors
Cholecystitis	626	9504
Not Cholecystitis	6693	192,060

[a]This table is adapted from Table 9 in Ref. 3.

The odds ratio for Table 10.5-1D is

$$\hat{\theta}_{2\times2}^{(D)} = \frac{626 \cdot 192,060}{9,504 \cdot 6,693} = 1.89.$$

Note that the value of $\hat{\theta}_{2\times2}^{(C)}$ is not different from the odds ratio in the source population (which is one), whereas the value of $\hat{\theta}_{2\times2}^{(D)}$ is very different from that of the source population. Through this example, Berkson showed that different disease selection rates could lead to an apparent association between pairs of diseases in the study population, even though they were independently distributed in the source population.

(b) In 1976, an example to show the possible existence of Berkson's bias is provided by Brown.[4] In reviewing the literature on the effect of Berkson's bias on the association of low birthweight and cerebral palsy, Brown noted that none of the previous investigators ever considered the possibility of this bias. Yet, he noted in his private practice that the apparent excess of neurologic disorders among girls is probably attributable to the different selection rates, since the sex ratio of boys to girls is about 4 to 1.

(c) In 1978, the first empirical evidence on the existence of Berkson's bias was provided by Roberts *et al.*[31] Based on the data from three separate community-based studies of 2784 non-institutionalized adults of age 25 or over, clinical data, health services utilization data and data about the use of drugs were obtained in household surveys of random samples of people living in Southern Ontario. Roberts *et al.* calculated the hospitalized rates for eight clinical conditions: (i) allergic, endocrine system, metabolic and nutritional disease (0.147), (ii) mental, psychoneurotic and personal disorders (0.128), (iii) disease of the circulatory system (0.187), (iv) disease of the respiratory system (0.089), (v) disease of the bones and organs of movement (0.114), (vi) injuries and adverse effects of chemicals, etc. (0.297), (vii) arthritic and rheumatic complaints (0.126), and (viii) fatigue (0.2), and for six medication groups: (i) A.S.A. (0.107), (ii) laxatives (0.131), (iii) sleeping pills (0.267), (iv) vitamins (0.056), (v) tranquilizers (0.171), and (vi) "heart" pills (0.143). Note that the hospitalization rates among these eight clinical conditions and six medications are unequal.

In order to retain all observations in each analysis, they chose those not affected by disease (ii) as the controls. Also, disease (i) was chosen as the suspected causal risk factor. All possible ($n = 28$) pairs of the eight clinical conditions and 48 ($= 6 \times 8$) clinical condition × medication were analyzed. They calculated the relative risk and odds ratio for both the source population and the study (hospitalization) population. Here I only considered a comparison of the odds ratio between the source population and its study population. If the ratio values of these two odds differ to a degree greater than that could be expected from a sampling variation alone, it could be reasonably attributed to Berkson's bias.

Out of the 28 comparisons for the paired clinical conditions 16 pairs do not meet the disease-independence assumption in the source population, because their odds ratio values are significantly deviant from the value of one. Out of the four pairs in which the odds ratio between the source population and the study population differs significantly at the level of 0.05, only one pair, disease (iv)–(v), meets the disease-independence assumption in the source population (see Table 5 in Ref. 28). Similarly, out of the five medical × clinical condition combinations in which the odds ratio between the source population and the study population differs significantly at the level of 0.05, only three pairs meet the disease-independence assumption in the source population. In general, it is hard to tell whether the independence assumption on the disease selection into the study population holds empirically. Yet, this assumption seems very likely to be not valid for the vitamins × allergy pair, because the odds ratio for the source population is 1.76, but 0.0 for the study population (see Table 6 in Ref. 31).

(d) In 1980, Walter[38] presented a theoretical model to analyze the existence of Berkson's bias in which the disease-independence assumption in the source population in Berkson's theory was dropped, though he retained the independence assumption on selecting the disease into the study population. He showed that Berkson's bias would not operate in the following two cases:

(i) When there are no hospitalizations due to exposure to the risk factor per se, and (a) the cases are all hospitalized, (b) a small fraction of controls is hospitalized, (c) there is no risk factor-control-disease association among the cases, or (d) few people have both the case and control diseases;
(ii) When there is no overlap between cases and controls and the two diseases are hospitalized in approximately the same rate.

Remarks

1. According to deductive logic, Berkson's bias is presented based on two assumptions: (i) the three diseases are independently distributed in the source population and (ii) the hospital selection rates are not equal. However, both of these two assumptions may not be valid empirically. In practice, the information on the source population is oftentimes unavailable. As a result, Berkson's bias is actually unobservable.
2. Indeed, the empirical result showed that even though neither the disease-independence assumption in the original population nor the assumption on the equal disease hospital selection were valid, it seemed that the bias still existed empirically. Of course, we do not know whether this empirical bias came solely from Berkson's bias. In fact, the empirical bias may, other than Berkson's bias, contain some components including clinical selection bias, other unknown biases and random errors.
3. By using the technique of causal modeling, Maclure and Schneeweiss[28] showed how different biases were combined across different domains into the final epidemiologic evidence.

Example 10.5-2

Feinstein and Horwitz[10] presented an algebraic analysis to show how the exclusion, susceptibility and protopathic bias might occur in case-control research. Let e and p denote the proportion of people exposed to an alleged causal agent and then develop the target disease, respectively. If the target disease occurs at a eate p_1 in the exposed group and at a rate p_2 in the non-exposed group, the two rates can be determined in a longitudinal cohort study and the relative risk is given by p_1/p_2. If no bias exists in the pathway that lies between exposure, hospitalization and selection for the case-control study, representatives of the four groups: (i) exposed and diseased, (ii) exposed and non-diseased, (iii) non-exposed and diseased, and (iv) non-exposed and non-diseased can be readily expressed in the following 2×2 table:

Table 10.5-2A. The distribution of exposed and nonexposed in a case-control study

	Cases	Controls
Exposed	ep_1	$e(1-p_1)$
Non-exposed	$(1-e)p_2$	$(1-e)(1-p_2)$

The odds ratio R for Table 10.5-2A is given by

$$R = \frac{ep_1 \cdot (1-e)(1-p_2)}{(1-e)p_2 \cdot e(1-p_1)} = \frac{p_1(1-p_2)}{p_2(1-p_1)} \qquad (10.5.1)$$

Under the rare disease assumption, namely, p_1 and p_2 are quite small, R of Eq. (10.5.1) is reduced approximately as the risk ratio. However, the observed odds ratio may not always accurately represent the true risk ratio. Distortions can be produced by the investigator who decides which people to choose as cases and controls, or by the physician or patient who makes the decision to initiate exposure with the suspected etiologic agent.

We are going to consider three possible biases:

Table 10.5-2B. The distribution of exposed and nonexposed as far as the exclusion bias is concerned

	Cases	Controls
Exposed	$(s_A e_A + s_B e_B)p_1$	$s_B e_B(1 - p_1)$
Non-exposed	$[s_A(1 - e_A) + s_B(1 - e_B)]p_2$	$s_B(1 - e_B)(1 - p_2)$

A. The Exclusion Bias

First, assume that only members of the potential control group are excluded inappropriately. An analogous but reverse set of problems would occur if the exclusions are made in the case group.

Suppose that the population at risk contains two strata A and B with and without a particular clinical condition, respectively. Let the proportion of A and B in the population be given respectively by s_A and s_B, while their exposure rates to an alleged etiologic agent are denoted by e_A and e_B, respectively. Assume that $e_A = c e_B$, where $c > 1$. Further, assume that the occurrence of the target disease is unaffected by the presence or absence of the underlying clinical condition. If people with or without the cited clinical condition are referred to the hospital at equal rates, the 2×2 table for this case-control study is given by Table 10.5-2B.

The odds ratio for Table 10.5-2B is

$$R_{EB} = \frac{(s_A e_A + s_B e_B)p_1 \cdot s_B(1 - e_B)(1 - p_2)}{s_B e_B(1 - p_1) \cdot [s_A(1 - e_A) + s_B(1 - e_B)]p_2}. \tag{10.5.2}$$

Again, under the rare disease assumption plus the fact that e_B^2 and $e_A e_B$ are substantially smaller than e_A and e_B, R_{EB} of Eq. (10.5.2) reduces by letting $s_A = k s_B$ to

$$R_{EB} = \frac{p_1}{p_2} \times \frac{kc + 1}{k + 1}. \tag{10.5.3}$$

Remarks

1. Since $c > 1$, Eq. (10.5.3) is falsely elevated than the true relative risk, p_1/p_2. The degree of elevation depends on the magnitude of k, the ratio of people who do or do not have the cited clinical condition, and also on the magnitude of c, the ratio of their exposure rates.
2. Equation (10.5.3) is illustrated by using an example of the reserpine–breast cancer relationship.[10] In that study, patients with cardiovascular disease were excluded from the control group but not from the cases.
3. The exclusion bias can be eliminated by insisting on using better criteria for these exclusions, and applying the criteria equally to both cases and controls.[10]

B. *The Susceptibility Bias*

The susceptibility bias occurs if people who are particularly susceptible to the development of a target disease are also particularly likely to be exposed to the alleged etiologic agent.

Let s_A and s_B be the proportion of two strata A and B in the total population at risk with stratum A having a higher susceptibility to the disease, namely, $s_A > s_B$. Under normal circumstances, the disease rate for A and B are denoted respectively by p_A and p_B. The rate of exposure to the susceptible etiologic agent are e_A in stratum A and e_B in stratum B, where $e_A > e_B$. The exposed patients develop the disease at a rate of $p_{A|E}$ in stratum A and $p_{B|E}$ in stratum B, where $p_{A|E} > p_{B|E}$. A 2×2 table for this case-control study is given by

Table 10.5-2C. The distribution of exposed and nonexposed as far as the susceptibility bias is concerned

	Cases	Controls
Exposed	$s_A e_A p_{A|E} + s_B e_B p_{B|E}$	$s_A e_A (1 - p_{A|E}) + s_B e_B (1 - p_{B|E})$
Non-exposed	$s_A (1 - e_A) p_A + s_B (1 - e_B) p_B$	$s_A (1 - e_A)(1 - p_A)|s_B(1 - e_B)p_B$

With an assumption that p_A, p_B, $p_{A|E}$ and $p_{B|E}$ are all very small relative to 1, the odds ratio for Table 10.5-2C is given by

$$R_{SB} = \frac{(s_A e_A p_{A|E}| + s_B e_B p_{B|E})[s_A(1 - e_A) + s_B(1 - e_B)]}{[s_A(1 - e_A)p_A + s_B(1 - e_B)p_B](s_A e_A + s_B e_B)}. \qquad (10.5.4)$$

To determine the bias that can occur in Eq. (10.5.4), assume that members of stratum B have no risk of disease and also have no exposure, that is, $p_B = p_{B|E} = e_B = 0$. With this assumption, Eq. (10.5.4) reduces to

$$R_{SB} = \frac{p_{A|E}}{p_A} \cdot \left[1 + \frac{s_B}{s_A(1 - e_A)}\right]. \qquad (10.5.5)$$

Since $s_B > s_A$ and the second term in the right side of Eq. (10.5.5) is much greater than 1, the odds ratio R_{SB} of Eq. (10.5.5) will falsely be elevated than the true relative risk $p_{A|E}/p_A$.

Remarks

1. Susceptibility bias can be managed under the following two situations: (i) the susceptibility factor is known, or (ii) if such factors are not known, then we need to know the reason why the agent is prescribed in the people who were exposed to it. Very often, this reason will point out the characteristic (such as bleeding, pain, etc.) of the clinical stratum to which the patient belonged at the time of prescription. Based upon this information, the investigator can stratify the cases and controls appropriately, and calculated the odds ratio separately for each stratum.
2. An example was given in Ref. 23 to illustrate the role of clinical susceptibility in the relationship of post-menopausal endometrial cancer.

C. The Protopathic Bias

The protopathic bias occurs if a pharmaceutic agent is inadvertently prescribed for an early manifestation of a disease that has not yet been diagnostically detected. When the disease is later discovered, it may then be fallaciously associated with the pharmaceutical agent.

Let p_1 and p_2 be the disease rate in patients with the respective rates of exposure and non-exposure being e_1 and $1 - e_1$. Among non-exposed cases, an additional exposure, e_2, takes place when the disease occurs. Thus, an additional increment, e_2, of the previously non-exposed cases becomes exposed, leaving $(1 - e_1)(1 - e_2)p_2$ as the non-exposed cases. A 2×2 table for this case-control study is then given by

Table 10.5-2D.   The distribution of exposed and nonexposed as far as the protopathic bias is concerned

	Cases	Controls
Exposed	$e_1 p_1 + e_2(1 - e_1)p_2$	$e_1(1 - p_1)$
Non-exposed	$(1 - e_1)(1 - e_2)p_2$	$(1 - e_1)(1 - p_2)$

Under the rare disease assumption, the odds ratio for Table 10.5-2D is

$$R_{PB} = \frac{[e_1 p_1 + e_2(1 - e_1)p_2](1 - e_1)(1 - p_2)}{e_1(1 - p_1)(1 - e_1)(1 - e_2)p_2}$$

$$= \frac{e_1 p_1 + e_2 p_2 - e_1 e_2 p_2}{e_1 p_2 - e_1 e_2 p_2}. \tag{10.5.6}$$

Since all the e_i and p_i terms are less than one, the term $e_1 e_2 p_2$ is substantially smaller than the terms in $e_i p_j$. If the $e_1 e_2 p_2$ term is regarded negligible, Eq. (10.5.6) reduces to

$$R_{PB} = \frac{p_1}{p_2} + \frac{e_2}{e_1}. \tag{10.5.7}$$

Remarks

1. Equation (10.5.7) shows that the true relative risk, p_1 / p_2, is elevated by an amount of e_2/e_1. If e_2 is relatively small compared to e_1, the bias may have only a minor effect on the results.

However, if e_2 is substantially larger than e_1, the true risk is much inflated.

2. An example dealing with the protopathic bias problem in a study of the estrogen-endometrial cancer relationship is given in Ref. 24.

10.6 Exercises

1. What is the effect of epidemiological transition on public health?
2. What is the issue of misclassification in case-control studies?
3. By using the log-odds-ratio test in Sec. 11.1B show that $\theta_{2\times2}^{(A)}$ and $\theta_{2\times2}^{(B)}$ are statistically significant.
4. What could be wrong in the argument for the empirical existence of Berkson's bias?

References

1. Austin H, Hill HA, Flanders WD, Greenberg RS. (1994) Limitations in the application of case-control methodology. *Epidemiol Rev* **16**: 65–76.
2. Bearman JE. (1975) Writing the protocol for a clinical trial. *Am J Ophthalmology* **79**: 775–778.
3. Berkson J. (1946) Limitations of the application of fourfold table to hospital data. *Biomet Bull* **2**: 47–53.
4. Brown GW. (1976) Berkson fallacy revisited. *Am J Dis Child* **130**: 56–60.
5. Comstock GW. (2001) Cohort analysis: W. H. Frost's Contribution to the epidemiology of tubercuolosis and chronic disease. *Soz.-Präventivmed* **46**: 7–12.
6. Delgado-Rodriguez M, Llorda J. (2004) Bias. *J Epidemiol Community Health* **58**: 635–641.
7. Dickson FG, Martin LW. (1956) Physician mortality, 1949–51. *J Am Med Asso* **162**: 1462–1468.
8. Dubin LI, Spiegelman M. (1947) The longevity and mortality of American physicians, 1938–1942. *J Am Med Asso* **134**: 1211–1215.
9. Emerson H, Hughes HE. (1926) Death rates of male white physicians in the United States, by age and cause. *Am J Public Health* **16**: 1088–1093.
10. Feinstein AR, Horwitz RI. (1981) An algebraic analysis of biases due to exclusion, susceptibility, and protopathic prescription in case-control research. *J Chron Dis* **34**: 393–403.

11. Feinstein AR, Horwitz RI. (1982) Double standards, scientific methods, and epidemiologic research. *New Engl J Med* **307**: 1611–1617.
12. Fleiss JL, Levin B, Paik MC. (2003) *Statistical Methods for Rates and Proportions*, 3rd ed. Wiley, New York.
13. Freiman JA, Chalmers TC, Smith H, Kuebler RR. (1978) The importance of beta, the type II error and sample size in the design and interpretation of the randomized controlled trial: Survey of 71 "negative" trials. *New Engl J Med* **299**: 690–694.
14. Freireich EJ, Gehan E, Frei E III, *et al.* (1963) The effect of 6-mercaptopurine on the duration of steroid-induced remissions in acute leukemia: A model for evaluation of other potentially useful therapy. *Blood* **21**: 699–716.
15. Geller NL. (1984) Design of phase I and II clinical trials in cancer: A statistician's view. *Cancer Investigation* **2**: 483–491.
16. Gerhard T. (2008) Bias: Considerations for research practice. *Am J Health-Syst Pharm* **65**: 2159–2168.
17. Gore SM. (1981) Assessing clinical trials: Why randomize? *Br Med J* **282**: 1958–1960.
18. Jaffe HW, Bregman DJ, Selik RM. (1983) Acquired immune deficiency syndrome in the United States: The first 1,000 cases. *J Infec Dis* **148**: 339–345.
19. Heyman A, Wilkinson WE, Hurwitz BJ, *et al.* (1983) Alzheimer's disease: Genetic aspects and associated clinical disorders. *Ann Neurol* **14**: 507–515.
20. Heyman A, Wilkinson WE, Stafford JA, *et al.* (1984) Alzheimer's disease: A study of epidemiological aspects. *Ann Neurol* **15**: 335–341.
21. Hill AB. (1952) The clinical trial, *New Engl J Med.* **247**: 113–119.
22. Horwitz RI, Feinstein AR. (1979) Methodologic standards and contradictory results in case-control research. *Am Int Med* **66**: 556–564.
23. Horwitz RI, Feinstein AR. (1979) Analysis of clinical susceptibility bias in case-control studies: Analysis as illustrated by the menopausal syndrome and the risk of endometrial cancer. *Arch J Med* **139**: 1111–1113.
24. Horwitz RI, Feinstein AR. (1980) The problem of "protopathic bias" in case-control studies. *Am J Med* **68**: 255–258.
25. Lee T-S, Hui Q. (2013) Testing the assumption of non-differential misclassification in case-control studies. *J Mod Appl Stat Methods* **12**: 211–230.
26. Lewis JA. (1983) Clinical trials: Statistical developments of practical benefits to the pharmaceutical industry. *J R Statist Soc A* **146**: 362–377.
27. Lewis SC, Warlow CP. (2004) How to spot bias and other potential problems in randomized controlled trials. *J Neurol Neurosurg Psychiatry* **75**: 181–187.
28. Maclure M, Schneeweiss S. (2001) Causation of bias: The episcope. *Epidemiology* **12**: 114–122.

29. Marshall G, Blacklock JWS, Hill AB, *et al.* (1948) Streptomycin treatment of pulmonary tuberculosis. *Br Med J* **2**: 769–782.
30. Oswald N. (1979) Tuberculosis. *Br Med J* **2**: 188–189.
31. Roberts R, Spitzer WO, Delmore T, Sackett DL. (1978) An empirical demonstration of Berkson's bias. *J Chron Dis* **31**: 119–128.
32. Sackett DL. (1979) Bias in analytic research. *J Chron Dis* **32**: 51–63.
33. Sanchez C, Lee T-S, Young S, *et al.* (2009) Risk factors for mortality during 2002 landslides in the State of Chuuk, Federated States of Micronesia. *Disasters* **33**: 705–720.
34. Schulz KF, Altman DG, Moher D for the CONSORT Group. (2010) CONSORT 2010 statement: Updated guidelines for reporting parallel group randomized trials. *PLOSmedicine* **7**: 1–7.
35. Sritara P, Cheepudomwit S, Woodward M, *et al.* (2003) Twelve-year changes in vascular risk factors and their associations with mortality in a cohort of 3499 Thais: The Electricity Generating Authority of Thailand Study. *Int J Epidemiol* **32**: 461–468.
36. Vineis P, McMichael AJ. (1998) Bias and confounding in molecular epidemiological studies: Special considerations. *Carcinogenesis* **19**: 2063–2067.
37. Waksman SA, Schatz A. (1945) Streptomycin: Origin, nature, and properties. *J Am Pharmaceut Asso* **34**: 273–291.
38. Walter SD. (1980) Berkson's bias and its control in epidemiologic studies. *J Chron Dis* **33**: 721–725.
39. Williams SV, Munford RS, Colton T, *et al.* (1971) Mortality among physicians: A cohort study. *J Chron Dis* **24**: 393–401.
40. Yang W, Lu J, Weng J, *et al.* (2010) Prevalence of diabetes among men and women in China. *New Engl J Med* **362**: 1090–1101.

11 Inference for Contingency Tables

Contingency (or cross-classification) tables are useful for the classification of two or more categorical random variables. Section 11.1 investigates the properties of 2×2 tables. Section 11.2 studies two-way ($I \times J$) tables. Section 11.3 describes three-way ($I \times J \times K$) tables. Incidentally, a bibliography of contingency table literature is given in Ref. 31.

11.1 2×2 Contingency Tables

A. *Pearson's Chi-squared Test on Independence*

Let X and Y be two dichotomous random variables. Suppose that the sample data of size n is randomly collected with respect to X and Y and are jointly cross-classified as given in the following form

Table 11.1A-1. The sample data of a 2 × 2 table

		Categories of Y		
		1	2	Row Total
Categories of X	1	n_{11}	n_{12}	n_{1+}
	2	n_{21}	n_{22}	n_{2+}
Column total		n_{+1}	n_{+2}	n

where $n_{i+} = \sum_{j=1}^{2} n_{ij}$, $n_{+j} = \sum_{i=1}^{2} n_{ij}$, and $n = \sum_{i=1}^{2} \sum_{j=1}^{2} n_{ij} = \sum_{i=1}^{2} n_{i+} = \sum_{j=1}^{2} n_{+j}$, $n_{ij} \geq 0$ for $i, j = 1, 2$.

Assume that the observed cell frequency $\{n_{ij}\}_{i,j=1}^2$ follow a multinomial distribution with the population parameters n being fixed and $\{p_{ij}\}_{i,j=1}^2$, where $m_{ij} \equiv E(n_{ij}) = np_{ij}$. Furthermore, the maximum likelihood estimator of p_{ij} is given by

$$\hat{p}_{ij} = n_{ij}/n. \tag{11.1A.1}$$

Consequently, the maximum likelihood estimator of m_{ij} is given by

$$\hat{m}_{ij} = n\hat{p}_{ij}, \tag{11.1A.2}$$

where $\hat{p}_{ij}$ is given by Eq. (11.1A.1).

To test whether X is independent of Y, we need to test the following pair of hypotheses:

$$H_0 : p_{ij} = p_{i+}p_{+j} \quad \text{versus} \quad H_1 : p_{ij} \neq p_{i+}p_{+j}, \tag{11.1A.3}$$

where $p_{i+} = \sum_{j=1}^2 p_{ij}$, and $p_{+j} = \sum_{i=1}^2 p_{ij}$. To test Eq. (11.1A.3), we use the Pearson chi-squared statistic given by

$$\chi_{\text{Pearson}} = \sum \frac{(\text{observed} - \text{expected})^2}{\text{expected}} = \sum_{i=1}^2 \sum_{j=1}^2 \frac{(n_{ij} - \hat{m}_{ij})^2}{\hat{m}_{ij}}$$

$$= n \left(\sum_{i=1}^2 \sum_{j=1}^2 \frac{n_{ij}^2}{n_{i+}n_{+j}} - 1 \right), \tag{11.1A.4}$$

where n_{i+} and n_{+j} are given in Table 11.1A-1. It can be shown that the sampling distribution of Eq. (11.1A.4) is a chi-squared distribution with one degree of freedom.[48]

The decision rule for testing Eq. (11.1A.3) is given as follows.

Decision Rule 11.1A-1 (Pearson's test on independence for 2 × 2 tables)

A two-tailed test for Eq. (11.1A.3) is to reject H_0 if the computed χ_{Pearson} of Eq. (11.1A.4) is greater than $\chi_{1;1-\frac{\alpha}{2}}^2$ or less than $\chi_{1;\frac{\alpha}{2}}^2$, where α is the level of significance.

Remarks

1. For a historical background on the use of cross classification to summarize counted data, see Sec. 1.3 in Ref. 19.
2. This test works only when the sample size is sufficiently large. When the sample size n is small, say < 5, it does not work because the chi-squared distribution of Eq. (11.1A.4) is only approximate and no longer valid. We need to use Fisher's exact test (see Sec. 11.1C) instead.
3. Equation (11.1A.4) is actually a special case of Eq. (11.2A.4) when $i = j = 2$. Also, see my remark below DR 11.2A.

Example 11.1A-1

Table 11.1A-2 is taken from Table 10.5-1A, in which X denotes whether a subject has cholecystitis (X = 1 if "Yes", X = 2 if "No"), and Y denotes whether a subject has diabetes (Y = 1 if "Yes", Y = 2 if "No").

Test if X and Y are independent at the significance level of 0.05.

Solution

From Table 11.1A-2,

$$n_{11} = 28, \quad n_{12} = 1{,}326, \quad n_{21} = 548, \quad n_{22} = 39{,}036, \quad n_{1+} = 1{,}354,$$

$$n_{2+} = 39{,}584, \quad n_{+1} = 576, \quad n_{+2} = 40{,}362, \quad \text{and} \quad n = 40{,}938.$$

$$(1)$$

Table 11.1A-2.   The sample data of cholecystitis (X) and diabetes (Y)

		Categories of Y		
		1	2	Row Total
Categories of X	1	28	1,326	1,354
	2	548	39,036	39,584
Column total		576	40,362	40,938

By substituting Eq. (1) into Eq. (11.1A.4),

$$\chi_{\text{Pearson}} = 40,938 \left(\frac{28^2}{1354 \cdot 576} + \frac{1326^2}{1354 \cdot 40362} + \frac{548^2}{39584 \cdot 1354} \right.$$

$$\left. + \frac{39036^2}{39584 \cdot 40362} - 1 \right) = 4.4097 \approx 4.41. \tag{2}$$

Since the computed χ_{Pearson} of Eq. (2) is not greater than $\chi^2_{1;0.975} = 5.024$, H_0 of Eq. (11.1A.1) is not rejected at the level of significance 0.05. Hence, whether a patient has cholecystitis or diabetes is independent.

Remarks

1. If the level of significance is chosen as 0.1, the computed χ_{Pearson} of Eq. (2) is greater than $\chi^2_{1;0.095} = 3.841$. It results in a decision to reject H_0 of Eq. (11.1A.1).
2. A lesson for an investigator is that he/she should not apply his/her decision in a mechanical way. Rather, he/she should base his/her professional judgment on the attained significance level of the computed statistic through a thorough understanding on all possible scenarios, or he/she should collect more data to settle the issue.

B. The Log-Odds-Ratio Test on First-Order Interaction

Let the joint distribution of two dichotomous random variables X and Y with the cell probabilities $\{p_{ij}\}$, $i, j = 1,2$, where $p_{ij} = \Pr(X = i, Y = j)$. The odds in the ith row of X is given by $odd_i = p_{i1}/p_{i2}$. The population odds ratio $\theta_{2\times2}$ for the joint distribution of X and Y is defined by

$$\theta_{2\times2} = \frac{odd_1}{odd_2} = \frac{p_{11}/p_{12}}{p_{21}/p_{22}} = \frac{p_{11}p_{22}}{p_{12}p_{21}}. \tag{11.1B.1}$$

In terms of Eq. (11.1B.1), the zero first-order interaction is defined as

Definition 11.1B.1. Two dichotomous random variables X and Y have a zero first-order (no two-factor) interaction if $\theta_{2\times2} = 1$, where $\theta_{2\times2}$ is given by Eq. (11.1B.1).

Remarks

1. If X and Y has a zero first-order (or no two-factor) interaction, it is equivalent to the independence of X and Y in Eq. (11.1A.3) (see Exercise 11.4-1).
2. If X and Y have a zero first-order interaction, it is said to be not associated between X and Y.[9]

To test whether two dichotomous random variables X and Y have a zero first-order interaction, we need to test the following pair of hypotheses:

$$H_0: \theta_{2\times2} = 1 \quad \text{versus} \quad H_1: \theta_{2\times2} \neq 1, \tag{11.1B.2}$$

where $\theta_{2\times2}$ is given by Eq. (11.1B.1).

By taking the natural logarithm of Eq. (11.1B.1), Eq. (11.1B.2) is equivalent to

$$H_0: \ln\theta_{2\times2} = 0 \quad \text{versus} \quad H_1: \ln\theta_{2\times2} \neq 0, \tag{11.1B.3}$$

where $\ln \equiv \log_e$ is the logarithmic function with base e.[35]

From the sample data collected in Table 11.1A-1, the population odds ratio of Eq. (11.1B.1) is estimated by the sample odds ratio given by

$$\hat{\theta}_{2\times2} = \frac{n_{11}n_{22}}{n_{12}n_{21}}. \tag{11.1B.4}$$

It can be shown that the estimated standard error of the logarithm of Eq. (11.1B.4) is given by[58]

$$\hat{\sigma}(\ln\hat{\theta}_{2\times2}) = \sqrt{n_{11}^{-1} + n_{12}^{-1} + n_{21}^{-1} + n_{22}^{-1}}. \tag{11.1B.5}$$

Remarks

1. Haldane[26] noticed that even though the logarithm of Eq. (11.1B.4) was an efficient estimate of $\ln\theta_{2\times2}$ in Eq. (11.1B.3), it had a bias that was not always negligible. He suggested to add $\frac{1}{2}$ to every cell entry in $\ln\hat{\theta}_{2\times2}$ to reduce the bias, namely, using

$$\ln\hat{\theta}^*_{2\times2} = \ln\left[\frac{\left(n_{11}+\frac{1}{2}\right)\left(n_{22}+\frac{1}{2}\right)}{\left(n_{12}+\frac{1}{2}\right)\left(n_{21}+\frac{1}{2}\right)}\right]. \qquad (11.1B.4^*)$$

and

$$\hat{\sigma}(\ln\hat{\theta}^*_{2\times2})$$

$$= \sqrt{\left(n_{11}+\frac{1}{2}\right)^{-1}+\left(n_{12}+\frac{1}{2}\right)^{-1}+\left(n_{21}+\frac{1}{2}\right)^{-1}+\left(n_{22}+\frac{1}{2}\right)^{-1}}. \qquad (11.1B.5^*)$$

2. Equations (11.1B.4*) and (11.1B.5*) are used by Fleiss *et al.*[22] But, for convenience, I will still use Eqs. (11.1B.4) and (11.1B.5) in this book.

A testing statistic for testing Eq. (11.1B.3) is given by

$$\chi_{OR} = [\ln\hat{\theta}_{2\times2}/\hat{\sigma}(\ln\hat{\theta}_{2\times2})]^2, \qquad (11.1B.6)$$

where $\hat{\theta}_{2\times2}$ and $\hat{\sigma}(\ln\hat{\theta}_{2\times2})$ are given by Eqs. (11.1B.4) and (11.1B.5), respectively. It can be shown[58] that the asymptotic sampling distribution of Eq. (11.1B.6) is a chi-squared distribution with one degree of freedom. A test for Eq. (11.1B.3) is thus given as follows.

Decision Rule 11.1B-1 (The log-odds-ratio test on first-order interaction for 2 × 2 tables)
A two-tailed test for Eq. (11.1B.3) is to reject H_0 at the level of significance α if the computed χ_{OR} of Eq. (11.1B.6) is greater than $\chi^2_{1;1-\frac{\alpha}{2}}$ or less than $\chi^2_{1;\frac{\alpha}{2}}$.

Remarks

1. If one of X and Y is a factor variable and the other is a response variable like the exposure factor and the disease variable in a case- control study, this test has an epidemiologic interpretation on the issue if there is an association between X and Y.
2. The zero first-order interaction for the general $I \times J$ tables will be covered in Sec. 11.2B.

To find the $100(1-\alpha)\%$ confidence interval for $\theta_{2\times2}$ is not trivial. The usual way is to find the confidence interval for $\ln\theta_{2\times2}$ first and then take the anti-logarithm operation to get back to the confidence interval for $\theta_{2\times2}$. The $100(1-\alpha)\%$ confidence interval for $\theta_{2\times2}$ is given as follows:

$$\exp[\ln\hat{\theta}_{2\times2} - z_{1-\frac{\alpha}{2}}\hat{\sigma}(\ln\hat{\theta}_{2\times2})] \leq \theta_{2\times2} \leq \exp[(\ln\hat{\theta}_{2\times2} + z_{1-\frac{\alpha}{2}}(\ln\hat{\theta}_{2\times2})].$$

$$(11.1B.7)$$

where $\hat{\sigma}(\ln\hat{\theta}_{2\times2})$ is given by Eq. (11.1B.5).

Remark

There are other more accurate ways to find the confidence interval for $\theta_{2\times2}$.[21] For example, a modification of Eq. (11.1B.7) proposed by O. Miettinen[42] is

$$\exp\left[\ln\hat{\theta}_{2\times2}\left(1 - \frac{z_{1-\frac{\alpha}{2}}}{\sqrt{\chi_{\text{Pearson}}}}\right)\right]$$

$$\leq \theta_{2\times2} \leq \exp\left[\ln\hat{\theta}_{2\times2}\left(1 + \frac{z_{1-\frac{\alpha}{2}}}{\sqrt{\chi_{\text{Pearson}}}}\right)\right].$$

$$(11.1B.8)$$

where χ_{Pearson} is defined by Eq. (11.1A.4).

Example 11.1B-1

(a) Test at the level of significance 0.05 if two random variables X and Y in Table 11.1A-2 have a zero first-order interaction.
(b) Find the 95% confidence interval for $\theta_{2\times2}$.

Solution

(a) From Table 11.1A-2,

$$n_{11} = 28 \quad n_{12} = 1,326, \quad n_{21} = 548 \quad n_{22} = 39,036. \tag{1}$$

By substituting Eq. (1) into Eq. (11.1B.4),

$$\hat{\theta}_{2 \times 2} = (28 \cdot 39,036)/(1,326 \cdot 548) = 1.504178 \approx 1.5042. \tag{2}$$

By substituting Eq. (1) into Eq. (11.1B.5),

$$\hat{\sigma}_{\ln \hat{\theta}_{2 \times 2}} = \sqrt{28^{-1} + 1326^{-1} + 548^{-1} + 39036^{-1}} \approx 0.1958. \tag{3}$$

By substituting Eqs. (2) and (3) into Eq. (11.1B.6),

$$\chi_{OR} = \left[\frac{\ln(1.5042)}{0.1958} \right]^2 = 2.08509^2 \approx 4.348. \tag{4}$$

Since the computed χ_{OR} of Eq. (4) is neither greater than $\chi^2_{1;0.975} = 5.024$ nor less than $\chi^2_{1;0.025} = 0.001$, H_0 of Eq. (11.1B.3) is not rejected at the level of significance 0.05. Hence, whether a patient has cholecystitis or diabetes has a zero first-order interaction.

(b) By substituting Eqs. (2) and (3) and $z_{0.975} = 1.96$ into Eq. (11.1B.7), the 95% confidence interval for $\theta_{2 \times 2}$ is

$$[\exp(\ln 1.5042 - 1.96 \cdot 0.1958), \exp(\ln 1.5042 + 1.96 \cdot 0.1958)]$$

$$= [1.025, 2.208]. \tag{5}$$

The 95% confidence interval of Eq. (5) indicates that the estimated odds ratio is greater than one.

Remarks

1. The confidence interval obtained from (b) somewhat contradicts the result in (a). This is probably attributed to the fact that Eq. (11.1B.7) is only an approximation.
2. Compare this result with that of using Eq. (11.1B.8) (see Exercise 11.4-2).

C.   *Fisher–Irwin's (Exact Conditional) Test*

If the expected cell count is less than 5, the Pearson's chi-squared test is not strictly applicable to test the independence of X and Y in Table 11.1A-1. We need to use Fisher's exact test.

Assume that the marginal row/column totals are fixed, out of the four random variables (r.v.s) $\{n_{ij}\}$, $i, j = 1, 2$ only one is independent. Without loss of generality, we designate n_{11} as this independent random variable. It can be shown that the conditional sampling distribution of n_{11}, given that the marginal row/column totals n_{i+} and n_{+j} are fixed, is a hypergeometric distribution that is given by[20]:

$$\Pr(n_{11} = x_{11}) = \frac{\dbinom{n_{1+}}{x_{11}}\dbinom{n_{2+}}{x_{+1} - x_{11}}}{\dbinom{n}{n_{+1}}}$$

$$= \frac{n_{+1}!\,n_{1+}!\,n_{+2}!\,n_{2+}!}{n!\,x_{11}!\,x_{12}!\,x_{21}!\,x_{22}!}, \quad n_- \le x_{11} \le n_+, \qquad (11.1C.1)$$

where $n_- = \max(0, n_{+1} - n_{2+})$, $n_+ = \min(n_{1+}, n_{+1})$, x_{11} is an integer, $x_{12} = n_{1+} - x_{11}$, $x_{21} = n_{+1} - x_{11}$, and $x_{22} = n_{2+} - n_{+1} + x_{11}$.

As shown in Exercise 11.4-1, independence is equivalent to the zero first-order interaction. For a two-tailed test on Eq. (11.1B.2), the p-value of the observed table is the sum of the hypergeometric probabilities of all tables that are more extreme than the observed one in either the upper or lower tails of the probability distribution.[23] Thus, the p-value of the Fisher–Irwin's test[28] of the observed table is given by

$$\sum_{x=n_-}^{n_+} \{\Pr(n_{11} = x) | \Pr(n_{11} = x) \le \Pr(n_{11} = x_{11})\}, \qquad (11.1C.2)$$

where $\Pr(n_{11} = x)$ is given by Eq. (11.1C.1).

Remarks

1. Since it is required that $\Pr(n_{11} = x) \le \Pr(n_{11} = x_{11})$, whether the x-values should be included in Eq. (11.1C.2) are those in the vicinity of either n_- or n_+.
2. Cormack and Mantel[12] used the experimental method to show that the model of fixed marginal totals was making more sense than the margins floating model.
3. Due to the discrete nature of the hypergeometric distribution, Fisher–Irwin's p-value is almost impossible to attain exactly the nominal significance level α. To compensate for this deficiency, the mid-p value given by

$$2\left[\frac{1}{2}\Pr(n_{11} = x_{11}) + \Pr(n_{11} < x_{11})\right], \quad \text{if } x_{11} < \frac{1}{2}(n_- + n_+),$$

$$(11.1C.3)$$

or

$$2\left[\frac{1}{2}\Pr(n_{11} = x_{11}) + \Pr(n_{11} > x_{11})\right], \quad \text{if } x_{11} > \frac{1}{2}(n_- + n_+),$$

is proposed to replace the usual p-value.[33]

A small-sample test for Eq. (11.1B.2) is given by the following decision rule.

Decision Rule 11.1C-1 (Fisher–Irwin's test)

Reject H_0 in Eq. (11.1B.2) if the p-value of the observed table of Eq. (11.1C.2) is less than the level of significance α. Otherwise, do not reject H_0.

Example 11.1C-1

By using the third table in Table 10.3-2B given by

Table 11.1C-1. The sample data of the structure of roof as an exposure factor in a case-control study

		Deaths	Controls	Row Total
Roof	**Concrete**	1	5	6
	Tin, Wood	21	15	36
Column Total		22	20	42

Since the observed value of of the random variable n_{11} is 1, test whether the structure of the roof is associated with landslide deaths by using Fisher–Irwin's exact test.

Solution

From Table 11.1C-1, we have

$$n_- = \max(0, 6 + 22 - 42) = \max(0, -14) = 0,$$

and

$$n_+ = \min(6, 22) = 6.$$

The possible range for x is $\{0, 1, 2, 3, 4, 5, 6\}$. Since $x_{11} = 1$, the possible extreme cases for x that need to be considered are $x = 0, 1, 5$ or 6. After calculation $x = 5$ is excluded from being used in Eq. (11.1C.2) because $\Pr(n_{11} = 5)$ is not less than $\Pr(n_{11} = 1)$ (see Exercise 11.4-3). Consequently, the p-value of the observed table is given by using Eq. (11.1C.2)

$$
\begin{aligned}
\sum_{x=0}^{1,6} \Pr(n_{11} = x) &= \Pr(n_{11} = 0) + \Pr(n_{11} = 1) + \Pr(n_{11} = 6) \\
&= \frac{6! \cdot 36! \cdot 22! \cdot 20!}{42! \cdot 0! \cdot 6! \cdot 22! \cdot 14!} + \frac{6! \cdot 36! \cdot 22! \cdot 20!}{42! \cdot 1! \cdot 5! \cdot 21! \cdot 15!} \\
&\quad + \frac{6! \cdot 36! \cdot 22! \cdot 20!}{42! \cdot 6! \cdot 0! \cdot 16! \cdot 20!} \\
&= \frac{9 \cdot 17 \cdot 4 \cdot 5}{7 \cdot 41 \cdot 39 \cdot 37} + \frac{22 \cdot 18 \cdot 17 \cdot 4}{7 \cdot 41 \cdot 39 \cdot 37} + \frac{11 \cdot 9 \cdot 17}{2 \cdot 41 \cdot 39 \cdot 37} \\
&= \frac{3,060}{414,141} + \frac{26,928}{414,141} + \frac{1,683}{118,326} \\
&= 0.00739 + 0.06502 + 0.01422 = 0.08639
\end{aligned}
$$

Since the p-value of the observed table is greater than 0.05, H_0 is not rejected at the level of significance 0.05. Hence, the landslide's death is not associated with the structure of the roof of the house.

Remarks

1. Since $n_{+1} = 22 \neq n_{+2} = 20$, this is an asymmetric case. Hence we need to calculate plausible probabilities from both tails to obtain the p-value.
2. By using Eq. (11.1C.3), the mid-p value is obtained as $2 \cdot (0.00739 + \frac{1}{2}0.06502) = 0.0798$.

If the alternative hypothesis in Eq. (11.1B.2) is replaced by $H_1^* : \theta_{2 \times 2} > 1$, the conditional distribution of n_{11} under H_1^*, given that n_{+1} is fixed,[20] is the non-central hypergeometric distribution given by

$$\Pr(n_{11} = x_{11}|\theta_{2 \times 2}) = \frac{\dbinom{n_{1+}}{x_{11}}\dbinom{n_{2+}}{n_{+1} - x_{11}}\theta_{2 \times 2}^{x_{11}}}{\displaystyle\sum_{x=n_-}^{n_+}\dbinom{n_{1+}}{x}\dbinom{n_{2+}}{n_{+1} - x}\theta_{2 \times 2}^{x}}, \qquad (11.1C.4)$$

where n_- and n_+ are the same as those given in Eq. (11.1C.1).

Let x_α be the critical value of n_{11} for the exact test of H_0 versus H_1^* at the level of significance α, that is,

$$\sum_{x=x_\alpha}^{n_+} \Pr(n_{11} = x|\theta_{2 \times 2} = 1) \leq \alpha$$

$$\text{and} \quad \sum_{x=x_\alpha - 1}^{n_+} \Pr(n_{11} = x|\theta_{2 \times 2} = 1) > \alpha,$$

the conditional power is thus given by

$$\beta(\theta_{2 \times 2}|n_{+1}) = \sum_{x=x_\alpha}^{n_+} \Pr(n_{11} = x|\theta_{2 \times 2}). \qquad (11.1C.5)$$

Similarly, if the two-tailed alternative hypothesis H_1 in Eq. (11.1B.4) is replaced by $H_1^{**} : \theta_{2 \times 2} < 1$, the conditional power under H_1^{**} is given by

$$\beta(\theta_{2\times2}|n_{+1}) = \sum_{x=n_-}^{x_\alpha^*} \Pr(n_{11} = x|\theta_{2\times2}), \qquad (11.1C.6)$$

where x_α^* is the critical value of n_{11} for the exact test of H_0 versus H_1^{**} at the level of significance α, that is,

$$\sum_{x=n_-}^{x_\alpha^*} \Pr(n_{11} = x|\theta_{2\times2} = 1) \le \alpha$$

$$\text{and} \quad \sum_{x=n_-}^{x_\alpha^*+1} \Pr(n_{11} = x|\theta_{2\times2} = 1) > \alpha.$$

Example 11.1C-2

By using Table 11.1C-1 in Example 11.1C-1, compute the conditional power at the significance level $\alpha = 0.05$ under $H_1^{**} : \theta_{2\times2} < 1$ for the sample estimate of the odds ratio.

Solution

The sample odds ratio for Table 11.1C-1 is obtained as follows:

$$\hat{\theta}_{2\times2} = (1 \cdot 15)/(5 \cdot 21) = 1/7 \approx 0.143.$$

The critical value is obtained as $x_{0.05}^* = 0$. By using Eq. (11.1C.6) with $n_- = 0$, $x_{0.05}^* = 0$, and $\theta_{2\times2} = \hat{\theta}_{2\times2} = 0.143$, we have

$$\beta(0.143|n_{+1} = 22) = \frac{\binom{6}{1}\binom{36}{22-1}0.143^1}{\sum_{x=0}^{6}\binom{6}{x}\binom{36}{22-x}0.143^x}$$

$$= 0.419853 \approx 0.42.$$

The conditional power at the significance level 0.05 under $H_1^{**} : \theta_{2\times2} < 1$ for the sample estimate of the odds ratio is 0.42.

Remark

The calculation of the conditional power is facilitated by using the combinatorial formula "COMBIN" available in the EXCEL spreadsheet.

D. McNemar's Test for Two Correlated Variables

There are many situations in which the two proportions are not based on independent samples. For example, p_1 may represent the proportion passing one test item while p_2 is another proportion of the same group passing a second item, and we wonder whether the items differ significantly in difficulty or the significance of the difference between the responses of a group of voters who approve or disapprove before and after a President's decision on a certain political issue.

Let X_A and X_B be two dichomous random variables (= 1 if favorable, = 2 otherwise) before and after tasting an ice cream of a certain brand. Assume that a random sample of voters of size n is randomly selected from customers who purchased it. Individual subjects are assessed with respect to their opinion on the flavor of this ice cream. The sample data are given in the following table.

Assume that the sample data $\{n_{ij}\}_{i,j=1}^2$ follow the multinomial distribution with the population parameters $\{p_{ij}\}_{i,j=1}^2$ and n, where $p_{ij} = \Pr[(X_A = i) \cap (X_B = j)]$, $i, j = 1, 2$. Let $p_A = \Pr(X_A = 1)$ and $p_B = \Pr(X_B = 1)$. For the correlated proportions, we would like

Table 11.1D-1. The sample data of before (X_A) and after (X_B) tasting ice cream

	$X_B = 1$	$X_B = 2$	Row Total
$X_A = 1$	n_{11}	n_{12}	n_{1+}
$X_A = 2$	n_{21}	n_{22}	n_{2+}
Column Total	n_{+1}	n_{+2}	n

where $n_{i+} = \sum_{j=1}^2 n_{ij}$, $n_{+j} = \sum_{i=1}^2 n_{ij}$, and $n = \sum_{i=1}^2 \sum_{j=1}^2 n_{ij} = \sum_{i=1}^2 n_{i+} = \sum_{j=1}^2 n_{+j}$, $n_{ij} > 0$ if $i \neq j$.

to test whether the difference between p_A and p_B is significantly nonzero, that is, we wish to test the margin homogeneity

$$H_0: p_A = p_B \quad \text{versus} \quad H_1: P_A \neq P_B. \tag{11.1D.1}$$

Since $p_A = p_{11} + p_{12}$ and $p_B = p_{11} + p_{21}$ (see Exercise 11.4-4), Eq. (11.1D.1) is equivalent to test the hypothesis of symmetry

$$H_0: p_{12} = p_{21} \quad \text{versus} \quad H_1: p_{12} \neq p_{21}. \tag{11.1D.2}$$

By setting $\delta = p_{12} - p_{21}$, Eq. (11.1D.2) is rewritten as

$$H_0: \delta = 0 \quad \text{versus} \quad H_1: \delta \neq 0. \tag{11.1D.3}$$

The sample estimate of δ is given by

$$\hat{\delta} = \hat{p}_{12} - \hat{p}_{21} = \frac{n_{12}}{n} - \frac{n_{21}}{n} = \frac{n_{12} - n_{21}}{n}. \tag{11.1D.4}$$

By applying the property of the multinomial distribution, the variance of $\hat{\delta}$ is given by (see Exercise 11.4-5):

$$\sigma^2(\hat{\delta}) = n^{-1}[(p_{12} + p_{21}) - (p_{12} - p_{21})^2]. \tag{11.1D.5}$$

The estimated standard error of $\hat{\delta}$ under H_0 is given by:

$$\hat{\sigma}(\hat{\delta}) = n^{-1}\sqrt{n_{12} + n_{21}}. \tag{11.1D.6}$$

The test statistic for Eq. (11.1D.2) is[39]

$$\chi_{McN} = z_{\hat{\delta}}^2 = \left[\frac{\hat{\delta}}{\hat{\sigma}(\hat{\delta})}\right]^2 = \frac{(n_{12} - n_{21})^2}{(n_{12} + n_{21})}. \tag{11.1D.7}$$

It can be shown[39] that the sampling distribution of Eq. (11.1D.7) is a chi-squared distribution with one degree of freedom.

Based on Eq. (11.1D.7), the decision rule for testing Eq. (11.1D.3) is given as follows:

Decision Rule 11.1D-1 (McNemar's test for two correlated variables)

Reject H_0 at the level of significance α if the computed χ_{McN} of Eq. (11.1D.7) is greater than $\chi_{1;1-\frac{\alpha}{2}}^2$ or less than $\chi_{1;\frac{\alpha}{2}}^2$. Otherwise, do not reject H_0.

Remarks

1. By adjusting for the continuity correction (See Refs. 16 and 60), Eq. (11.1D.7) is modified to become

$$\chi^*_{McN} = Z^2_{\hat{\delta}} = \left[\frac{|\hat{\delta}| - \frac{1}{n}}{\hat{\sigma}(\hat{\delta})} \right]^2 = \frac{(|n_{12} - n_{21}|)^2}{n_{12} + n_{21}}. \qquad (11.1D.8)$$

2. Incidentally, if we consider using the ratio in Eq. (11.1D.2) by letting $\varphi = p_{12}/p_{21}$ rather than the difference δ and wish to test

$$H_0 : \varphi = 1 \quad \text{versus} \quad H_1 : \varphi \neq 1, \qquad (11.1D.9)$$

the test for Eq. (11.1D.9) ends up exactly in the same form as Eq. (11.1E.14), provided that the maximum likelihood estimation is used to estimate all the unknown parameters.

3. For a $I \times I$ table, where $I > 2$, the marginal homogeneity is not equivalent to symmetry.[10]

Example 11.1D-1

Suppose that the same 100 patients have all been treated on two different occasions with the same dose for drug A and drug B.[45] The collected data could be mishandled in the following table

Table 11.1D-2.   The Data are Mishandled

	Nausea	Not-Nausea	Row Total
Drug A	18	82	100
Drug B	10	90	100
Column Total	28	172	200

The primary reason is that a subject experiencing nausea after being treated with drug A is likely to experience nausea with drug B and vice versa. Consequently, the data are correlated. The correct way is reclassification of the data using patients as the unit. This reclassification leads to the correct table (see Table 11.1.D-3).

Table 11.1.D-3.   The Data are Correctly Classified

		Drug B		
		Nausea	Not-Nausea	Row Total
Drug A	**Nausea**	9	9	18
	Not-Nausea	1	81	82
Column Total		10	90	100

By substituting $n_{12} = 9$ and $n_{21} = 1$ from Table 11.1.D-3 into Eq. (11.1D.7), we have

$$\chi_{McN} = \frac{(9-1)^2}{(9+1)} = 6.4.$$

Since the computed $\chi_{McN} = 6.4$ is greater than the critical value $\chi^2_{1;0.975} = 5.024$, H_0 is rejected at the significance level 0.05. The response of nausea for drug A and drug B is not the same.

Remarks

1. If the continuity correction formula for McNemar's test (Eq. 11.1D.8) is used, the computed χ^*_{McN} is

$$\chi^*_{McN} = \frac{(|9-1|-1)^2}{10} = 4.9.$$

   Since the computed $\chi^*_{McN} = 4.9$ is not greater than $\chi^2_{1;0.975} = 5.024$, but is greater than $\chi^2_{1;0.95} = 3.841$, H_0 is rejected at the significance level 0.05 when the alternative hypothsis is replaced by the one-sided hypothesis, $H_1 : \delta > 1$.
2. The second problem in Ref. 45 is involved with that of placebo relief in the comparative testing of two analgesics, aspirin and morphine/codeine. As a group, the results suggest strongly that placebo reactors do not differentiate well between aspirin and morphine/codine at the dosage used, but that the placebo non-reactors can differentiate the effect between the studied two analgesics.

E. *Ejigou–McHugh's Test for Matched-pair Data*

One-to-one matching is frequently used to increase the precision of a comparison. Let D denote the disease status with $D = 1$ if a subject has the disease; otherwise, $D = 0$. Suppose that a sample data of size n is collected from the population free of disease ($D = 0$: control) is matched on the covariate X that has K categories one-to-one to a random sample of size n taken from the population which has the disease ($D = 1$: case) and a certain risk factor A, where $A = 1$ if A is present, otherwise $A = 0$, and is given in Table 11.1E-1.

Assume that the sample data $\{a_{ij}\}_{i,j=0}^{1}$ follow the multinomial distribution with the population parameters $\{p_{ij}\}_{i,j=0}^{1}$ and n, where $p_{ij} = \sum_{k=1}^{K} \Pr[A = 1|D = i, X = k) \cap (A = 0|D = j, X = k)]$, $i, j = 0, 1$. For such a matched-pair design, it is natural to compare if the marginal proportion of the case population is the same as that of the control population, that is, $p_{i+} = p_{+i}$, $i = 1, 0$, called the hypothesis of margin homogeneity. Interestingly, the margin homogeneity is equivalent to symmetry because $p_{1+} = p_{+1}$ implies $p_{10} = p_{01}$. To test the hypothesis of margin homogeneity, we turn to test that of symmetry, that is,

$$H_0 : p_{10} = p_{01} \quad \text{versus } H_1 : p_{10} \neq p_{01}. \tag{11.1E.1}$$

Table 11.1E-1. The sample data of one-to-one mapping in a case-control study

		Control (D=0)		
		A = 1	A = 0	Row Total
Case (D=1)	A = 1	a_{11}	a_{10}	a_{1+}
	A = 0	a_{01}	a_{00}	a_{0+}
Column Total		a_{+1}	a_{+0}	n

where $n = \sum_{i=0}^{1}\sum_{j=0}^{1} a_{ij}$. Incidentally, a_{ii} and $a_{ij} = (i \neq j)$ $i, j = 0, 1$ are called the concordant and discordant observations. Note that the nature of Table 11.1E-1 is intrinsically different from that of Table 11.1D-1. Table 11.1D-1 involves two correlated random variables with n individual subjects, whereas Table 11.1E-1 is concerned with n pairs of matched data.

Now, for $i = 0, 1$, $k = 1, 2, \ldots, K$, let

$$c_{ik} = \Pr(A = 1 | D = i, \ X = k), \qquad (11.1\text{E}.2)$$

and

$$b_k = \Pr(X = k | D = 1). \qquad (11.1\text{E}.3)$$

As a consequence of the design, the conditional probabilities $\Pr(A | D = 1, X = k)$ and $\Pr(A | D = 0, X = k)$, given $X = k$ fixed, are independent. It follows that

$$p_{11} = \sum_{k=1}^{K} \Pr(A = 1 | D = 1, X = k) \Pr(A = 0 | D = 1, X = k)$$

$$\Pr(X = k | D = 1) \qquad (11.1\text{E}.4)$$

$$p_{10} = \sum_{K=1}^{K} \Pr(A = 1 | D = 1, X = k) \Pr(A = 0 | D = 0, X = k)$$

$$\Pr(X = k | D = 1) = \sum_{k=1}^{K} c_{1k}(1 - c_{0k}) b_k, \qquad (11.1\text{E}.5)$$

$$p_{01} = \sum_{k=1}^{K} \Pr(A = 1 | D = 0, X = k) \Pr(A = 0 | D = 1, X = k)$$

$$\Pr(X = k | D = 1) = \sum_{k=1}^{K} (1 - c_{1k}) c_{0k} b_k, \qquad (11.1\text{E}.6)$$

and

$$p_{00} = \sum_{k=1}^{K} \Pr(A = 1 | D = 0, X = k) \Pr(A = 0 | D = 0, X = k)$$

$$\Pr(X = k | D = 1) = \sum_{k=1}^{K} (1 - c_{1k})(1 - c_{0k}) b_k, \qquad (11.1\text{E}.7)$$

where c_{ik} and b_k are given by Eqs. (11.1E.2) and (11.1E.3), respectively. If the odds ratio

$$\psi_k \equiv \frac{c_{1k}(1 - c_{0k})}{(1 - c_{1k}) c_{0k}} \quad k = 1, 2, \ldots, K, \qquad (11.1\text{E}.8)$$

is constant over k, say equal to ψ, we have the common odds ratio ψ that can be obtained from Eqs. (11.1E.5) and (11.1E.6) as

$$\psi = p_{10}/p_{01}. \qquad (11.1E.9)$$

In terms of this common odds ratio, Eq. (11.1E.1) can be rewritten as

$$H_0 : \psi = 1 \quad \text{versus} \quad H_1 : \psi \neq 1. \qquad (11.1E.10)$$

The maximum likelihood estimator of Eq. (11.1E.9) (see Exercise 11.4-6) is given by

$$\hat{\psi} = a_{10}/a_{01}, \qquad (11.1E.11)$$

where a_{10} and a_{01} are the discordant observations given in Table 11.1E-1. The asymptomatic variance of Eq. (11.1E.11) is shown to be given by[17]

$$\sigma^2(\hat{\psi}) = n^{-1}\psi^2(p_{10}^{-1} + p_{01}^{-1}). \qquad (11.1E.12)$$

The estimated standard error of $\hat{\psi}$ is obtained from Eq. (11.1E.12)

$$\hat{\sigma}(\hat{\psi}) = \hat{\psi}\sqrt{a_{10}^{-1} + a_{01}^{-1}}. \qquad (11.1E.13)$$

where $\hat{\psi}$ is given by Eq. (11.1E.11).

The testing statistic for Eq. (11.1E.10) is given by

$$\chi_{EMc} = \left[\frac{\hat{\psi} - 1}{\hat{\sigma}(\hat{\psi})}\right]^2 = \frac{a_{01}(a_{10} - a_{01})^2}{a_{10}(a_{10} + a_{01})}. \qquad (11.1E.14)$$

It can be shown that the sampling distribution of Eq. (11.1E.14) is a chi-squared distribution with one degree of freedom. The decision rule for testing Eq. (11.1E.10) is given as follows.[17]

Decision Rule 11.1E-1 (Ejigou–McHugh's Test for 1-1 Matched samples)

Reject H_0 at the significance level α if the computed χ_{EMc} of Eq. (11.1E.14) is greater than $\chi^2_{1;1-\frac{\alpha}{2}}$ or less than $\chi^2_{1;\frac{\alpha}{2}}$. Otherwise, do not reject H_0.

Remarks

1. Equation (11.1E.14) only holds for one-to-one matched pair design. For an m-to-one design, where $m > 1$ (see Ref. 18).
2. If the sample size for the sum of discordant observations, namely, $n^* = n_{10} + n_{01}$, is small, a conditional test given n^* fixed can be used instead.[40]

Example 11.1E-1

A researcher wishes to test if the hypothesis that induced abortions increase the risk of tubal implantation in subsequent pregnancies is true.[41] Eighteen married women who had tubal pregnancies following at least one earlier pregnancy were matched individually to one married control woman each. The covariate used for matching was based on order and age of the case woman and degree of the husband's education. The history of induced abortion in cases with tubal pregnancy and matched controls are given in qualitative terms in Table 11.1E-2, where "+" means that a woman has induced abortion, otherwise it is denoted by "−".

Let the risk factor of having induced abortion be A in which $A = 1$ if a woman has an abortion, otherwise, $A = 0$. By collecting these information from Table 11.1E-2, the total numbers of (case, control) = $(+,+)$, $(+,-)$, $(-,+)$ and $(-, -)$ are given in Table 11.1E-3, respectively.

At the level of significance 0.05, test whether the hypothesis that an induced abortion has increased the risk of women having tubal implantation in a subsequent pregnancy is true.

Use Ejigou–McHugh's test (DR 11.1E-1) to test Eq. (11.1E.10) at the significance level 0.05.

Table 11.1E-2. The sample data of 18 women with the tubal implantation in a case-control study

	Subject								
	1	2	3	4	5	6	7	8	9
Case	−	+	+	−	−	+	+	−	+
Control	−	−	−	−	+	−	−	−	+

	Subject								
	10	11	12	13	14	15	16	17	18
Case	+	+	−	+	+	+	+	−	+
Control	−	−	−	+	−	−	+	−	+

Table 11.1E-3. The summarized data of Table 11.1E-2

		Control		
		A = 1	A = 0	Row Total
Case	A = 1	4	8	12
	A = 0	1	5	6
Column Total		5	13	18

Solution

By substituting $a_{10} = 8$ and $a_{01} = 1$ into Eq. (11.1E.14), the computed χ_{EMc} is

$$\chi_{EMc} = \frac{1 \cdot (8-1)^2}{8 \cdot (8+1)} = \frac{49}{72} \approx 0.68.$$

Since the computed $\chi_{EMc} = 0.68$ is neither greater than $\chi^2_{1;0.975} = 5.024$ nor less than $\chi^2_{1;0.025} = 0.001$, H_0 is not rejected at the significance level 0.05. Hence, the hypothesis that the history of induced abortion increases the risk of women having tubal implanation in a subsequent pregnancy is not true.

Remark

Table 11.1E-3 is adapted from Ref. 40 by using only the data from case and the first control group.

11.2   Two-Way Contingency Tables

This section is basically an extension of the result from 2×2 tables in Sec. 11.1 to a general case of $I \times J$ tables.

A.   *Pearson's Test on Independence*

Let X and Y be two unordered categorical random variables having I and J categories with the nominal data, respectively, where both I and J are greater than two. A random sample of size n is collected from a certain population and jointly cross-classified with respect to X and Y as given in Table 11.2A-1.

Assume that $\{n_{ij}\}$, $i = 1, \ldots, I$, $j = 1, \ldots, J$ in Table 11.2A-1, follow a multinomial distribution with the parameters n and $\{p_{ij}\}$, where $m_{ij} = E(n_{ij}) = n \cdot p_{ij}$. The maximum likelihood estimator of p_{ij} is given by

$$\hat{p}_{ij} = n_{ij}/n. \tag{12.2A.1}$$

Table 11.2A-1.   The sample data of two-way table for X and Y

		\multicolumn{4}{c}{**Categories of Y**}		
		1	**2**	$\cdots$	**J**	**Row Total**
Categories of X	1	n_{11}	n_{12}	$\cdots$	n_{1J}	n_{1+}
	2	n_{21}	n_{22}	$\cdots$	n_{2J}	n_{2+}
	$\vdots$	$\vdots$	$\vdots$	$\vdots$	$\vdots$	$\vdots$
	I	n_{I1}	n_{I2}	$\cdots$	n_{IJ}	n_{I+}
Column Total		n_{+1}	n_{+2}	$\cdots$	n_{+J}	n

where $n_{i+} = \sum_{j=1}^{J} n_{ij}$, $n_{+j} = \sum_{i=1}^{I} n_{ij}$, and $n = \sum_{i=1}^{I} n_{i+} = \sum_{j=1}^{J} n_{+j} = \sum_{i=1}^{I} \sum_{j=1}^{J} n_{ij}$.

Thus, the maximum likelihood estimator of m_{ij} is obtained as

$$\hat{m}_{ij} = n \cdot \hat{p}_{ij}, \tag{12.2A.2}$$

where $\hat{p}_{ij}$ is given by Eq. (12.2A.1).

To test if X is independent of Y in Table 12.2A-1, we need to test the following pair of hypotheses:

$$H_0 : p_{ij} = p_{i+} \cdot p_{+j} \quad \text{versus} \quad H_1 : p_{ij} \neq p_{i+} \cdot p_{+j}, \tag{12.2A.3}$$

where $p_{i+} = \sum_{j=1}^{J} p_{ij}$, and $p_{+j} = \sum_{i=1}^{I} p_{ij}$. To test Eq. (12.2A.3), we use Pearson's chi-squared statistics as follows:

$$\chi_{2-way} = \sum \frac{*(\text{observd-expected})^2}{\text{expected}} = \sum_{i=1}^{I} \sum_{j=1}^{J} \frac{(n_{ij} - \hat{m}_{ij})^2}{\hat{m}_{ij}}$$

$$= n \left(\sum_{i=1}^{I} \sum_{j=1}^{J} \frac{n_{ij}^2}{n_{i+} \cdot n_{+j}} \right). \tag{12.2A.4}$$

The decision rule is given below.

Decision Rule 11.2A-1 (Pearson's test on independence for two-way tables with the nominal data)

A two-tailed test for Eq. (11.2A.3) is to reject H_0 if the computed χ_{2-way} of Eq. (11.2A.4) is greater than $\chi^2_{(I-1)(J-1);1-\frac{\alpha}{2}}$ or less than $\chi^2_{(I-1)(J-1);\frac{\alpha}{2}}$, where α is the level of significance.

Remarks

1. Mirkin[43] presented eleven definitions of Eq. (11.2A.4) as either an independence/homogeneity test statistic or summary association measure for Table 11.2A-1.
2. SS Wilks[58] derived Eq. (11.2A.4) from using the likelihood ratio test.

Example 11.2A-1

The data in Table 11.2A-2 are taken from Yates,[61] in which they were obtained in the course of a pilot inquiry on how conditions

Table 11.2A-2. **The sample data of the grade given by two teachers X and Y on the quality of the students' homework**

		Y					
		1	2	3	4	5	Row Total
X	1	141	67	114	79	39	440
	2	131	66	143	72	35	447
	3	36	14	38	28	16	132
Column Totals		308	147	295	179	90	1019

affect schoolchildren doing their homework. Let X and Y denote the grade given by the teacher on the quality of their homework and the conditions that homeworks were carried out in, respectively. Note that X has three categories: X = 1 if the grade received was A, X = 2 if the grade was B, and X = 3 if the grade was C, while Y has five categories: Y = 1 if his/her homework condition was the best, Y = 2 if the condition was second-best, Y = 3 if the condition was ok, Y = 4 if the condition was bad, and Y = 5 if the condition was the worst.

Are the conditions under which homework was carried out and the teacher rating their homework independent?

Solution

By substituting $n_{11} = 141$, $n_{12} = 67$, $n_{13} = 114$, $n_{14} = 79$, $n_{15} = 39$, $n_{21} = 131$, $n_{22} = 66$, $n_{23} = 143$, $n_{24} = 72$, $n_{25} = 35$, $n_{31} = 36$, $n_{32} = 14$, $n_{33} = 38$, $n_{34} = 28$, $n_{35} = 16$, $n_{1+} = 440$, $n_{2+} = 447$, $n_{3+} = 132$, $n_{+1} = 308$, $n_{+2} = 147$, $n_{+3} = 295$, $n_{+4} = 179$, $n_{+5} = 90$ and $n = 1,019$ into Eq. (11.2A.4), we have

$$\chi_{2\text{-}way} = 1019 \left[\left(\frac{141^2}{440 \cdot 308} + \frac{67^2}{440 \cdot 147} + \frac{114^2}{440 \cdot 295} + \frac{79^2}{440 \cdot 179} \right. \right.$$

$$\left. + \frac{39^2}{440 \cdot 90} + \frac{131^2}{447 \cdot 308} + \frac{66^2}{447 \cdot 147} + \frac{143^2}{447 \cdot 295} \right.$$

$$+ \frac{72^2}{447 \cdot 179} + \frac{35^2}{447 \cdot 90} + \frac{36^2}{132 \cdot 308} + \frac{14^2}{132 \cdot 147}$$

$$+ \frac{38^2}{132 \cdot 295} + \frac{28^2}{132 \cdot 179} + \frac{16^2}{132 \cdot 90} \bigg) - 1 \bigg]$$

$$= 1{,}019(1.008923 - 1) = 9.0928 \approx 9.09. \tag{1}$$

Since the value of $\chi_{2\text{-}way}$ of Eq. (1) is not greater than the critical value of the chi-squared distribution with $8 (= (3-1)(5-1))$ degrees of freedom, $\chi^2_{8;0975} = 17.54$, H_0 of Eq. (11.2A.1) is not rejected at the level of significance 0.05. Hence, the homework condition and the grade received on the homework are independent.

Remark

Yates[61] pointed out that both X and Y had ordered categories. Yet, Pearson's test (DR 11.2A-1) did not take into account the information on the ordinal data. He was therefore proposing a trend test for incorporating this information, which is covered in Sec. 11.2C.

B. A Test on First-Order Interaction for Two-Way Tables

In this section we are going to generalize the odds ratio test for the first-order interaction for the general $I \times J$ tables, where both I and J are greater than two.

Definition 11.2B.1. Two categorical random variables X and Y given in Table 11.2A-1 are said to have a zero first-order (or no two-factor) interaction if $\theta^{ij}_{i^*j^*} = 1$ for all pairs (i, i^*) and (j, j^*) such that $i \neq i^*$ and $j \neq j^*$, where $\theta^{ij}_{i^*j^*}$ is defined by[33]:

$$\theta^{ij}_{i^*j^*} = \frac{p_{ij}\, p_{i^*j^*}}{p_{i^*j}\, p_{ij^*}}, \tag{11.2B.1}$$

where $\{p_{k\ell}\}$, $k = 1, 2, \ldots, I$ and $\ell = 1, 2, \ldots J$, are defined in Sec. 11.2A.

To test if X and Y has a zero first-order interaction, we need to test the following pair of hypothses that

$$H_0^{(XY)} : \theta_{i^*j^*}^{ij} = 1, \text{ for all pairs } (i, i^*) \text{ and } (j, j^*) \text{ such that } i \neq i^*$$

$$\text{and } j \neq j^*, \tag{11.2B.2}$$

versus

$$H_1^{(XY)} : \theta_{i^*j^*}^{ij} \neq 1, \text{ for at least one of the pairs } (i, i^*) \text{ and } (j, j^*)$$

such that

$$i \neq i^* \text{ and } j \neq j^*,$$

where $\theta_{i^*j^*}^{ij}$ is defined by Eq. (11.2B.1).

It has been shown that Table 11.2A-1 has $(I - 1)(J - 1)$ independent 2×2 tables. The maximum likelihood estimator of Eq. (11.2B.1) is

$$\hat{\theta}_{i^*j^*}^{ij} = \frac{n_{ij}n_{i^*j^*}}{n_{i^*j}n_{ij^*}}, \tag{11.2B.3}$$

where $\{n_{ij}\}$ are given in Table 11.2A-1. To test each $\theta_{i^*j^*}^{ij}$ of Eq. (11.2B.2), we can apply the odds ratio test for 2×2 tables (DR 11.1B-1) to Eq. (11.2B.3), given by:

$$\chi_{\hat{\theta}_{i^*j^*}}^{ij} = \left[\frac{\ln(\hat{\theta}_{i^*j^*}^{ij})}{\hat{\sigma}\ln(\hat{\theta}_{i^*j^*}^{ij})} \right]^2, \tag{11.2B.4}$$

where $\hat{\sigma}(\ln\hat{\theta}_{i^*j^*}^{ij})$ is given by

$$\hat{\sigma}(\ln\hat{\theta}_{i^*j^*}^{ij}) = \sqrt{n_{ij}^{-1} + n_{i^*j}^{-1} + n_{ij^*}^{-1} + n_{i^*j^*}^{-1}}. \tag{11.2B.5}$$

Thus, the decision rule for testing Eq. (11.2B.2) is given as follows.

Decision Rule 11.2B-1 (The log-odds-ratio test on first-order interaction for $I \times J$ tables)

A two-tailed test for Eq. (11.2B.2) is to reject H_0 if the computed $\chi_{\hat{\theta}_{i^*j^*}^{ij}}$ of Eq. (11.2B.4) is greater than $\chi_{1;1-\frac{\alpha}{2}}^2$ or less than $\chi_{1;\frac{\alpha}{2}}^2$ for at least one of the pairs (i, i^*) and (j, j^*) such that $i \neq i^*$ and $j \neq j^*$, where α is the level of significance.

Example 11.2B-1

The data in Table 11.2B-1 is taken from Table 11.3A-2 when $Z = 1$. Test at the level of significance 0.05 if X and Y given in Table 11.2B-1 have no two-factor interaction.

Solution

Since Table 11.2B-1 is a 2×3 table, there are only two independent 2×2 tables that are obtained from it. Without loss of generality, we form two independent 2×2 tables by choosing $\{Y = 1, Y = 2\}$ and $\{Y = 2, Y = 3\}$ associated with $\{X = 1, X = 2\}$ as follows: By applying Eqs. (11.2B.3) and (11.2B.5) to the data in Table 11.2B-2,

$$\hat{\theta}_{12}^{21} = (58 \cdot 19)/(11 \cdot 75) \approx 1.336, \tag{1}$$

Table 11.2B-1. The sample data of litters of mice treated by two different ways (X) and the number of deaths (Y)

	Y = 1	Y=2	Y=3
X=1	58	11	5
X=2	75	19	7

Table 11.2B-2. The sample data of X and two categories of Y = 1 and Y = 2

	Y = 1	Y = 2
X=1	58	11
X=2	75	19

Table 11.2B-3.   The sample data of X and
two categories of $Y = 2$ and $Y = 3$

	$Y = 2$	$Y = 3$
$X = 1$	11	5
$X = 2$	19	7

and

$$\hat{\sigma}(\ln\hat{\theta}_{12}^{21}) = \sqrt{58^{-1} + 11^{-1} + 75^{-1} + 19^{-1}} \approx 0.417. \qquad (2)$$

By substituting Eqs. (1) and (2) into Eq. (11.2B.4),

$$\chi_{\hat{\theta}_{12}^{21}} = (\ln(1.336)/0.417)^2 \approx 0.481. \qquad (3)$$

Similarly, by applying Eqs. (11.2B.3) and (11.2B.5) to the data in Table 11.2B-3,

$$\hat{\theta}_{12}^{23} = (11 \cdot 7)/(5 \cdot 19) \approx 0.811, \qquad (4)$$

and

$$\hat{\sigma}(\ln\hat{\theta}_{12}^{23}) = \sqrt{11^{-1} + 5^{-1} + 19^{-1} + 7^{-1}} \approx 0.697. \qquad (5)$$

By substituting Eqs. (4) and (5) into Eq. (11.2B.4),

$$\chi_{\hat{\theta}_{12}^{23}} = (\ln(0.811)/0.697)^2 \approx 0.091. \qquad (6)$$

Since both of the computed value of Eqs. (3) and (6) are neither greater than $\chi_{1;0.975}^2 = 5.024$ nor less than $\chi_{1;0.025}^2 = 0.001$, H$_0$ of Eq. (11.2B.2) is not rejected at the level of significance 0.05. Hence, X and Y have no two-factor interaction.

Remarks

1. Since the categories of Y are ordered, it is preferable to choose two adjacent columns of Y to form two independent 2 × 2 tables.
2. Since the data in Table 11.2B-1 is only taken from Table 11.3A-2 when Z=1 for the illustrative purpose within the context of two-way tables, we will come back to Table 11.3A-2 again in Sec. 11.3B to show how to calculate the first-order interaction within three-way contingency tables.

C. *Yates' Test on Linear Trend*

If both the categories of X and Y in Table 11.2A-1 are ordered, it is possible that there exists a linear trend between X and Y. Suppose that we are interested in testing whether the column marginal probabilities is a linear function of the observed column marginal total, namely,

$$p_{+j} = a + b \cdot n_{+j}, \qquad (11.2C.1)$$

where a and b are two unknown parameters to be determined. We need to test the following hypotheses

$$H_0 : b = 0 \quad \text{versus} \quad H_1 : b \neq 0, \qquad (11.2C.2)$$

where b is given in Eq. (11.2C.1).

The appropriate way to test Eq. (11.2C.2) is by assigning the row/column score to each of the categories for X and Y. Without loss of generality, we assign the equally-spaced row score u_i to be specified later to the ith row of X, in which $\{u_i\}$ satisfy the inequality of $u_1 < u_2 < \cdots < u_I$. Let the average column score $\{y_j\}$ of the jth column be defined by

$$y_j = \sum_{i=1}^{I} u_i^* n_{ij} / I, \quad j = 1, 2, \ldots, J \qquad (11.2C.3)$$

where u_i^* is the standardized row score of the ith row of X, which is defined by $u^* = (u_i - \bar{u})/s_u$, $\bar{u} = \sum_{i=1}^{I} u_i / I$, $s_u = \sqrt{\sum_{i=1}^{I} (u_i - \bar{u})^2 / (I - 1)}$ and n_{ij} are the observed frequency in the $(i,j)^{\text{th}}$ cell in Table 11.2A-1.

Let us regress y_j on the jth column marginal $x_j \equiv n_{+j}$ by assuming that y_j is a linear equation in x_j, namely,

$$y_j = a + b x_j + e_j, \quad j = 1, 2, \ldots, J \qquad (11.2C.4)$$

where a and b are unknown parameters to be determined, $\{e_j\}$ denote the uncorrelated random errors with $E(e_j) = 0$, $\text{var}(e_j) = \sigma^2$ and $\text{cov}(e_j, e_k) = 0$ if $j \neq k$.

From Eq. (7.2A.2), the least square estimator for b in Eq. (11.2C.4) is

$$\hat{b} = \left(\sum_{j=1}^{J} x_j y_j - J\bar{x}\bar{y} \right) \Big/ \left(\sum_{j=1}^{J} x_j^2 - J\bar{x}^2 \right), \qquad (11.2C.5)$$

where $\bar{x}$ and $\bar{y}$ are tha sample average of $\{x_j\}_{j=1}^{J}$ and $\{y\}_{j=1}^{J}$. The estimated variance of Eq. (11.2C.5) is

$$\hat{\sigma}_{\hat{b}}^2 = \hat{\sigma}^2 \Big/ \left(\sum_{j=1}^{J} x_j^2 - J\bar{x}^2 \right), \qquad (11.2C.6)$$

where $\hat{\sigma}^2$ is given by applying Eq. (7.2A.8)

$$\hat{\sigma}^2 = (J-2)^{-1} \left[\sum_{j=1}^{J} y_j^2 - J\bar{y}^2 - \hat{b}^2 \left(\sum_{j=1}^{J} x_j^2 - J\bar{x}^2 \right) \right]. \qquad (11.2C.7)$$

The test statistic for testing Eq. (11.2C.2) is

$$\chi_{Yates} = \left(\frac{\hat{b}}{\hat{\sigma}_{\hat{b}}} \right)^2 = \frac{\hat{b}^2 \left(\sum_{j=1}^{J} x_j^2 - J\bar{x}^2 \right)}{\hat{\sigma}^2}, \qquad (11.2C.8)$$

where $\hat{\sigma}^2$ is given by Eq. (11.2C.7). It is easily seen that the asymptotic sampling distribution of Eq. (11.2C.8) is a chi-squared distribution with one degree of freedom. Thus, the decision rule for testing Eq. (11.2C.2) is given as follows.[60]

Decision Rule 11.2C-1 (Yates' test on linear trend for two-way tables)
Reject H_0 of Eq. (11.2C.2) at the level of significance α if the computed χ_{Yates} of Eq. (11.2C.8) is greater than $\chi_{1;1-\frac{\alpha}{2}}^2$ or less than $\chi_{1;\frac{\alpha}{2}}^2$. Otherwise, do not reject H_0.

Remarks

1. The row (or column) scores are ordinarily chosen to be symmetric with respect to the central row (or column) category. When the number of categories is odd, the score for the central

category is chosen to be zero and the rest scores are chosen as positive and negative integers symmetric with respect to the central category (see Example 11.2C-1), whereas the scores are chosen to be positive and negative integers symmetric with respect to two central categories if the number of categories is even, e.g., $u_1 = 2$, $u_2 = 1$, $u_3 = -1$ and $u_4 = -2$ for $I = 4$.

2. A similar test can be formulated accordingly for testing if there exists a linearly increasing or decreasing trend among the row marginal probabilities $\{p_{i+}\}_{i=1}^{I}$.

3. When I=2, the Yates' test is reduced to the Armitage's test.[5]

Example 11.2C-1

With the data given in Table 11.2A-2, test if there exists a linear trend among the column marginal probability $\{p_{+j}\}_{j=1}^{J}$.

Solution

Because Table 11.2A-2 has three categories, the row scores are chosen as $u_1 = +1$, $u_2 = 0$, and $u_3 = -1$. Since the mean and standard deviation of the row score are computed as

$$\bar{u} = \sum_{i=1}^{2} u_i/3 = [1 + 0 + (-1)]/3 = 0$$

and

$$s_u = \sqrt{[(1-0)^2 + (0-0)^2 + (-1-0)^2]/(3-1)} = 1.$$

Therefore, the standardized row score is the same as the original row score, namely, $u^* = u_i$. From Table 11.2A-2,

$$x_1 \equiv n_{+1} = 308, \quad x_2 \equiv n_{+2} = 147, \quad x_3 \equiv n_{+3} = 295,$$

$$x_4 \equiv n_{+4} = 179, \quad \text{and} \quad x_5 \equiv n_{+5} = 90. \tag{1}$$

By using Eq. (11.2C.3), five column average scores are

$$y_1 = [1 \cdot 141 + 0 \cdot 131 + (-1) \cdot 36]/3 = 105/3 \approx 35,$$

$$y_2 = [1 \cdot 67 + 0 \cdot 66 + (-1) \cdot 14]/3 = 53/3 \approx 17.67,$$

$$y_3 = [1 \cdot 114 + 0 \cdot 143 + (-1) \cdot 38]/3 = 76/3 \approx 25.33, \qquad (2)$$

$$y_4 = [1 \cdot 79 + 0 \cdot 72 + (-1) \cdot 28]/3 = 51/3 \approx 17,$$

$$y_5 = [1 \cdot 39 + 0 \cdot 35 + (-1) \cdot 16]/3 = 23/3 \approx 7.67.$$

From Eqs. (1) and (2),

$$\bar{x} = (308 + 147 + 295 + 179 + 90)/5 = 203.8. \qquad (3)$$

and

$$\bar{y} = (35 + 17.67 + 25.33 + 17 + 7.67)/5 = 20.53. \qquad (4)$$

By substituting Eqs. (1) to (4) into Eq. (11.2C.5),

$$\hat{b} = [(308 \cdot 35 + 147 \cdot 17.67 + 295 \cdot 25.33 + 179 \cdot 17 + 90 \cdot 7.67)$$

$$- 5 \cdot 203.8 \cdot 20.53]/[(308^2 + 147^2 + 295^2 + 179^2 + 90^2)$$

$$- 5 \cdot 203.8^2] = 0.101757 \approx 0.102. \qquad (5)$$

By substituting Eqs. (1) to (4) into Eq. (11.2C.7),

$$\hat{\sigma}^2 = (5-2)^{-1}[(35^2 + 17.67^2 + 25.33^2 + 17^2 + 7.67^2 - 5 \cdot 20.53^2$$

$$- 0.102^2 \cdot (308^2 + 147^2 + 295^2 + 179^2 + 90^2 - 5 \cdot 203.8^2)]$$

$$= 15.38715 \approx 15.39. \qquad (6)$$

By substituting Eqs. (1), (3), (5) and (6) into Eq. (11.2C.8),

$$\chi_{Yates} = \frac{0.102^2(308^2 + 147^2 + 295^2 + 179^2 + 90^2 - 5 \cdot 203.8^2)}{15.39}$$

$$= 24.20308 \approx 24.2. \qquad (7)$$

Since the computed χ_{Yates} of Eq. (7) is greater than $\chi^2_{1;0.975} = 5.024$, H_0 of Eq. (11.2C.2) is rejected at the level of significance 0.05. Hence, there is a linear trend among the column marginal probabilities of the homework conditions.

Remarks

1. You may want to test if there exists any linear trend among the row marginal probabilities of the teacher's rating (see Exercise 11.4-7).
2. Yate's test only works in one direction and is unable to test nonlinear trends in both (row and column) directions of the entire table. To test any nonlinear trend for the entire table, we need to turn to the correlation test (DR 11.2C-2), which is presented below.

To test any (nonlinear) trend for the entire table, we need to test the following pair of hypotheses:

$$H_0: p_{ij} = p_{i^*j^*} \text{ for all pairs of } (i, j) \text{ and } (i^*, j^*),$$
$$\text{where } i < i^*, \; j < j^* \tag{11.2C.9}$$

versus

$$H_1: p_{ij} < p_{i^*j^*} \text{ or } p_{ij} > p_{i^*j^*} \text{ for at least one of the pairs of } (i, j)$$
and (i^*, j^*), where $i < i^*, \; j < j^*$.

The test statistic for Eq. (11.2C.9) is given by

$$\rho = \sum_{i=1}^{I} \sum_{j=1}^{J} u_i^* p_{ij} v_j^*, \tag{11.2C.10}$$

where u_i^* and v_j^* denote, respectively, the standardized version of the row and column score u_i and v_j. The maximum likelihood estimator for Eq. (11.2C.10) is

$$\hat{\rho} = n^{-1} \sum_{i=1}^{I} \sum_{j=1}^{I} u_i^* n_{ij} v_j^*, \tag{11.2C.11}$$

where n_{ij} is given in Table 11.2A-1.

The estimated standard error of Eq. (11.2C.11) is

$$\hat{\sigma}(\hat{\rho}) = \sqrt{ n^{-2} \left[\begin{array}{c} \sum\limits_{i=1}^{I} \sum\limits_{j=1}^{J} u_i^{*2} n_{ij} (n - n_{ij}) v_j^{*2} \\ -2 \sum\limits_{i=1}^{I} \sum\limits_{k=1}^{I} \sum\limits_{j=1}^{J} \sum\limits_{\ell=j+1}^{J} u_i^* n_{ij} v_j^* u_k^* n_{k\ell} v_\ell^* \end{array} \right] },$$

$$(11.2C.12)$$

where I < J.

The test statistic for Eq. (11.2C.9) is

$$\chi_{Corr} = [\hat{\rho} / \hat{\sigma}(\hat{\rho})]^2, \qquad (11.2C.13)$$

where $\hat{\rho}$ and $\hat{\sigma}_{\hat{\rho}}$ are given by Eqs. (11.2C.11) and (11.2C.12), respectively. It is easily seen that the asymptotic sampling distribution of Eq. (11.2C.13) is a chi-squared distribution with one degree of freedom. The decision rule for testing Eq. (11.2C.9) is thus given as follows.

Decision Rule 11.2C-2 (The correlation test on nonlinear trend for two-way tables)

Reject H_0 of Eq. (11.2C.9) at the level of significance α if the computed χ_{Corr} of Eq. (11.2C.13) is greater than $\chi^2_{1;1-\frac{\alpha}{2}}$ or less than $\chi^2_{1;\frac{\alpha}{2}}$ Otherwise, do not reject H_0.

Remarks

1. The correlation test of DR 11.2C-2 is different from that of the Mantel's test,[38] in which he only considers the case when I = 2.
2. If the row/column scores are chosen to be constrained by the marginal totals,[47] Eq. (11.2C.12) no longer holds.

Example 11.2C-2

With the data given in Table 11.2A-2, test if there exists any nonlinear trend in the entire table.

Solution

The row scores are chosen to be the same as given in Example 11.3C-1, namely, $u_1 = +1$, $u_2 = 0$, and $u_3 = -1$, while the column scores are chosen as $v_1 = 2$, $v_2 = 1$, $v_3 = 0$, $v_4 = -1$ and $v_5 = -2$. Their standardized scores are:

$$u_i^* \equiv u_i \quad \text{and} \quad (v_1^*, v_2^*, v_3^*, v_4^*, v_5^*)$$

$$= (1.2649, 0.6325, 0, -0.6325, -1.2649) \tag{1}$$

By substituting $n_{11} = 141$, $n_{12} = 67$, $n_{13} = 114$, $n_{14} = 79$, $n_{15} = 39$, $n_{21} = 131$, $n_{22} = 66$, $n_{23} = 143$, $n_{24} = 72$, $n_{25} = 35$, $n_{31} = 36$, $n_{32} = 14$, $n_{33} = 38$, $n_{34} = 28$, $n_{35} = 16$ and $n = 1,019$, and Eq. (1) into Eq. (11.2C.11), we have

$$\hat{\rho} = [1 \cdot 141 \cdot 1.2649 + 1 \cdot 67 \cdot 0.6325 + 1 \cdot 114 \cdot 0$$

$$+ 1 \cdot 79 \cdot (-0.6325) + 1 \cdot 39 \cdot (-1.2649) + 0 \cdot 131 \cdot 1.2649$$

$$+ 0 \cdot 66 \cdot 0.6325 + 0 \cdot 143 \cdot 0 + 0 \cdot 72 \cdot (-0.6325)$$

$$+ 0 \cdot 35 \cdot (-1.2649) + (-1) \cdot 36 \cdot 1.2649 + (-1) \cdot 14 \cdot 0.6325$$

$$+ (-1) \cdot 38 \cdot 0 + (-1) \cdot 28 \cdot (-0.6325)$$

$$+ (-1) \cdot 16 \cdot (-1.2649)]/1019 = 0.103029 \approx 0.1. \tag{2}$$

By using Eq. (11.2C.12), the estimated standard error of Eq. (2) is

$$\hat{\sigma}_{\hat{\rho}} = \sqrt{\{405.7569 - 2 \cdot [-12.8406 + (-4.813) + 0 + 3.2251}$$

$$\sqrt{+0.3674 + 0 + 0 + 0 + 0 + 0 + (-1.3) + (-0.3297)}$$

$$\sqrt{+0]\}/1,019^2}$$

$$= \sqrt{436.4352/1,019^2} = 0.0205 \approx 0.021. \tag{3}$$

By substituting Eqs. (2) and (3) into Eq. (11.2C.13),

$$\chi_{Corr} = (0.1/0.021)^2 = 25.2551 \approx 25.26. \tag{4}$$

Since the computed χ_{Corr} of Eq. (4) is greater than $\chi_{1;0.975}^2 = 5.024$, H_0 of Eq. (11.2C.9) is rejected at the level of significance 0.05.

Hence, there exists a nonlinear trend between the teacher's rating and the homework conditions.

Remarks

1. To calculate Eq. (3), we treat it as computing from the expansion of $(\sum_{i=1}^{2} \sum_{j=1}^{5} a_{ij})^2$, where $a_{ij} \equiv u_i^* n_{ij} v_j^*$.
2. The computed values of χ_{Yates} and χ_{Corr} for Table 11.1A-2 are comparable.

D. *Stuart's Test on the Marginal Homogeneity in Unordered Square Tables*

Let Y_A and Y_B be correlated categorical random variables having the same K categories with the nominal data, where $K > 2$. A sample data is collected over n subjects and jointly cross-classified with respect to Y_A and Y_B as given in Table 11.2D-1.

Assume that the sample data follow a multinomial distribution with the parameters $\{p_{ij}\}_{i,j=1}^{K}$ and n, where $p_{ij} = \Pr(Y_A = i, Y_B = j)$.

To test the marginal homogeneity of Y_A and Y_B, we need to test the following pair of hypotheses:

$$H_0 : p_{i+} = p_{+i} \quad \text{versus} \quad H_1 : p_{i+} \neq p_{+i}, \quad i = 1, \ldots, K \quad (11.2D.1)$$

Table 11.2D-1. The sample data of two correlated categorical variables Y_A and Y_B

		Categories of Y_B				
		1	2	$\cdots$	K	Row Total
Categories of Y_A	1	n_{11}	n_{12}	$\cdots$	n_{1K}	n_{1+}
	2	n_{21}	n_{22}	$\cdots$	n_{2K}	n_{2+}
	$\vdots$	$\vdots$	$\vdots$	$\vdots$	$\vdots$	$\vdots$
	K	n_{K1}	n_{K2}	$\cdots$	n_{KK}	n_{K+}
Column Total		n_{+1}	n_{+2}	$\cdots$	n_{+K}	n

where $n_{i+} = \sum_{j=1}^{K} n_{ij}$, $n_{+j} = \sum_{i=1}^{K} n_{ij}$ and $n = \sum_{i=1}^{K} n_{i+} = \sum_{j=1}^{K} n_{+j} = \sum_{i=1}^{K} \sum_{j=1}^{K} n_{ij}$.

where $p_{i+} = \sum_{j=1}^{K} p_{ij}$, and $p_{+j} = \sum_{i=1}^{K} p_{ij}$. Let $\vec{\eta} = [\eta_1, \eta_2, \ldots, \eta_K]^T$, where η_i is defined by

$$\eta_i = p_{i+} - p_{+i}, \quad i = 1, \ldots, K, \tag{11.2D.2}$$

where $\sum_{i=1}^{K} \eta_i = \sum_{i=1}^{K} (p_{i+} - p_{+i}) = \sum_{i=1}^{K} p_{i+} - \sum_{i=1}^{K} p_{+i} = 1 - 1 = 0$. Thus, Eq. (11.2D.1) can be re-written as

$$H_0 : \vec{\eta} = \vec{0} \quad \text{versus} \quad H_1 : \vec{\eta} \neq \vec{0}. \tag{11.2D.3}$$

The maximum likelihood estimator of η_i is given by

$$\hat{\eta}_i = \hat{p}_{i+} - \hat{p}_{+i} = n^{-1}(n_{i+} - n_{+i}). \tag{11.2D.4}$$

Under H_0 of Eq. (11.2D.3), the variance of $\hat{\eta}_i$ and covariance between $\hat{\eta}_i$ and $\hat{\eta}_j$ are given, respectively, by

$$\sigma^2(\hat{\eta}_i) = n(p_{i+} p_{+i} - 2p_{ii}), \tag{11.2D.5}$$

and

$$\text{cov}(\hat{\eta}_i, \hat{\eta}_j) = -n(p_{ij} + p_{ji}), \quad \text{if } i \neq j. \tag{11.2D.6}$$

Since $\sum_{i=1}^{K} \eta_i = 0$, only $K - 1$ variables out of $\{\eta_i\}_{i=1}^{K}$ are independent.

Without loss of generality, we use the first $K - 1$ variables by dropping the last variable η_K. The test statistic for Eq. (11.2D.3) is then given by[56]

$$\chi_{Stuart} = \hat{\vec{\eta}}^{*T} W^{-1} \hat{\vec{\eta}}^* = \sum_{i=1}^{K-1} \sum_{j=1}^{K-1} v_{ij} \hat{\eta}_i \hat{\eta}_j, \tag{11.2D.7}$$

where W is the estimated variance-covariance matrix of $\hat{\vec{\eta}}^* = (\hat{\eta}_1, \hat{\eta}_2, \ldots, \hat{\eta}_{K-1})^T$ given by

$$W = \begin{bmatrix} n_{1+} + n_{+1} - 2n_{11} & \cdots & \cdots & -(n_{1,K-1} + n_{K-1,1}) \\ -(n_{21} + n_{12}) & \cdots & \cdots & -(n_{2,K-1} + n_{K-1,2}) \\ \vdots & \vdots & \vdots & \vdots \\ -(n_{K-1,1} + n_{1,K-1}) & \cdots & \cdots & n_{K-1,+} + n_{+,K-1} - 2n_{K-1,K-1} \end{bmatrix} \tag{11.2D.8}$$

and $V = [v_{ij}]_{i,j=1}^K \equiv W^{-1}$ is the inverse matrix of W of Eq. (11.2D.8), provided that W is nonsingular.

It can be shown that the asymptotic sampling distribution of Eq. (11.2D.8) is a chi-squared distribution with $K-1$ degrees of freedom. The decision rule for testing Eq. (11.2D.3) is given as follows.[56]

Decision Rule 11.2D-1 (Stuart's test on the margin homogeneity with the nominal data)
Reject H_0 of Eq. (11.2D.3) at the level of significance α if the computed χ_{Stuart} of Eq. (11.2D.8) is greater than $\chi^2_{K-1;1-\frac{\alpha}{2}}$ or less than $\chi^2_{K-1;\frac{\alpha}{2}}$. Otherwise, do not reject H_0.

Remarks

1. Stuart's test can be regarded as an extension of McNemar's test to the case of $K \times K$ contingency tables for $K > 2$.
2. It makes no difference which one is deleted from $\{\eta_i\}_{i=1}^K$ in formulating Eq. (11.2D.7), so long as W of Eq. (11.2D.8) is formed accordingly.

Example 11.2D-1

Table 11.2D-2 is the data[57] in which 227 Merino ewes are cross-classified by the number of lambs born to them in two consecutive years: 1952 (Y_A) and 1953 (Y_B). Both Y_A and Y_B have three

Table 11.2D-2. The sample data of lambs born in 1952 (Y_A) and 1953 (Y_B)

		Y_B			
		1	2	3	Row Total
Y_A	1	58	52	1	111
	2	26	58	3	87
	3	8	12	9	29
Column Total		92	122	13	227

categories: = 1 if no lamb was born, = 2 if one lamb was born, and = 3 if two lambs were born.

Does the marginal homogeneity hold for Table 11.2D-2?

Solution

To test the marginal homogeneity of Table 11.2D-2, we need to calculate the test statistic χ_{Stuart} of Eq. (11.2D.7). Since K = 3, we need only to calculate $\{\hat{\eta}_i\}_{i=1}^2$ by dropping $\hat{\eta}_3$. By substituting $n_{1+} = 111$, $n_{2+} = 87$, $n_{+1} = 92$, $n_{+2} = 122$ and $n = 227$ obtained from Table 11.2D-2 into Eq. (11.2C.4),

$$\hat{\eta}_1 = (111 - 92)/227 = 19/227 \approx 0.0837, \tag{1}$$

and

$$\hat{\eta}_2 = (87 - 122)/227 = -35/227 \approx -0.1542. \tag{2}$$

By using Eq. (11.2D.8), the estimated variance-covariance matrix W is obtained as

$$W = \begin{bmatrix} 111 + 92 - 2 \cdot 58 & -(52 + 26) \\ -(52 + 26) & 87 + 122 - 2 \cdot 58 \end{bmatrix} = \begin{bmatrix} 87 & -78 \\ -78 & 93 \end{bmatrix} \tag{3}$$

By applying Theorem 17.5.4 (Formula for the 2×2 matrix) in Ref. 35,

$$V = W^{-1} = \frac{1}{2007} \begin{bmatrix} 93 & 78 \\ 78 & 87 \end{bmatrix} = \begin{bmatrix} 0.0463 & 0.0389 \\ 0.0389 & 0.0433 \end{bmatrix} \tag{4}$$

By substituting Eqs. (1), (2) and (4) into Eq. (11.2D.7),

$$\chi_{Stuart} = [0.0837 - 0.1542] \begin{bmatrix} 0.0463 & 0.0389 \\ 0.0389 & 0.0433 \end{bmatrix} \begin{bmatrix} 0.0837 \\ -0.1542 \end{bmatrix}$$

$$\approx 0.00035. \tag{5}$$

Since the computed χ_{Stuart} of Eq. (5) is less than the critical value of chi-squared distribution with 2(= 3 − 1) degrees of freedom $\chi^2_{2;0.025} = 0.051$, H_0 is rejected at the level of significance 0.05.

Hence, there is no marginal homogeneity between the number of the lambs born in 1952 and 1953, respectively.

Remarks

1. Show that it makes no difference in inference if the second term $\hat{\eta}_2$ is dropped from consideration in forming Eq. (11.2D.7) instead of the third term $\hat{\eta}_3$ (see Exercise 11.4-8).
2. Note that Table 11.2D-2 is the ordinal data rather than the nomial data. Yet, Stuart's test is only good for the nominal data. Strictly, we need to apply Kendall's test (DR 11.2E-1) in Sec. 11.2E to analyze Table 11.2D-2 (see Exercise 11.4-9).

E.   *Kendall's Test for Independence for Two-Way Ordered Tables*

Let X and Y be two categorical random variables having I and J ordered categories, denoted by $x_1 < x_2 < \cdots < x_I$ and $y_1 < y_2 < \cdots < y_J$, respectively, where both I and J are greater than two. A random sample of size m is collected from a certain population and jointly cross-classified with respect to X and Y as given in Table 11.2E-1.

Assume that the sample data $\{m_{ij}\}_{i,j=1}^{I,J}$ follow a multinomial distribution with the parameters $\{p_{ij}\}_{i,j=1}^{I,J}$ and n, where

Table 11.2E-1.   The sample ordinal data of two categorical variables X and Y

		Categories of Y				
		y_1	y_2	$\cdots$	Y_J	Row Total
Categories of X	x_2	m_{11}	m_{12}	$\cdots$	m_{1J}	m_{1+}
	x_2	m_{21}	m_{22}	$\cdots$	m_{2J}	m_{2+}
	$\vdots$	$\vdots$	$\vdots$	$\vdots$	$\vdots$	$\vdots$
	x_I	m_{I1}	m_{I2}	$\cdots$	m_{IJ}	m_{I+}
Column Total		m_{+1}	m_{+2}	$\cdots$	m_{+J}	m

where $m_{i+} = \sum_{j=1}^{J} m_{ij}$, $m_{+j} = \sum_{i=1}^{I} m_{ij}$ and $m = \sum_{i=1}^{I} m_{i+} = \sum_{j=1}^{J} m_{+j} = \sum_{i=1}^{I} \sum_{j=1}^{J} m_{ij}$.

$p_{ij} = \Pr(X = x_i, Y = y_j)$. To test the independence of X and Y, we need to test the following pair of hypotheses:

$$H_0 : p_C = p_D \quad \text{versus} \quad H_1 : p_C \neq p_D, \tag{11.2E.1}$$

where $p_C = \sum_{i<k}\sum_{j<\ell} p_{ij}p_{k\ell} \equiv \frac{1}{2}P_C$, $p_D = \sum_{i<k}\sum_{j>\ell} p_{ij}p_{k\ell} \equiv \frac{1}{2}P_D$, P_C and P_D denote respectively the number of concordant pairs for which the higher X also has the higher Y, and discordant pairs for which the higher X has the lower Y. By setting $\Delta = p_C - p_D$, Eq. (11.2E.1) can be rewritten as

$$H_0 : \Delta = 0 \quad \text{versus} \quad H_1 : \Delta \neq 0. \tag{11.2E.2}$$

The maximum likelihood estimator of Δ is

$$\hat{\Delta} = \hat{p}_C - \hat{p}_D = m^{-2}\left[\sum_{i<k}\sum_{j<\ell} m_{ij}m_{k\ell} - \sum_{i<k}\sum_{j>\ell} m_{ij}m_{k\ell}\right], \tag{11.2E.3}$$

where m_{ij} and $m_{k\ell}$ are given in Table 11.2E-1. It can be shown[3] that the variance of $\hat{\Delta}$ is

$$\sigma^2(\hat{\Delta}) = \frac{4(1 - \sum_{i=1}^{I} p_{i+}^3)(1 - \sum_{j=1}^{J} p_{+j}^3)}{9m} \tag{11.2E.4}$$

By substituting $\hat{p}_{i+} = m_{i+}/m$ and $\hat{p}_{+j} = m_{+j}/m$ into Eq. (11.2E.4) for p_{i+} and p_{+j}, respectively, the estimated standard error of $\hat{\Delta}$ is

$$\hat{\sigma}(\hat{\Delta}) = \frac{2}{3}\sqrt{m^{-7}\left[\left(m^3 - \sum_{i=1}^{I} m_{i+}^3\right)\left(m^3 - \sum_{j=1}^{J} m_{+j}^3\right)\right]}. \tag{11.2E.5}$$

The test statistic for Eq. (11.2E.2) is

$$\chi_{Kendall} = \left[\frac{\hat{\Delta}}{\hat{\sigma}(\hat{\Delta})}\right]^2. \tag{11.2E.6}$$

It can be shown[3] that Eq. (11.2E.6) is a chi-squared distribution wth one degree of freedom. The decision rule for testing Eq. (11.2E.2) is given as follows.

Decision Rule 11.2E-1 (Kendall's test for independence in ordinal data)

Reject H_0 of Eq. (11.2E.2) at the level of significance α if the computed χ_{Kendall} of Eq. (11.2E.6) is greater than $\chi^2_{1;1-\frac{\alpha}{2}}$ or less than $\chi^2_{1;\frac{\alpha}{2}}$ Otherwise, do not reject H_0.

Example 11.2E-1

Table 11.2E-2 is taken from that of Table 11.3A-2 after X is pooled. Both Y and Z have three and five-ordered categories, respectively. Test at the level of significance 0.05 if Y and Z are independent.

Solution

By first calculating $\hat{p}_c$ and $\hat{p}_D$ in Eq. (11.2E.3),

$$
\begin{aligned}
\hat{p}_C = 657^{-2}[&133(31+40+35+27+18+25+33+25) \\
&+ 107(40+35+27+25+33+25) + 78(35+27+33+25) \\
&+ 54(27+25) + 30(18+25+33+25) + 31(25+33+25) \\
&+ 40(33+25) + 35 \cdot 25] = 0.166531,
\end{aligned}
\tag{1}
$$

and

$$
\begin{aligned}
\hat{p}_D = 657^{-2}[&9(30+31+40+35+12+18+25+33) \\
&+ 54(30+31+40+12+18+25) + 78(30+31+12+18) \\
&+ 107(30+12) + 27(12+18+25+33) + 35(12+18 \\
&+ 25) + 40(12+18) + 31 \cdot 12] = 0.05104.
\end{aligned}
$$

Table 11.2E-2.   The sample data from Table 11.3A-2 after X is pooled

	z_1	z_2	z_3	z_4	z_5	**Row Total**
y_1	133	107	78	54	9	381
y_2	30	31	40	35	27	163
y_3	12	18	25	33	25	113
Column Total	175	156	143	122	61	657

After substituting Eq. (1) into Eq. (11.2E.3),

$$\hat{\Delta} = 0.166531 - 0.064647 = 0.101884. \tag{2}$$

From Table 11.2E-2, we have

$$m_{1+} = 381, \quad m_{2+} = 163, \quad m_{3+} = 113, \quad m_{+1} = 175,$$

$$m_{+2} = 156, \quad m_{+3} = 143, \quad m_{+4} = 122, \quad m_{+5} = 61$$

$$\text{and} \quad m = 657. \tag{3}$$

After substituting Eq. (3) into Eq. (11.2E.5),

$$\hat{\sigma}(\hat{\Delta}) = \frac{2}{3}\sqrt{657^{-7}\{[657^3 - (381^3 + 163^3 + 113^3)][657^3 - (175^3 + 156^3}$$

$$+ 143^3 + 122^3 + 61^3)]\} = 0.022458. \tag{4}$$

After substituting Eqs. (2) and (4) into Eq. (11.2E.6),

$$\chi_{Kendall} = \left[\frac{0.101884}{0.022458}\right]^2 = 20.58174 \approx 20.58. \tag{5}$$

Since the computed $\chi_{Kendall}$ of Eq. (5) is greater than $\chi^2_{1;0.975} = 5.024$, H_0 of Eq. (11.2E.2) is rejected at the level of significance 0.05. Hence, Y and Z are not independent.

Remark

For a comparison with the result of Pearson's test, do Exercise 11.4-10.

F. Wilcoxon–Mann–Whitney's (WMW's) Test for Marginal Homogeneity for Two-way Ordered Tables

Let Z_A and Z_B be the correlated categorical random variables having the same K ordered categories, $z_1 < z_2 < \cdots < z_K$, where $K > 2$. A sample data is collected over n subjects and jointly cross-classified with respect to Z_A and Z_B as given in Table 11.2F-1.

Table 11.2F-1.   The sample data of two correlated variables Z_A and Z_B

		Categories of Z_B				
		z_1	z_2	$\cdots$	z_K	**Row Total**
Categories of Z_A	z_1	n_{11}	n_{12}	$\cdots$	n_{1K}	n_{1+}
	z_2	n_{21}	n_{22}	$\cdots$	n_{2K}	n_{2+}
	$\vdots$	$\vdots$	$\vdots$	$\vdots$	$\vdots$	$\vdots$
	z_K	n_{K1}	n_{K2}	$\cdots$	n_{KK}	n_{K+}
Column Total		n_{+1}	n_{+2}	$\cdots$	n_{+K}	n

where $n_{i+} = \sum_{j=1}^{K} n_{ij}$, $n_{+j} = \sum_{i=1}^{K} n_{ij}$ and $n = \sum_{i=1}^{K} n_{i+} = \sum_{j=1}^{K} n_{+j} = \sum_{i=1}^{K} \sum_{j=1}^{K} n_{ij}$.

Assume that the sample data follow a multinomial distribution with the parameters of cell probabilities $\{p_{ij}\}_{1,j=1}^{K}$ and n, where $p_{ij} = \Pr(Z_A = z_i, Z_B = z_j)$.

To test the marginal homogeneity of Z_A and Z_B, we need to test the following pair of hypotheses:

$$H_0:\ p_A = p_B \quad \text{versus} \quad H_1:\ p_A \neq p_B, \tag{11.2F.1}$$

where

$$p_A = \sum_{i<j} p_{i+} p_{+j} = \sum_{i=1}^{K=1} \sum_{j=i+1}^{K} p_{i+} p_{+j},$$

$$p_B = \sum_{i>j} p_{i+} p_{+j} = \sum_{i=1}^{K} \sum_{j=1}^{i-1} p_{i+} p_{+j}.$$

By letting $\delta = p_A - p_B$, Eq. (11.2F.1) can be re-written as

$$H_0:\ \delta = 0 \quad \text{versus} \quad H_1:\ \delta \neq 0. \tag{11.2F.2}$$

The maximum likelihood estimator of δ is

$$\hat{\delta} = \hat{p}_A - \hat{p}_B = n^{-2} \left(\sum_{i=1}^{K-1} n_{i+} n_{i+}^{*} - \sum_{i=2}^{K} n_{i+} n_{+i}^{**} \right), \tag{11.2F.3}$$

where $n_{K+}^* = n_{+1}^{**} \equiv 0$, $n_{i+}^* = \sum_{j=i+1}^K n_{+j}$, $n_{+j}^{**} = \sum_{j=1}^{i-1} n_{+j}$, n_{i+} and n_{+j} are given in Table 11.2F-1. It can be shown that the estimated standard error of $\hat{\delta}$ is[1]

$$\hat{\sigma}(\hat{\delta}) = \sqrt{n^{-1}\left[\sum_{i,j=1}^K s_{ij}^{*2} n_{ij} - \left(\sum_{i,j=1}^K s_{ij}^* n_{ij}\right)^2\right]}, \qquad (11.2F.4)$$

where $s_{ij}^* = n^{-1}(n_{j+}^* + n_{j-1,+}^* - n_{+i}^{**} - n_{+,i-1}^{**})$, and n_{i+}^* and n_{+i}^{**} are given in Eq. (11.2F.3). Thus, the test statistic for Eq. (11.2F.2) is

$$\chi_{WMW} = \left[\frac{\hat{\delta}}{\hat{\sigma}(\hat{\delta})}\right]^2 = \frac{\left(\sum_{i=1}^{K-1} n_{i+} n_{i+}^* - \sum_{i=2}^K n_{i+} n_{+i}^{**}\right)^2}{n^2\left[\sum_{i,j=1}^K n_{ij} s_{ij}^{*2} - \left(\sum_{i,j=1}^K n_{ij} s_{ij}^*\right)^2\right]},$$

$$(11.2F.5)$$

where s_{ij}^* is given in Eq. (11.2F.4).

It is easily shown that the asymptotic sampling distribution of Eq. (11.2F.5) is a chi-squared distribution with one degree of freedom. As a consequence, the decision rule for testing Eq. (11.2F.2) is given as follows.[1]

Decision Rule 11.2F-1 (WMW's test on margin homogeneity for ordinal data)
Reject H_0 of Eq. (11.2F.2) at the level of significance α if the computed χ_{WMW} of Eq. (11.2F.5) is greater than $\chi_{1;1-\frac{\alpha}{2}}^2$ or less than $\chi_{1;\frac{\alpha}{2}}^2$. Otherwise, do not reject H_0.

Remarks

1. The test statistic χ_{WMW} of Eq. (11.2F.5) is actually the square of the Mann–Whitney z-statistic, $z_{WMW} = \hat{\delta}/\hat{\sigma}(\hat{\delta})$.
2. The power of χ_{Stuart} of Eq. (11.2D.8) is uniformly smaller than that of the Wilcoxon–Mann–Whitney z-statistic, z_{WMW}, for all combinations of α (type I errors = 0.001, 0.01, 0.02, 0.05, 0.1 or 0.2), δ (shift in marginal probability = 0.1 or 0.2), ρ (correlation of bivariate normal distribution = 0.2 or 0.8), n (sample size = 200 or 400), and K (= 3 or 6) considered in Ref. 1.

Table 11.2F-2.   7477 Women Aged 30–39: Unaided Distance Vision

		Left Eye			
		z_1	z_2	z_3	z_4	Row Total
Right Eye	z_1	1520	266	124	66	1976
	z_2	234	1512	432	78	2256
	z_3	117	362	1772	205	2456
	z_4	36	82	179	492	789
Column Total		1907	2222	2507	841	7477

Example 11.2F-1

Table 11.2F-2 is based on eye test case records of female employees in Royal Ordnance factories in 1943-1946.[55] Let Z_A and Z_B be the graded levels of an employee's eyesight in her right and left-eye: z_1 = highest grade, z_2 = second grade, z_3 = third grade, and z_4 = lowest grade.

Is the eyesight between an employee's right and left-eye marginal homogeneous?

Solution

From Table 11.2F-2,

$$n_{1+} = 1976, \quad n_{2+} = 2256, \quad n_{3+} = 2456, \quad n_{4+} = 789,$$

$$n_{+1} = 1907 \quad n_{+2} = 2222, \quad n_{+3} = 2507, \quad n_{+4} = 841, \qquad (1)$$

$$\text{and} \quad n = 7477.$$

From Eq. (11.2F.3) by using Eq. (1),

$$n_{1+}^* = n_{+2} + n_{+3} + n_{+4} = 2222 + 2507 + 841 = 5570,$$

$$n_{2+}^* = n_{+3} + n_{+4} = 2507 + 841 = 3348,$$

$$n_{3+}^* = n_{+4} = 841, \quad n_{4+}^* = 0,$$

$$n_{+1}^{**} = 0, \quad n_{+2}^{**} = n_{+1} = 1907,$$

$$n_{+3}^{**} = n_{+1} + n_{+2} = 1907 + 2222 = 4129,$$ (2)

$$n_{+4}^{**} = n_{+1} + n_{+2} + n_{+3} = 1907 + 2222 + 2507 = 6636.$$

By substituting Eqs. (1) and (2) into Eq. (11.2F.3),

$$\hat{\delta} = 7477^{-2}[(1976 \cdot 5570 + 2256 \cdot 3348 + 2456 \cdot 841)$$

$$- (2256 \cdot 1907 + 2456 \cdot 4129 + 789 \cdot 6636)]$$

$$= 0.016923 \approx 0.0169.$$ (3)

By substituting Eqs. (1) and (2) into s_{ij}^* in Eq. (11.2F.4),

$$s_{11}^* = 7477^{-1}(5570 + 0 - 0 - 0) = 0.744951184 \approx 0.745,$$

$$s_{12}^* = 7477^{-1}(3348 + 5570 - 0 - 0) = 1.192724 \approx 1.1927,$$

$$s_{13}^* = 7477^{-1}(841 + 3348 - 0 - 0) = 0.560251 \approx 0.5603,$$

$$s_{14}^* = 7477^{-1}(0 + 841 - 0 - 0) = 0.112478 \approx 0.1125,$$

$$s_{21}^* = 7477^{-1}(5570 + 0 - 1907 - 0) = 0..489902367 \approx 0.4899,$$

$$s_{22}^* = 7477^{-1}(3348 + 5570 - 1907 - 0) = 0.937676 \approx 0.9377,$$

$$s_{23}^* = 7477^{-1}(841 + 3348 - 1907 - 0) = 0.305203 \approx 0.3052,$$

$$s_{24}^* = 7477^{-1}(0 + 841 - 1907 - 0) = -0.14257 \approx -0.1426,$$

$$s_{31}^* = 7477^{-1}(5570 + 0 - 4129 - 1907)$$

$$= -0.06232446 \approx -0.0623,$$

$$s_{32}^* = 7477^{-1}(3348 + 5570 - 4129 - 1907)$$

$$= 0.385449 \approx 0.3855,$$

$$s_{33}^* = 7477^{-1}(841 + 3348 - 4129 - 1907)$$

$$= -0.24702 \approx -0.247,$$

$$s_{34}^* = 7477^{-1}(0 + 841 - 4129 - 1907) = -0.6948,$$

$$s_{41}^* = 7477^{-1}(5570 + 0 - 6636 - 4129)$$

$$= -0.69479738 \approx -0.6948,$$

$$s_{42}^* = 7477^{-1}(3348 + 5570 - 6636 - 4129)$$

$$= -0.24702 \approx -0.247,$$

$$s_{43}^* = 7477^{-1}(841 + 3348 - 6636 - 4129) = -0.8795,$$

$$s_{44}^* = 7477^{-1}(0 + 841 - 6636 - 4129) = -1.32727 \approx -1.3273.$$

(4)

By substituting Eqs. (1) and (4) into Eq. (11.2F.4),

$$\hat{\sigma}(\hat{\delta}) = \sqrt{\begin{array}{l} 7477^{-1} \cdot \{[0.745^2 \cdot 1520 + 0.4478^2 \cdot 266 \\ + \cdots + (-1.3273)^2 \cdot 492] \end{array}}$$

$$- [0.745 \cdot 1520 + 0.4478 \cdot 266 + \cdots + (-1.3273) \cdot 492]^2\}$$

$$= 0.007920619 \approx 0.0079.$$

(5)

By substituting Eqs. (3) and (5) into Eq. (11.2F.5),

$$\chi_{WMW} = [0.0169/0.0079]^2 = 4.564903626 \approx 4.565.$$

(6)

Since the computed χ_{WMW} of Eq. (6) is not greater than $\chi_{1;0.975}^2 = 5.024$, H_0 of Eq. (11.2F.2) is not rejected at the level of significance 0.05. Hence, the grades of the right and left eye are marginal homogeneous.

Remark

The result $Q = 11.96$ in Ref. 56 contradicts a conclusion drawn by using the Wilcoxon–Mann–Whitney test. This shows that failing to taking the ordinal nature of the data into consideration could lead to an invalid conclusion.

11.3   Three-Way Contingency Tables

The inference on three-way $(I \times J \times K)$ contingency tables is much more versatile than that of two-way $(I \times J)$ tables. There are many different hypotheses to be set up in Sec. 11.3A. Second-order interaction in three-way tables (see Sec. 11.3B) is more complex than the first-order interaction in two-way tables. Mantel–Haenszel estimation of a common odds ratio (see Sec. 11.3C) is a challenging topic that attracts attention from researchers. Simpson's paradox (see Sec. 11.3D) is indeed an interesting paradoxical phenonmenon.

A. Pearson's Test on Mutual Independence for Three-Way Unordered Tables

Let X (or row), Y (or column) and Z (or layer) be three categorical random variables having I, J and K categories with the nominal data, respectively. Assume that a random sample of size n is collected and cross-classified into Table 11.3A-1.

Assume that the observed sample frequency $\{n_{ijk} > 0\}_{i=1,j=1,k=1}^{I,J,K}$ follows a multinomial distribution with the parameters of cell probabilities $\{p_{ijk} > 0\}_{i=1,j=1,k=1}^{I,J,K}$, where $p_{ijk} = \Pr(X = i, Y = j, Z = k)$.

To test the mutual independence among X, Y and Z, we need to test the following hypotheses:

$$H_{0(XYZ)}: \ p_{ijk} = p_{i++}p_{+j+}p_{++k},$$
$$\text{for all pairs of (i, j, k)} \tag{11.3A.1}$$

versus

$$H_{1(XYZ)}: \ p_{ijk} \neq p_{i++}p_{+j+}p_{++k},$$
$$\text{for at least one pair of (i, j, k)}$$

where $p_{i++} = \sum_{j=1}^{J}\sum_{k=1}^{K} p_{ijk}, p_{+j+} = \sum_{i=1}^{I}\sum_{k=1}^{K} p_{ijk}$ and $p_{++k} = \sum_{i=1}^{I}\sum_{j=1}^{J} p_{ijk}$.

Furthermore, the maximum likelihood estimator of p_{ijk} is given by

$$\hat{p}_{ijk} = n_{ijk}/n. \tag{11.3A.2}$$

Consequently, the maximum likelihood estimator of $m_{ijk} = E(n_{ijk}) = np_{i++}p_{+j+}p_{++k}$ is given by

$$\hat{m}_{ijk} = n\hat{p}_{i++}\hat{p}_{+j+}\hat{p}_{++k} = n^{-2}n_{i++}n_{+j+}n_{++k}, \tag{11.3A.3}$$

where n_{i++}, n_{+j+}, and n_{++k} are given in Table 11.3A-1.

Table 11.3A-1. The sample data of X, Y and Z for 3-way tables

$Z = 1$

		\multicolumn{4}{c}{Categories of Y}	
		1	2	$\cdots$	J	Row Total
Categories of X	1	n_{111}	n_{121}	$\cdots$	n_{1J1}	n_{1+1}
	2	n_{211}	n_{221}	$\cdots$	n_{2J1}	n_{2+1}
	$\vdots$	$\vdots$	$\vdots$	$\vdots$	$\vdots$	$\vdots$
	I	n_{I11}	n_{I21}	$\cdots$	n_{IJ1}	n_{I+1}
Column Total		n_{+11}	n_{+21}	$\vdots$	n_{+J1}	n_{++1}

$Z = 2$

		\multicolumn{4}{c}{Categories of Y}	
		1	2	$\cdots$	J	Row Total
Categories of X	1	n_{112}	n_{122}	$\cdots$	n_{1J2}	n_{1+2}
	2	n_{212}	n_{222}	$\cdots$	n_{2J2}	n_{2+2}
	$\vdots$	$\vdots$	$\vdots$	$\vdots$	$\vdots$	$\vdots$
	I	n_{I12}	n_{I22}	$\cdots$	n_{IJ2}	n_{I+2}
Column Total		n_{+12}	n_{+22}	$\vdots$	n_{+J2}	n_{++2}

$\vdots$

$Z = K$

		\multicolumn{4}{c}{Categories of Y}	
		1	2	$\cdots$	J	Row Total
Categories of X	1	n_{11K}	n_{12K}	$\cdots$	n_{1JK}	n_{1+K}
	2	n_{21K}	n_{22K}	$\cdots$	n_{2JK}	n_{2+K}
	$\vdots$	$\vdots$	$\vdots$	$\vdots$	$\vdots$	$\vdots$
	I	n_{I1K}	n_{I2K}	$\cdots$	n_{IJK}	n_{I+K}
Column Total		n_{+1K}	n_{+2K}	$\vdots$	n_{+JK}	n_{++K}

where $n = \sum_{i=1}^{I} \sum_{j=1}^{J} \sum_{k=1}^{K} n_{ijk} = \sum_{k=1}^{K} n_{++k} = \sum_{j=1}^{J} n_{+j+} = \sum_{i=1}^{I} n_{i++} = \sum_{j=1}^{J} \sum_{k=1}^{K} n_{+jk} = \sum_{i=1}^{I} \sum_{k=1}^{K} n_{i+k} = \sum_{i=1}^{I} \sum_{j=1}^{J} n_{ij+}$, and the total sample size n.

To test Eq. (11.3A.1), we use the Pearson's chi-squared statistic given by

$$\chi_{3-way} = \sum \frac{(\text{observed-expected})^2}{\text{expected}} = \sum_{i=1}^{I} \sum_{j=1}^{J} \sum_{k=1}^{K} \frac{(n_{ijk} - \hat{m}_{ijk})^2}{\hat{m}_{ijk}}$$

$$= n \left[n \sum_{i=1}^{I} \sum_{j=1}^{J} \sum_{k=1}^{K} \frac{n_{ijk}^2}{n_{i++} n_{+j+} n_{++k}} - 1 \right], \qquad (11.3A.4)$$

where n_{i++}, n_{+j+} and n_{++k} are given in Table 11.3A-1. It can be shown that the sampling distribution of Eq. (11.3A.4) is a chi-squared distribution with $(I-1)(J-1)(K-1)$ degrees of freedom.[48]

The decision rule for testing Eq. (11.3A.1) is given as follows.

Decision Rule 11.3A-1 (Pearson's test on mutual independence for three-way unordered tables with the nominal data)

A two-tailed test for Eq. (11.3A.1) is to reject H_0 if the computed χ_{3-way} of Eq. (11.3A.4) is greater than $\chi^2_{(I-1)(J-1)(K-1);\ 1-\frac{\alpha}{2}}$ or less than $\chi^2_{(I-1)(J-1)(K-1);\ \frac{\alpha}{2}}$, where α is the level of significance.

Remarks

1. Unlike the two-way table, there only exist two null hypotheses of independence and zero first-order interaction. For three-way tables, there are at least four other null hypothesis of interest, in addition to the mutual independence, to be tested that are given as follows[8]:

    (i) $H_{0(XY)}^{(Z)}$: Z is independent of X and Y together, namely,

$$p_{ijk} = p_{ij+} p_{++k}; \qquad (11.3A.5)$$

(ii) $H_{0(XY)}^{(Z+)}$: X and Y are independent marginally, given that Z is pooled, namely,

$$p_{ij+} = p_{i++}p_{+j+} / p_{+++}; \qquad (11.3A.6)$$

(iii) $H_{0(XY)}^{(Z=k)}$: X and Y are independent in each layer of $Z = k$, namely, $p_{ijk} = p_{i+k}p_{+jk}/p_{+++}$; and $\qquad$ (11.3A.7)

(iv) $H_0^{(XYZ)}$: there is no three-factor interaction among X, Y and Z, which will be defined in the next section. $\qquad$ (11.3A.8)

2. In a $2 \times 2 \times 2$ table, Simpson[54] shows that Eq. (11.3A.6) and Eq. (11.3A.8) may both be true while Eq. (11.3A.7) is not. Further, if Eqs. (11.3A.6) and (11.3A.7) are both true, then one of $H_{0(YZ)}^{(X)}$ or $H_{0(XZ)}^{(Y)}$ is true. In other words, independence in both layers marginally implies that X is independent of Y and Z together, or Y is independent of X and Z together. In addition, Eq. (11.3A.7) implies Eq. (11.3A.8) since Eq. (11.3A.8) means that the association in each layer of Z is the same from layer to layer, while Eq. (11.3A.7) means that the association in each layer is zero.

3. That neither Eq. (11.3A.6) implies Eq. (11.3A.8) nor vice versa is called the Simpson's paradox, which will be covered in Sec. 11.3D.

4. A warning to any practitioner is that one has to know where the data come from before being able to analyze a three-way contingency table properly.

Example 11.3A-1

The data in Table 11.3A-2 are taken from Ref. 29. It represents a portion of an experiment performed at the Oak Ridge National Laboratory. For this experiment litters of mice of various sizes (Z: five categories) were treated in either one of two different ways (X: two categories) and the number of deaths per litter before weaning was observed (Y: three categories).

Are X, Y and Z mutually independent of one another?

Table 11.3A-2. The sample data of three variables X (treatment), Y (number of depletion) and Z (Litter size)

	Z = 1			
	Y=1	Y=2	Y=3	Row Total
X = 1	58	11	5	74
X = 2	75	19	7	101
Column Total	133	30	12	175

	Z = 2			
	Y = 1	Y = 2	Y = 3	Row Total
X = 1	49	14	10	73
X = 2	58	17	8	83
Column Total	107	31	18	156

	Z = 3			
	Y = = 1	Y = 2	Y = 3	Row Total
X = 1	33	18	15	66
X = 2	45	22	10	77
Column Total	78	40	25	143

	Z = 4			
	Y = 1	Y = 2	Y = 3	Row Total
X = 1	15	13	15	43
X = 2	39	22	18	79
Column Total	54	35	33	122

	Z = 5			
	Y = 1	Y = 2	Y = 3	Row Total
X = 1	4	12	17	33
X = 2	5	15	8	28
Column Total	9	27	25	61

Solution

Table 11.3A-2 is a $2 \times 3 \times 5$ contingency table. To test whether X, Y and Z are independent of one another, we need to calculate the test statistic of Eq. (11.3A.4). From Table 11.3A-2, we get

$$
\begin{aligned}
&n_{111} = 58, \ n_{121} = 11, \ n_{131} = 5, \ n_{211} = 75, \\
&n_{221} = 19, \ n_{231} = 7, \\
&n_{112} = 49, \ n_{122} = 14, \ n_{132} = 10, \ n_{212} = 58, \\
&n_{222} = 17, \ n_{232} = 8, \\
&n_{113} = 33, \ n_{123} = 18, \ n_{133} = 15, \ n_{213} = 45, \\
&n_{223} = 22, \ n_{233} = 10, \\
&n_{114} = 15, \ n_{124} = 13, \ n_{134} = 15, \ n_{214} = 39, \\
&n_{224} = 22, \ n_{234} = 18, \\
&n_{115} = 4, \ n_{125} = 12, \ n_{135} = 17, \ n_{215} = 5, \\
&n_{225} = 15, \ n_{235} = 8, \\
&n_{1++} = 289, \ n_{2++} = 368, \ n_{+1+} = 381, \\
&n_{+2+} = 163, \ n_{+3+} = 113, \\
&n_{++1} = 175, \ n_{++2} = 156, \ n_{++3} = 143, \\
&n_{++4} = 122, \ n_{++5} = 61, \ \text{and} \ n = 657.
\end{aligned}
\tag{1}
$$

By substituting Eq. (1) into Eq. (11.3A.4), we obtain

$$
\begin{aligned}
\chi_{3\text{-}way} = 657 \Bigg\{ 657 \Bigg[& \left(\frac{58^2}{289 \cdot 381 \cdot 175} + \frac{11^2}{289 \cdot 163 \cdot 175} + \frac{5^2}{289 \cdot 113 \cdot 175} \right. \\
& + \frac{75^2}{368 \cdot 381 \cdot 175} + \frac{19^2}{368 \cdot 163 \cdot 175} + \frac{7^2}{368 \cdot 113 \cdot 175} \\
& + \frac{49^2}{289 \cdot 381 \cdot 156} = + \cdots + \frac{5^2}{368 \cdot 381 \cdot 61} \\
& \left. + \frac{5^2}{368 \cdot 163 \cdot 61} + \frac{5^2}{368 \cdot 113 \cdot 61} \right) - 1 \Bigg] \Bigg\} \\
= 657(1.178057 - 1) & = 116.9835 \approx 116.98.
\end{aligned}
\tag{2}
$$

Since the computed $\chi_{3\text{-}way}$ of Eq. (2) is greater than the critical value of the chi-squared distribution with $8(= (2-1)(3-1)(5-1))$ degrees of freedom, $\chi^2_{8;0.975} = 17.54$ (see Table A-3), H_0 of Eq. (11.3A.1) is rejected at the level of significance 0.05. Hence, the treatment, the number of depletions and the litter sizes are not independent.

B. A Test for First/Second-Order Interaction in Three-Way Tables

By following along the lines of Sec. 11.2B, the first-order interaction in three-way tables is given as follows.

Definition 11.3B.1. Given that Z is pooled in Table 11.3A-1, X and Y are said to have zero first-order (or no two-factor) interaction if $\theta^{i^* j^*}_{ij|Z} = 1$ for all pairs (i, i^*) and (j, j^*) such that $i \neq i^*$ and $j \neq j^*$, where $\theta^{i^* j^*}_{ij|Z+}$ is the odds ratio of the 2×2 table formed by using two distinct rows of X ($X = i$ and $X = i^*$) and two distinct columns of Y ($Y = j$ and $Y = j^*$), and is defined by

$$\theta^{i^* j^*}_{ij|Z+} = \frac{p_{ij+}p_{i^* j^*+}}{p_{i^* j+}p_{ij^*+}}, \tag{11.3B.1}$$

where $\{p_{ij+}\}$, $i = 1,2,\ldots,I$ and $j = 1,2,\ldots J$ are defined in Sec. 11.3A.

Note that when X (or Y) is pooled, $\theta^{j^* k^*}_{jk|X+}$ *(or $\theta^{i^* k^*}_{ik|Y+}$) is defined accordingly.

Given that Z is pooled, test if X and Y has a zero first-order interaction, thus we need to test the following pair of hypothses:

$$H^{Z+}_{0(XY)} : \theta^{i^* j^*}_{ij|Z+} = 1, \text{ for all pairs } (i, i^*) \text{ and } (j, j^*) \text{ such that}$$

$$i \neq i^* \text{ and } j \neq j^*, \tag{11.3B.2}$$

versus

$$H_{1(XY)}^{(Z+)} : \theta_{ij|Z+}^{i^*j^*} \neq 1, \text{ for at least one of the pairs } (i, i^*) \text{ and}$$

$$(j, j^*) \text{ such that } i \neq i^* \text{ and } j \neq j^*,$$

where $\theta_{ij|Z+}^{i^*j^*}$ is defined by Eq. (11.3B.1)

Again, it is well known that Table 11.3A-1 has $(I-1)(J-1)$ independent 2×2 tables, given that Z is pooled. The maximum likelihood estimator of Eq. (11.3B.1) is

$$\hat{\theta}_{ij|Z+}^{i^*j^*} = \frac{n_{ij+}n_{i^*j^*+}}{n_{i^*j+}n_{ij^*+}}, \qquad (11.3B.3)$$

where $\{n_{ij+}\}$ are given in Table 11.3A-1. To test each of $\theta_{ij|i^*j^*(Z)}$ of Eq. (11.3B.2), we can apply the odds ratio test for 2×2 tables (DR 11.1B-1) to Eq. (11.3B.3) given by

$$\chi_{\hat{\theta}_{ij|Z}^{i^*j^*}} = \left[\frac{\ln \hat{\theta}_{ij|Z}^{i^*j^*}}{\hat{\sigma}_{\ln \hat{\theta}_{ij|Z}^{i^*j^*}}} \right]^2, \qquad (11.3B.4)$$

where $\hat{\sigma}_{\ln \hat{\theta}_{ij|Z}}^{i^*j^*}$ is given by

$$\hat{\sigma}_{\ln \hat{\theta}_{ij|Z}}^{i^*j^*} = \sqrt{n_{ij}^{-1} + n_{i^*j}^{-1} + n_{ij^*}^{-1} + n_{i^*j^*}^{-1}}. \qquad (11.3B.5)$$

Thus, the decision rule for testing Eq. (11.3B.2) is given as follows.

Decision Rule 11.3B-1 (The log-odds-ratio test on first-order interaction for X and Y given that Z is pooled)
A two-tailed test for Eq. (11.3B.2) is to reject H_0 if the computed $\chi_{ij|Z}^{i^*j^*}$ of Eq. (11.3B.4) for at least one of the pairs (i, i^*) and (j, j^*) such that $i \neq i^*$ and $j \neq j^*$ is greater than $\chi_{1;1-\frac{\alpha}{2}}^2$ or less than $\chi_{1;\frac{\alpha}{2}}^2$, where α is the level of significance. Otherwise, do not reject H_0.

Before we consider the general case of second-order interaction in three-way tables. Let us consider first the simplest three-way tables, that is, the $2 \times 2 \times 2$ tables. When $I = J = K = 2$, Bartlett[7] defined the condition for no three-factor interaction as follows.

Definition 11.1B.2. A $2 \times 2 \times 2$ contingency table is said to have a zero second-order (no three-factor) interaction if $\theta_{2 \times 2 \times 2} = 1$, where $\theta_{2 \times 2 \times 2}$ is defined by

$$\theta_{2 \times 2 \times 2} = \frac{p_{111} p_{221} p_{122} p_{212}}{p_{121} p_{211} p_{112} p_{222}}, \tag{11.3B.6}$$

where $\{p_{ijk}\}$, $i = j = k = 1$ or 2, are the cell probabilities for Table 11.3A-1.

Remarks

1. Note that the right side of Eq. (11.3B.6) represents, respectively, the ratio of the odds ratio for X and Y across the levels of $Z = 1$ and 2. This implies that a $2 \times 2 \times 2$ contingency table has zero second-order interaction if the odds ratios between X and Y are constants across the levels of Z.
2. Simpson[54] discussed the paradox arising from this definition, which will be covered in Sec. 11.4.

To test whether a $2 \times 2 \times 2$ contingency table has zero second-order interaction, we need to test the following pair of hypotheses

$$H_0 : \theta_{2 \times 2 \times 2} = 1 \quad \text{versus} \quad H_1 : \theta_{2 \times 2 \times 2} \neq 1. \tag{11.3B.7}$$

Assume that the marginal totals with respect to Z in Table 11.3A-1 are fixed. Since there is only one degree of freedom, we are free to choose the deviation x from the expectation in each of 8 cells, such that the value of x has to satisfy the following cubic equation in x

$$(n_{111} + x)(n_{221} + x)(n_{122} + x)(n_{212} + x)$$
$$= (n_{121} - x)(n_{211} - x)(n_{112} - x)(n_{222} - x). \tag{11.3B.8}$$

The test statistic for testing Eq. (11.3B.7) is

$$\chi_{Bart} = x^2 \left\{ \sum_{i=1}^{2} [(n_{ii1} + x)^{-1} + (n_{ii2} - x)^{-1}] \right.$$
$$\left. + \sum_{i \neq j}^{2} [(n_{ij1} - x)^{-1} + (n_{ij2} + x)^{-1}] \right\} \tag{11.3B.9}$$

where x is the root obtained from Eq. (11.3B.8). The decision rule is thus given as follows. With the Yates' correction for continuity, Eq. (11.3B.9) is rewritten as[7]

$$\chi^*_{Bart} = \left(|x| - \frac{1}{2}\right)^2 \left\{ \sum_{i=1}^{2} [(n_{ii1} + x)^{-1} + (n_{ii2} - x)^{-1}] \right.$$
$$\left. + \sum_{i \neq j} [(n_{ij1} - x)^{-1} + (n_{ij2} + x)^{-1}] \right\} \qquad (11.3B.10)$$

Thus, the decision rule for testing Eq. (11.3B.2) is given as follows.

Decision Rule 11.3B-2 (Bartlett's test on second-order interaction for $2 \times 2 \times 2$ tables)
Reject H_0 of Eq. (11.3B.7) at the level of significance α if the computed χ^*_{Bart} of Eq. (11.3B.10) is greater than $\chi^2_{1;1-\frac{\alpha}{2}}$ or less than $\chi^2_{1;\frac{\alpha}{2}}$. Otherwise, do not reject H_0.

Remarks

1. It was proved by Lancaster[32] that the cubic equation of Eq. (11.3B.8) has a unique real root. In practice, the closed form formula for the real root of Eq. (11.3B.8) is given by Theorem 14.5.4 (Tartaglia– Cardano's formula for cubic equations).[35]
2. An extension of Bartlett's test for a $2 \times 2 \times 2$ table to the $2 \times 2 \times K(K > 2)$ table is given in Norton.[46]
3. Without the need of the assumption that the marginal totals are fixed, Roy and Kastenbaum[51] assume that only the total sample size is fixed and show that x in Eq. (11.3B.8) is the same as the Lagrangian multiplier λ associated with the constraint of Eq. (11.3B.7).
4. By following the log-odds-ratio test in Sec. 11.1B, an alternative test statistic to Eq. (11.3B.10) is given by

$$\chi_{\hat{\theta}_{2 \times 2 \times 2}} = \left(\frac{\ln \hat{\theta}_{2 \times 2 \times 2}}{\hat{\sigma}_{\hat{\theta}_{2 \times 2 \times 2}}}\right)^2, \qquad (11.3B.11)$$

where $\hat{\theta}_{2\times2\times2}$ and $\hat{\sigma}_{\ln\hat{\theta}_{2\times2\times2}}$ are given, respectively, by

$$\hat{\theta}_{2\times2\times2} = \frac{n_{111}\,n_{221}\,n_{122}\,n_{212}}{n_{121}\,n_{211}\,n_{112}\,n_{222}}, \tag{11.3B.12}$$

and

$$\hat{\sigma}(\ln\hat{\theta}_{2\times2\times2})$$
$$= \sqrt{n_{111}^{-1} + n_{221}^{-1} + n_{122}^{-1} + n_{212}^{-1} + n_{121}^{-1} + n_{211}^{-1} + n_{112}^{-1} + n_{222}^{-1}}. \tag{11.3B.13}$$

An alternative decision rule by using Eq. (11.3B.10) is given as follows.[49]

Decision Rule 11.3B-3 (The log-odds-ratio's test on second-order interaction for 2 × 2 × 2 tables)
Reject H_0 of Eq. (11.3B.7) at the level of significance α if the computed $\chi_{\hat{\theta}_{2\times2\times2}}$ of Eq. (11.3B.11) is greater than $\chi^2_{1;1-\frac{\alpha}{2}}$ or less than $\chi^2_{1;\frac{\alpha}{2}}$. Otherwise, do not reject H_0.

Example 11.3B-1

The data in Table 11.3B-1 are taken from Crane *et al.*[13] A case-control study was conducted to examine the hypothesis that fenoterol in a metered dose inhaler increases the risk of death in patients with asthma. Cases were drawn from the National Asthma Mortality Survey, which identified all asthma deaths in New Zealand from August 1981 to July 1983. Of the 271 asthma deaths identified in the survey, 125 occurred in patients aged 5–45 years, and these formed the case group. For each case, 4 controls, matched for age and ethnic group, were selected from asthma admissions to hospitals to which the cases themselves would have been admitted, had they survived. Controls were obtained for 124 out of the 125 cases. Seven cases were subsequently excluded because they died after admission to hospitals. Therefore the analysis pertains to 117 cases and 468 matched controls.

Table 11.3B-1. The sample data of X (use of fenoterol), Y (dose of corticosteroids) and Z (asthma death)

	Z = 1		Z = 2	
	Y = 1	Y = 2	Y = 1	Y = 2
X = 1	26	34	38	151
X = 2	7	50	66	213

In terms of symbols, let X = use of prescribed fenoterol (X = 1 if "Yes", X = 2 if "No"), Y = dose of corticosteroids (Y = 1 if "used", Y = 2 if "not used") , and Z = asthma deaths (Z = 1 if "outpatient deaths", Z = 2 if "hospitalized control").

Test at the level of significance 0.05 if Table 11.3B-1 has a zero second-order interaction by applying two different decision rules, (a) DR 11.3B-2 and (b) DR 11.3B-3, respectively.

Solution

(a) By substituting $n_{111} = 26$, $n_{121} = 34$, $n_{211} = 7$, $n_{221} = 50$, $n_{112} = 38$, $n_{122} = 151$, $n_{212} = 66$ and $n_{222} = 213$, obtained from Table 11.3B-1, into Eq. (11.3B.8), we have after simplification

$$(26 + x)(50 + x)(151 + x)(66 + x)$$

$$= (34 - x)(7 - x)(38 - x)(213 - x)$$

$$\Rightarrow x^3 + 15.6154x^2 + 2446.3385x + 18853.7231 = 0. \qquad (a.1)$$

To solve Eq. (a.1) for x, I am going to use a closed form formula in Theorem 14.5.4 (Tartaglia–Cardano's formula for cubic equations).[35] I will use the symbols provided there. From Eq. (a.1), $b_2^* = 15.6145$, $b_1^* = 2446.3385$ and $b_0^* = 18853.7231$. Then, by substituting the value of $\{b_j^*\}$ into c_0^* and c_1^*, we have

$$c_0^* = b_0^* - \frac{1}{3}b_1^* b_2^* + \frac{2}{27}b_2^{*3} = 6402.2547, \qquad (a.2)$$

and

$$c_1^* = b_1^* - \frac{1}{3}b_2^{*2} = 2365.0583. \qquad (a.3)$$

By substituting Eqs. (a.2) and (a.3) into Δ^*, we obtain

$$\Delta^* = 4c_1^{*3} + 27c_0^{*2} = 5.402252 \cdot 10^{10}.\tag{a.4}$$

Since Eq. (a.4) is greater than zero, Eq. (a.1) has one real root and a pair of two complex roots. By substituting Eqs. (a.2) and (a.4) into A and B, we get

$$A = -\frac{1}{2}c_0^* + \frac{1}{6}\sqrt{\frac{1}{2}\Delta^*} = 19164.2148,\tag{a.5}$$

and

$$B = -\frac{1}{2}c_0^* + \frac{1}{6}\sqrt{\frac{1}{3}\Delta^*} = -22566.4695.\tag{a.6}$$

By substituting Eqs. (a.5) and (a.6) into x_1, we obtain

$$x_1 = -\frac{1}{3}b_2^* + \sqrt[3]{A} + \sqrt[3]{B} = -7.9038 \approx -7.9.\tag{a.7}$$

After substituting Eq. (a.7) for x and $\{n_{ijk}\}$ obtained from Table 11.3B-1 into Eq. (11.3B.10), we get

$$\begin{aligned}
\chi_{Bart}^* = &\left(|-7.9| - \frac{1}{2}\right)^2 [(26-7.9)^{-1} + ((7+7.9)^{-1}\\
&+ (34+7.9)^{-1} + (50-7.9)^{-1} + (38+7.9)^{-1}\\
&+ (151-7.9)^{-1} + (66-7.9)^{-1} + (213+7.9)^{-1}]\\
= &\ 12.0746 \approx 12.07.
\end{aligned}\tag{a.8}$$

Since the computed χ_{Bart}^* of Eq. (a.8) is greater than $\chi_{1;0.975}^2 = 5.024$, H_0 of Eq. (11.3B.2) is rejected at the level of significance 0.05. Hence, there exists a three-factor interaction for Table 11.3B-1.

(b) By substituting $n_{111} = 26$, $n_{121} = 34$, $n_{211} = 7$, $n_{221} = 50$, $n_{112} = 38$, $n_{122} = 151$, $n_{212} = 66$ and $n_{222} = 213$, obtained from

Table 11.3B-1, into Eqs. (11.3B.12) and (11.3B.13),

$$\hat{\theta}_{2\times2\times2} = \frac{26\cdot50\cdot151\cdot66}{34\cdot7\cdot38\cdot213} = 6.725492 \approx 6.725, \qquad \text{(b.1)}$$

and

$$\hat{\sigma}\,(\ln\hat{\theta}_{2\times2\times2}$$

$$= \sqrt{26^{-1} + 34^{-1} + 7^{-1} + 50^{-1} + 38^{-1} + 151^{-1} + 66^{-1} + 213^{-1}}$$

$$= 0.532461 \approx 0.532. \qquad \text{(b.2)}$$

By substituting Eqs. (b.1) and (b.2) into Eq. (11.3B.11),

$$\chi_{\hat{\theta}_{2\times2\times2}} = (\ln 6.725/0.532)^2 = 12.81225 \approx 12.81. \qquad \text{(b.3)}$$

Since the computed $\chi_{\hat{\theta}_{2\times2\times2}}$ of Eq. (b.3) is greater than $\chi^2_{1;0.975} = 5.024$, H_0 of Eq. (11.3B.2) is rejected at the level of significance 0.05. Hence, there exists a three-factor interaction for Table 11.3B-1.

Remarks

1. It is not surprising to see that the computed χ^*_{Bart} of Eq. (a.8) and the computed $\chi_{\hat{\theta}_{2\times2\times2}}$ of Eq. (b.3) are comparable, because the total sample size ($n = 585$) is large and both DR 11.3B-2 and DR 11.3B-3 are large sample tests.
2. DR 11.3B-3 is preferable to DR 11.3B-2 for two reasons: (i) there is no need of the assumption that the marginal totals are fixed and (ii) there is no need to solve the required cubic equation.

Definition 11.3B.2 is generalized to the full three-way ($I \times J \times K$) tables as follows.[34]

Definition 11.3B.3. Three categorical r.v.s X, Y and Z, given in a $I \times J \times K$ contingency table of Table 13.3A-1, are said to have a zero second-order (or no three-factor) interaction if $\theta^{i^* j^* k^*}_{ijk}$ for all pairs (i, i^*), (j, j^*) and (k, k^*) such that $i \neq i^*$, $j \neq j^*$ and $k \neq k^*$ where

$\theta_{i^*j^*k}^{ijk}$ is defined by

$$\theta_{ijk}^{i^*j^*k^*} = \frac{p_{ijk}p_{i^*jk}p_{i^*jk^*}p_{ij^*k^*}}{p_{i^*jk}p_{ij^*k}p_{ijk^*}p_{i^*j^*k^*}}, \tag{11.3B.14}$$

where $\{p_{ijk}\}$, $i = 1, 2, \ldots, I$, $j = 1, 2, \ldots J$, $k = 1, 2, \ldots, K$ are defined in Sec. 11.3A.

To test if X, Y and Z have a zero second-order interaction, we need to test the following pair of hypothses that

$$H_0: \theta_{i^*j^*k^*}^{ijk} = 1 \text{ for all pairs } (i, i^*), (j, j^*) \text{ and } (k, k^*)$$

$$\text{such that } i \neq i^*, \, j \neq j^* \text{ and } k \neq k, \tag{11.3B.15}$$

versus

$$H_1: \theta_{ijk}^{i^*j^*k^*} \neq 1 \text{ for at least one of the pairs } (i, i^*), (j, j^*)$$

$$\text{and } (k, k^*) \text{ such that } i \neq i^*, \, j \neq j^* \text{ and } k \neq k^*,$$

where $\theta_{ijk}^{i^*j^*k^*}$ is defined by Eq. (11.3B.14).

It has been shown[51] that Table 11.3A-1 has $(I - 1)(J - 1)(K - 1)$ independent $2 \times 2 \times 2$ tables. The maximum likelihood estimator of Eq. (11.3B.14) is

$$\hat{\theta}_{ijk}^{i^*j^*k^*} = \frac{n_{ijk}n_{i^*jk}n_{i^*jk^*}n_{ij^*k^*}}{n_{i^*jk}n_{ij^*k}n_{ijk^*}n_{i^*j^*k^*}}, \tag{11.3B.16}$$

where $\{n_{ijk}\}$ are given in Table 11.3A-1. To test each of $\theta_{i^*j^*k^*}^{ijk}$ of Eq. (11.3B.14), we can apply the log-odds-ratio test (DR 11.3B-3) for $2 \times 2 \times 2$ tables to Eq. (11.3B.14) given by

$$\chi_{\hat{\theta}_{ijk}}^{i^*j^*k^*} = \left[\frac{\ln(\hat{\theta}_{ijk}^{i^*j^*k^*})}{\hat{\sigma}_{\ln(\hat{\theta}_{ijk}^{i^*j^*k^*})}} \right]^2, \tag{11.3B.17}$$

where $\hat{\sigma}\left(\ln\hat{\theta}_{ijk}^{i^*j^*k^*}\right)$ is given by

$$\hat{\sigma}\left(\ln\hat{\theta}_{ijk}^{i^*j^*k^*}\right)$$

$$= \sqrt{n_{ijk}^{-1} + n_{i^*jk}^{-1} + n_{i^*jk^*}^{-1} + n_{ij^*k^*}^{-1} + n_{i^*jk}^{-1} + n_{ij^*k}^{-1} + n_{ijk^*}^{-1} + n_{i^*j^*k^*}^{-1}}$$

$$(11.3B.18)$$

Thus, the decision rule for testing Eq. (11.3B.13) is given as follows.

Decision Rule 11.3B-4 (The test on a second-order interaction for $I \times J \times K$ tables)
A two-tailed test for Eq. (11.3B.15) is to reject H_0 if the computed $\chi_{\hat{\theta}_{i^*j^*k^*}^{ijk}}$ of Eq. (11.3B.17) for at least one of the pairs (i, i^*), (j, j^*) and (k, k^*) such that $i \neq i^*$, $j \neq j^*$ and $k \neq k^*$ is greater than $\chi_{1;1-\frac{\alpha}{2}}^2$ or less than $\chi_{1;\frac{\alpha}{2}}^2$, where α is the level of significance. Otherwise, do not reject H_0.

Remark

Equation (11.3B.14) is the multiplicative definition of the second-order interaction. Yet, it was criticized[32] that the multiplicative definition of no three-factor interaction is not almalgation invariant, that is, it cannot be reduced to that of a no two-factor interaction (see Definition 11.3B.1) by pooling the marginal totals except in trivial cases; hence the use of his additive definition presented in Ref. 34 is advocated. However, after a comparison, Darroch[15] shows that the multiplicative version is preferable by a small margin, since both versions of the three-factor interaction test under the additive or multiplicative definition fall short of the ideal.

Example 11.3B-2

By using the data given in Table 11.3A-2, test at the level of significance 0.05 if there exists (a) a first-order interaction between X and Y, given that Z is pooled, and (b) a second-order interaction between X, Y and Z.

Table 11.3B-2. The sample data of X and Y after Z is pooled

	Y = 1	Y = 2	Y = 3
X = 1	159	68	62
X = 2	222	95	51

Solution

(a) By pooling the data in the five levels of Z,

$$n_{11+} = n_{111} + n_{112} + n_{113} + n_{114} + n_{115}$$
$$= 58 + 49 + 33 + 15 + 4 = 159,$$

$$n_{12+} = n_{121} + n_{122} + n_{123} + n_{124} + n_{125}$$
$$= 11 + 14 + 18 + 13 + 12 = 68,$$

$$n_{13+} = n_{131} + n_{132} + n_{133} + n_{134} + n_{135}$$
$$= 5 + 10 + 15 + 15 + 17 = 62,$$

$$n_{21+} = n_{211} + n_{212} + n_{213} + n_{214} + n_{215}$$
$$= 75 + 58 + 45 + 39 + 5 = 222,$$

$$n_{22+} = n_{221} + n_{222} + n_{223} + n_{224} + n_{225}$$
$$= 19 + 17 + 22 + 22 + 15 = 95,$$

and

$$n_{23+} = n_{231} + n_{232} + n_{233} + n_{234} + n_{235} = 7 + 8 + 10 + 18 + 8 = 51.$$

By assembling Table 11.3A-2 after Z is pooled into a 2×3 table, we have Table 11.3B-2 that has two independent 2×2 tables.

By using Eqs. (11.3B.3) and (11.3B.5) in calculating the odds ratio and its estimated standard error of the logarithmic odds ratio for case 1 in Table 11.3B-3,

$$\hat{\theta}^{21}_{12|Z} = (159 \cdot 95)/(68 \cdot 222) \approx 1.001, \tag{1}$$

Table 11.3B-3.   Two independent 2 × 2 tables are obtained from Table 11.3B-2

	Case 1			Case 2	
	Y = 1	Y = 2		Y = 2	Y = 3
X = 1	159	68	X = 1	68	62
X = 2	222	95	X = 2	95	51

and

$$\hat{\sigma}_{\ln\hat{\theta}^{21}_{12|Z}} = \sqrt{159^{-1} + 68^{-1} + 222^{-1} + 95^{-1}} \approx 0.1898.$$

By substituting Eq. (1) into Eq. (11.3B.4),

$$\chi_{\hat{\theta}^{21}_{12|Z}} = (\ln 1.001/0.1898)^2 = 9.86 \cdot 10^{-6}. \tag{2}$$

Similarly, the odds ratio and its estimated standard error of the logarithmic odds ratio for case 2 in Table 11.3B-3 are obtained as follows:

$$\hat{\theta}^{32}_{23|Z} = (68 \cdot 51)/(62 \cdot 95) \approx 0.5889, \tag{3}$$

and

$$\hat{\sigma}_{\ln\hat{\theta}^{32}_{23|Z}} = \sqrt{68^{-1} + 62^{-1} + 95^{-1} + 51^{-1}} \approx 0.2469.$$

By substituting Eq. (3) into Eq. (11.3B.4),

$$\chi_{\hat{\theta}^{32}_{23|Z}} = (\ln 0.5889/0.2469)^2 = 4.6017. \tag{4}$$

Although Eq. (4) is not greater than $\chi^2_{1;0.975} = 5.024$, Eq. (2) is less than $\chi^2_{1;0.025} = 0.001$. By applying DR 11.3B-1, H_0 of Eq. (11.3B.2) is rejected at the level of significance 0.05. Hence there exists a first-order interaction between X and Y when Z is pooled.

(b) Since Table 11.3A-2 is a 2 × 3 × 5 table, there are 8(= (2 − 1) (3 − 1)(5 − 1)) independent 2 × 2 × 2 tables. Since all three random variables have ordered categories, we are going to select the adjacent rows/columns/layers to form these 8 independent 2 × 2 × 2 tables.

Table 11.3B-4. The sample data of 8 2 × 2 × 2 tables formed from Table 11.3A-2

Case 1

	Z = 1			Z = 2	
	Y = 1	Y = 2		Y = 1	Y = 1
X = 1	58	11	X = 1	49	14
X = 2	75	19	X = 2	58	17

Case 2

	Z = 1			Z = 2	
	Y = 2	Y = 3		Y = 2	Y = 3
X = 1	11	5	X = 1	14	10
X = 2	19	7	X = 2	17	8

Case 3

	Z = 2			Z = 3	
	Y = 1	Y = 2		Y = 1	Y = 2
X = 1	49	14	X = 1	33	18
X = 2	58	17	X = 2	45	22

Case 4

	Z = 2			Z = 3	
	Y = 2	Y = 3		Y = 2	Y = 3
X = 1	14	10	X = 1	18	15
X = 2	17	8	X = 2	22	10

Case 5

	Z = 3			Z = 4	
	Y = 1	Y = 2		Y = 1	Y = 2
X = 1	33	18	X = 1	15	13
X = 2	45	22	X = 2	39	22

Table 11.3B-4. (*Continued*)

Case 6

	Z = 3			Z = 4	
	Y = 2	Y = 3		Y = 2	Y = 3
X = 1	58	15	X = 1	13	15
X = 2	22	10	X = 2	22	18

Case 7

	Z = 4			Z = 5	
	Y = 1	Y = 2		Y = 1	Y = 2
X = 1	15	13	X = 1	4	12
X = 2	39	22	X = 2	5	15

and

Case 8

	Z = 4			Z = 5	
	Y = 2	Y = 3		Y = 2	Y = 3
X = 1	13	15	X = 1	12	17
X = 2	22	18	X = 2	15	18

By using Eqs. (11.3B.6), (11.3B.11) and (11.3B.12), the estimated odds ratio $(\hat{\theta}_{2\times2\times2}^{(i)})$, the standard error of logarithmic odds-ratio $\hat{\sigma}(\ln(\hat{\theta}_{2\times2\times2}^{(i)}))$, and the chi-squared statistic $(\chi_{\hat{\theta}_{2\times2\times2}^{(i)}})$ for each of the ith case in Table 11.3B-4 are calculated as follows.

Case 1:

$$\hat{\theta}_{2\times2\times2}^{(1)} = \frac{58 \cdot 19 \cdot 14 \cdot 58}{11 \cdot 75 \cdot 49 \cdot 17} \approx 1.302,$$

$$\hat{\sigma}\left(\ln\hat{\theta}_{2\times2\times2}^{(1)}\right) = \sqrt{58^{-1} + 11^{-1} + 75^{-1} + 19^{-1} + 49^{-1} + 14^{-1} + 58^{-1} + 17^{-1}}$$

$$\approx 0.585,$$

$$\chi_{\hat{\theta}_{2\times2\times2}^{(1)}} = [\ln(1.302)/0.585]^2 \approx 0.204. \tag{1}$$

Case 2:

$$\hat{\theta}^{(2)}_{2\times2\times2} = \frac{11\cdot7\cdot10\cdot17}{5\cdot19\cdot14\cdot8} \approx 1.23,$$

$$\hat{\sigma}\left(\ln\hat{\theta}^{(2)}_{2\times2\times2}\right) = \sqrt{11^{-1}+5^{-1}+19^{-1}+7^{-1}+14^{-1}+10^{-1}+17^{-1}+8^{-1}}$$
$$\approx 0.917,$$

$$\chi_{\hat{\theta}^{(2)}_{2\times2\times2}} = [\ln(1.23)/0.917]^2 \approx 0.051. \tag{2}$$

Case 3:

$$\hat{\theta}^{(3)}_{2\times2\times2} = \frac{49\cdot17\cdot18\cdot45}{14\cdot58\cdot33\cdot22} \approx 1.145,$$

$$\hat{\sigma}\left(\ln\hat{\theta}^{(3)}_{2\times2\times2}\right) = \sqrt{49^{-1}+14^{-1}+58^{-1}+17^{-1}+33^{-1}+18^{-1}+45^{-1}+22^{-1}}$$
$$\approx 0.567,$$

$$\chi_{\hat{\theta}^{(3)}_{2\times2\times2}} = [\ln(1.145)/0.567]^2 \approx 0.057. \tag{3}$$

Case 4:

$$\hat{\theta}^{(4)}_{2\times2\times2} = \frac{14\cdot8\cdot15\cdot22}{10\cdot17\cdot18\cdot10} \approx 1.208,$$

$$\hat{\sigma}\left(\ln\hat{\theta}^{(4)}_{2\times2\times2}\right) = \sqrt{14^{-1}+10^{-1}+17^{-1}+8^{-1}+18^{-1}+15^{-1}+22^{-1}+10^{-1}}$$
$$\approx 0.789,$$

$$\chi_{\hat{\theta}^{(4)}_{2\times2\times2}} = [\ln(1.208)/0.789]^2 \approx 0.057. \tag{4}$$

Case 5:

$$\hat{\theta}^{(5)}_{2\times2\times2} = \frac{33\cdot22\cdot13\cdot39}{18\cdot45\cdot15\cdot22} \approx 1.377,$$

$$\hat{\sigma}\left(\ln\hat{\theta}^{(5)}_{2\times2\times2}\right) = \sqrt{33^{-1}+22^{-1}+15^{-1}+22^{-1}+13^{-1}+39^{-1}+18^{-1}+45^{-1}}$$
$$\approx 0.607,$$

$$\chi_{\hat{\theta}^{(5)}_{2\times2\times2}} = [\ln(1.377)/0.607]^2 \approx 0.278. \tag{5}$$

Case 6:

$$\hat{\theta}^{(6)}_{2\times2\times2} = \frac{18\cdot10\cdot15\cdot22}{15\cdot22\cdot13\cdot18} \approx 2.479,$$

$$\hat{\sigma}\left(\ln\hat{\theta}^{(6)}_{2\times2\times2}\right) = \sqrt{18^{-1}+15^{-1}+22^{-1}+10^{-1}+13^{-1}+15^{-1}+22^{-1}+18^{-1}}$$

$$\approx 0.688,$$

$$\chi_{\hat{\theta}^{(6)}_{2\times2\times2}} = [\ln(2.479)/0.688]^2 \approx 1.738. \tag{6}$$

Case 7:

$$\hat{\theta}^{(7)}_{2\times2\times2} = \frac{15\cdot22\cdot12\cdot5}{13\cdot39\cdot4\cdot15} \approx 0.651,$$

$$\hat{\sigma}\left(\ln\hat{\theta}^{(7)}_{2\times2\times2}\right) = \sqrt{15^{-1}+13^{-1}+39^{-1}+22^{-1}+4^{-1}+12^{-1}+5^{-1}+15^{-1}}$$

$$\approx 0.903,$$

$$\chi_{\hat{\theta}^{(7)}_{2\times2\times2}} = [\ln(0.651)/0.903]^2 \approx 0.226. \tag{7}$$

Case 8:

$$\hat{\theta}^{(8)}_{2\times2\times2} = \frac{13\cdot18\cdot17\cdot15}{15\cdot22\cdot12\cdot8} \approx 1.884,$$

$$\hat{\sigma}(\ln\hat{\theta}^{(8)}_{2\times2\times2}) = \sqrt{13^{-1}+15^{-1}+22^{-1}+18^{-1}+12^{-1}+17^{-1}+15^{-1}+8^{-1}}$$

$$\approx 0.791,$$

$$\chi_{\hat{\theta}^{(8)}_{2\times2\times2}} = [\ln(1.884)/0.761]^2 \approx 0.693. \tag{8}$$

Since all of Eqs. (1) to (8) are neither greater than $\chi^2_{1;0.975} = 5.024$ nor less than $\chi^2_{1;0.025} = 0.001$, H_0 of Eq. (11.3B.15) is not rejected at the level of significance 0.05. Hence, there exists no second-order interaction among treatment, number of depletions and litter sizes.

Remarks

1. By using the Bartlett's test, Kastenbaum and Lamphiear[29] solved eight simultaneous third degree equations in eight unknowns to obtain $\chi_{Bart} = 3.158$, which is neither greater than $\chi^2_{8;0.975} = 17.54$ nor less than $\chi^2_{8;0.025} = 2.18$.
2. This example provides empirical evidence to confirm that the multiplicative definition of second-order interaction is not an amalgamation invariant[14] (see Exercise 11.4-12).

C. Mantel–Haenszel's Estimator for a Common Odds Ratio

In a $2 \times 2 \times K(K > 2)$ contingency table, assume that the observed cell frequencies $\{n_{ijk}\}$, $i,j = 1,2$ in the kth 2×2 table follow a multinomial distribution with the cell probability parameters $\{p_{ijk}\}$ and the sample size n_{++k}, where $E(n_{ijk}) = n_{++k}p_{ijk}$ and it has a constant common odds ratio among K 2×2 tables, that is, it satisfies the following pair of hypotheses:

$$H_0: \theta^{(k)}_{2\times2} = \theta^{(j)}_{2\times2} \text{ for all pairs of } (j,k), \ j \neq k, \tag{11.3C.1}$$

versus

$$H_1: \theta^{(k)}_{2\times2} \neq \theta^{(j)}_{2\times2} \text{ for at least one pair of } (j,k), \ j \neq k,$$

where $\theta^{(k)}_{2\times2}$ is the odds ratio of the kth 2×2 table defined by

$$\theta^{(k)}_{2\times2} = p_{11k}p_{22k}(p_{12k}p_{21k})^{-1}. \tag{11.3C.2}$$

By multiplying the denominator of Eq. (11.3C.2) to the right side for H_0 in Eq. (11.3C.1) and summing up all K equations, the Mantel–Haenszel parameter for a common odds ratio is

$$\theta_{MH} = \frac{\sum_{k=1}^{K} p_{11k}p_{22k}}{\sum_{k=1}^{K} p_{12k}p_{21k}}. \tag{11.3C.3}$$

From Eq. (11.3C.3), the Mantel–Haenszel estimator of θ is given by[37]

$$\hat{\theta}_{MH} = \frac{\sum_{k=1}^{K} \hat{p}_{11k}\hat{p}_{22k}}{\sum_{k=1}^{K} \hat{p}_{12k}\hat{p}_{21k}}, \qquad (11.3C.4)$$

where $\{\hat{p}_{ijk}\}_{i,j=1;k=1}^{2;K}$ are the maximum likelihood estimator of $\{p_{ijk}\}_{i,j=1;k=1}^{2;K}$ in Table 11.3A-1 when $I = J = 2$.

To simplify the derivation of the large sample variance of Eq. (11.3C.4), let us consider a simple practical case, that is, for each 2×2 table there are two independent binomial random variables Y_{1k} and Y_{2k} with their respective probability p_{1k} and p_{2k}, and their sample sizes n_{1+k} and n_{2+k}, in which $\hat{p}_{ik} = n_{i1k}/n_{i+k}$, $\hat{q}_{ik} = 1 - \hat{p}_{ik}$, $E(\hat{p}_{ik}) = n_{i+k}p_{ik}$ and $\sigma^2(\hat{p}_{ik}) = n_{i+k}p_{ik}q_{ik}$, $i = 1, 2, k = 1, \ldots, K$. In this case, Eq. (11.3C.3) is given by

$$\theta_{MH} = \frac{\sum_{k=1}^{K} p_{1k}q_{2k}}{\sum_{k=1}^{K} p_{2k}q_{1k}}, \qquad (11.3C.5)$$

where $q_{ik} = 1 - p_{ik}$, $i = 1, 2$. Since Eq. (11.3C.5) is a nonlinear function of $2K$ independent variables $(p_{11}, p_{21}, \ldots, p_{1K}, p_{2K})$, we need to apply the delta's method[2] to find the sample variance for the corresponding Mantel–Haenszel's estimator of Eq. (11.3C.4) given by

$$\hat{\theta}_{MH} = \frac{\sum_{k=1}^{K} \hat{p}_{1k}\hat{q}_{2k}}{\sum_{k=1}^{K} \hat{p}_{2k}\hat{q}_{1k}}, \qquad (11.3C.6)$$

where $\hat{p}_{ik} = n_{1ik}/n_{ik}$, n_{1ik} is the number of success in n_{ik} independently repeated Bernoulli trials for the Binomial random variable Y_{ik}, $\hat{q}_{ik} = 1 - \hat{p}_{ik}$.

By taking the partial derivative of Eq. (11.3C.5) with respect to p_{ik} (see Exercise 11.4-13), $i = 1, 2$, and $k = 1, \ldots, K$, the large-sample estimated standard error of Eq. (11.3C.4) is

$$\hat{\sigma}(\hat{\theta}_{MH}) = \sqrt{\sum_{k=1}^{K} \sum_{i=1}^{2} \hat{c}_{ik}^2 \hat{\sigma}^2(\hat{p}_{ik})}, \qquad (11.3C.7)$$

where for $i = 1, 2$, $k = 1, \ldots, K$, $\hat{\sigma}^2(\hat{p}_{ik}) = n_{ik}\hat{p}_{ik}\hat{q}_{ik}$, $\hat{\theta}_{MH}$ is given by Eq. (11.3C.6), and $\hat{c}_{ik}$ s are given respectively by

$$\hat{c}_{1k} = \left[(\hat{q}_{2k} + \hat{\theta}_{MH}\hat{p}_{2k}) \bigg/ \left(\sum_{k=1}^{K} \hat{p}_{2k}\hat{q}_{1k} \right) \right], \qquad (11.3C.8)$$

and

$$\hat{c}_{2k} = \left[(\hat{p}_{1k} + \hat{\theta}_{MH}\hat{q}_{1k}) \bigg/ \left(\sum_{k=1}^{K} \hat{p}_{2k}\hat{q}_{1k} \right) \right]. \qquad (11.3C.9)$$

Remarks

1. Note that $\theta_{MH} \neq \theta$ since Eq. (11.3C.3) holds only when H_0 in Eq. (11.3C.1) is true, but the converse is not true. In other words, Eq. (11.3C.3) is a necessary, but not a sufficient condition for the validity of H_0 in Eq. (11.3C.1). As a result, the Mantel–Haenszel estimator $\hat{\theta}_{MH}$ Eq. (11.3C.4) is valid only when the homogeneity of the odds ratio holds for the entire $2 \times 2 \times K$ table, or equivalently, it has a zero second-order interaction.
2. To test the validity of Eq. (11.3C.1), we can apply the log-odds-ratio test (DR 11.3B-3) on the given $2 \times 2 \times K$ table for the zero second-order ineraction.
3. Unlike my derivation of Eq. (11.3C.7), Hauck[27] fails to take the nonlinear nature of Eq. (11.3C.5) into consideration to derive his large sample variance of the Mantel–Haenszel estimator.
4. The $100(1 - \alpha)\%$ confidence interval for θ_{MH} is given by

$$\hat{\theta}_{MH} - z_{1-\frac{\alpha}{2}}\hat{\sigma}_{\hat{\theta}MH} \leq \theta_{MH} \leq \hat{\theta}_{MH} + z_{1-\frac{\alpha}{2}}\hat{\sigma}_{\hat{\theta}_{MH}}, \qquad (11.3C.10)$$

where $\hat{\theta}_{MH}$ and $\hat{\sigma}_{\hat{\theta}_{MH}}$ are defined respectively by Eqs. (11.3C.6) and (11.3C.7).
5. For the general case in which the multinomial distribution is assumed for each 2×2 table, Eq. (11.3C.7) has to be derived differently.
6. If Eq. (11.3C.1) does not hold, it is inappropriate to use the Mantel–Haenszel's estimator of Eq. (11.3C.6) any more.

7. In addition to Mantel–Haenszel's estimator, an alternative estimate for the entire population odds ratio θ is the Woolf's estimator $\hat{\theta}_W$ given by[59]

$$\ln \hat{\theta}_W = \sum_{k=1}^{K} v_k \ln \hat{\theta}_{2 \times 2}^{(k)} \Big/ \sum_{k=1}^{K} v_k, \qquad (11.3\text{C}.11)$$

where $v_k \equiv \hat{\sigma}^2 (\ln \hat{\theta}_{2 \times 2}^{(k)}) = [n_{11k}^{-1} + n_{12k}^{-1} + n_{21k}^{-1} + n_{22k}^{-1}]^{-1}$. The $100(1 - \alpha)\%$ confidence interval for θ is given by[21]

$$\exp \left[\ln \hat{\theta}_W - Z_{1-\frac{\alpha}{2}} \hat{\sigma} (\ln \hat{\theta}_W) \right] \leq \theta \leq \exp \left[\ln \hat{\theta}_W - Z_{1-\frac{\alpha}{2}} \hat{\sigma} (\ln \hat{\theta}_W) \right], \qquad (11.3\text{C}.12)$$

where $\hat{\theta}_W$ is given by Eq. (11.3C.11) and $\hat{\sigma} (\ln \hat{\theta}_W)$ is given by

$$\hat{\sigma} (\ln \hat{\theta}_W) = \left(\sum_{k=1}^{K} v_k \right)^{-\frac{1}{2}}. \qquad (11.3\text{C}.13)$$

Example 11.3C-1

The data in Table 11.3C-1 is taken partially from Table 4 in Ref. 52 by collapsing the original four levels of alcohol use into two levels: yes and no.

(a) Does Table 11.3C-1 have a common odds ratio?
(b) If the answer to (a) is affirmative, then find the 95% confidence interval for θ_{MH}.

Table 11.3C-1.   The sample data of three variables smoking (X), alcoholic use (Y) and age (Z)

					Cases	Controls
Age < 60		No		Yes	8	18
				No	3	20
	Alcohol use	Yes	Smoker	Yes	225	166
				No	6	12
Age ≥ 60		No		Yes	25	7
				No	52	18

(c) Also, find the 95% confidence interval for Woolf's estimator $\hat{\theta}_W$.

Solution

(a) To see if Table 11.3C-1 has a common odds ratio, we need to examine whether it has a zero second-order interaction. Since Table 11.3C-1 has three independent 2×2 tables, it has two independent $2 \times 2 \times 2$ tables. We are going to apply the log-odds-ratio test on second-order interaction (see DR 11.3B-3) to the combination of the first and second, and second and third 2×2 tables. Let $\theta_{2 \times 2 \times 2}^{(i)}$, $i = 1, 2$, denote the ith combination defined as above. Thus,

$$\theta_{2 \times 2 \times 2}^{(1)} = \frac{8 \cdot 20 \cdot 166 \cdot 6}{18 \cdot 3 \cdot 225 \cdot 12} \approx 1.093, \tag{a.1}$$

$$\theta_{2 \times 2 \times 2}^{(2)} = \frac{225 \cdot 12 \cdot 7 \cdot 52}{166 \cdot 6 \cdot 25 \cdot 18} \approx 2.1928. \tag{a.2}$$

Their respective estimated standard errors are

$$\hat{\sigma}\left(\ln\hat{\theta}_{2 \times 2 \times 2}^{(1)}\right) = \sqrt{8^{-1} + 18^{-1} + 3^{-1} + 20^{-1} + 225^{-1} + 166^{-1} + 6^{-1} + 12^{-1}}$$

$$= 0.907941 \approx 0.9079, \tag{a.3}$$

$$\hat{\sigma}\left(\ln\hat{\theta}_{2 \times 2 \times 2}^{(2)}\right) = \sqrt{225^{-1} + 166^{-1} + 6^{-1} + 12^{-1} + 25^{-1} + 7^{-1} + 52^{-1} + 18^{-1}}$$

$$= 0.7198. \tag{a.4}$$

By substituting Eqs. (a.1) to (a.4) into Eq. (11.3B.11),

$$\chi_{\hat{\theta}_{2 \times 2 \times 2}^{(1)}} = \left[\frac{\ln(1.093)}{0.9079}\right]^2 = 0.009594 \approx 0.0096, \tag{a.5}$$

$$\chi_{\hat{\theta}_{2 \times 2 \times 2}^{(2)}} = \left[\frac{\ln(2.1928)}{0.7198}\right]^2 = 1.18957 \approx 1.1896. \tag{a.6}$$

Since both Eqs. (a.5) and (a.6) are neither greater than $\chi_{1;0.975}^2 = 5.024$ nor less than $\chi_{1;0.025}^2 = 0.001$, the $3 \times 2 \times 2$ table given in Table 11.3C-1 has a zero second-order interaction.

(b) Since Table 11.3C-1 has a zero second-order interaction and it is reasonable to assume that the sampling data in each 2×2 table are obtained from two independent Binomial random variables, we can use the Mantel–Haenszel estimator of Eq. (11.3C.6) to estimate the common odds ratio and Eq. (11.3C.7) for its estimated standard error.

First, we calculate, respectively, the probability of success [X (smoker) = yes] and variance for $Y = 1$ (cases) and $Y = 2$ (controls) for each 2×2 table:

$$\hat{p}_{11} = \frac{8}{8+3} \approx 0.7273, \quad \hat{q}_{11} = 1 - 0.7273 = 0.2727,$$

$$\hat{\sigma}^2(\hat{p}_{11}) = (8+3) \cdot 0.7273 \cdot (1 - 0.7273) \approx 2.1818;$$

$$\hat{p}_{21} = \frac{18}{18+20} \approx 0.4737, \quad \hat{q}_{21} = 1 - 0.4737 = 0.5263;$$

$$\hat{\sigma}^2(\hat{p}_{21}) = (18+20) \cdot 0.4737 \cdot (1 - 0.4737) \approx 9.4737;$$

$$\hat{p}_{12} = \frac{225}{225+6} \approx 0.974, \quad \hat{q}_{12} = 1 - 0.974 = 0.026,$$

$$\hat{\sigma}^2(\hat{p}_{12}) = (225+6) \cdot 0.974 \cdot 0.026 \approx 5.8441;$$

(b.1)

$$\hat{p}_{22} = \frac{166}{166+12} \approx 0.9326, \quad \hat{q}_{22} = 1 - 0.9326 = 0.0674,$$

$$\hat{\sigma}^2(\hat{p}_{22}) = (166+12) \cdot 0.9326 \cdot 0.0674 \approx 11.191;$$

$$\hat{p}_{13} = \frac{25}{25+52} = 0.3247, \quad \hat{q}_{13} = 1 - 0.3247 = 0.6753,$$

$$\hat{\sigma}^2(\hat{p}_{13}) = (25+52) \cdot 0.3247 \cdot 0.6753 \approx 16.8831;$$

$$\hat{p}_{23} = \frac{7}{7+18} = 0.28, \quad \hat{q}_{23} = 1 - 0.28 = 0.72,$$

$$\hat{\sigma}^2(\hat{p}_{23}) = (7+18) \cdot 0.28 \cdot 0.72 \approx 5.04.$$

By substituting Eq. (b.1) into Eqs. (11.3C.6), (11.3C.8) and (11.3C.9),

$$\hat{\theta}_{MH} = \frac{0.7273 \cdot 0.5263 + 0.974 \cdot 0.0674 + 0.3247 \cdot 0.72}{0.4737 \cdot 0.2727 + 0.9326 \cdot 0.026 + 0.28 \cdot 0.6753}$$

$$= \frac{0.6822}{0.3425} \approx 1.9918.$$

$$\hat{c}_{11} = \frac{0.5263 + 1.9918 \cdot 0.4737}{0.3425} \approx 4.2914,$$

$$\hat{c}_{12} = \frac{0.0674 + 1.9918 \cdot 0.9326}{0.3425} = 5.6201,$$

$$\hat{c}_{13} = \frac{0.6753 + 1.9918 \cdot 0.3247}{0.3425} \approx 3.8598,$$

$$\hat{c}_{21} = -\frac{0.7273 + 1.9918 \cdot 0.2727}{0.3425} \approx -3.7094, \qquad \text{(b.2)}$$

$$\hat{c}_{22} = -\frac{0.9326 + 1.9918 \cdot 0.0674}{0.3425} \approx -3.1149,$$

$$\hat{c}_{23} = -\frac{0.28 + 1.9918 \cdot 0.72}{0.3425} \approx -5.0045$$

$$n = \sum_{k=1}^{3} \sum_{i=1}^{2} n_{ik} = 11 + 38 + 231 + 178 + 77 + 25 = 560.$$

By substituting Eq. (b.2) into Eq. (11.3C.7),

$$\hat{\sigma}(\hat{\theta}_{MH}) = \sqrt{[4.2914^2 \cdot 2.1818 + (-3.7094)^2 \cdot 9.4737}$$
$$\overline{\sqrt{+5.6204^2 \cdot 5.8441 + (-3.1149)^2 \cdot 11.191}}$$
$$\overline{\sqrt{+3.7306^2 \cdot 16.8831 + (-4.8754)^2 \cdot 5.04]/560}}$$
$$\approx 1.2258. \qquad \text{(b.3)}$$

By substituting $\hat{\theta}_{MH} = 1.9918$ and Eq. (b.3) into Eq. (11.3C.10), 95% confidence for θ_{MH} is

$$1.9918 - 1.96 \cdot 1.2258 \leq \theta_{MH} \leq 1.9918 + 1.96 \cdot 1.2258,$$

$$\Rightarrow -0.4108 \leq \theta_{MH} \leq 4.3944. \qquad \text{(b.4)}$$

Since Eq. (b.4) includes the number one, $\theta_{MH} = 1$ is not rejected at the level of significance 0.05.

(c) Let $\theta_{2\times2}^{(k)}$ denote the odds ratio of the kth 2×2 table, $k = 1, 2, 3$. Thus, from the data given in Table 11.3C-1,

$$\hat{\theta}_{2\times2}^{(1)} = (8 \cdot 20)/(18 \cdot 3) = 2.962963 \approx 2.963,$$

$$\hat{\theta}_{2\times2}^{(2)} = (225 \cdot 12)/(166 \cdot 6) = 2.710843 \approx 2.7108, \qquad \text{(c.1)}$$

$$\hat{\theta}_{2\times2}^{(3)} = (25 \cdot 18)/(7 \cdot 52) = 1.236264 \approx 1.2363.$$

By using Eq. (11.3C.13),

$$w_1 = (8^{-1} + 20^{-1} + 18^{-1} + 3^{-1})^{-1} = 1.77399015 \approx 1.774,$$
$$w_2 = (225^{-1} + 12^{-1} + 166^{-1} + 6^{-1})^{-1} = 3.839235 \approx 3.8392,$$

$$\text{(c.2)}$$

$$w_3 = (25^{-1} + 18^{-1} + 7^{-1} + 52^{-1})^{-1} = 3.88133264 \approx 3.8813;$$
$$\hat{\sigma}(\ln\hat{\theta}_W) = (\sqrt{1.774 + 3.8392 + 3.8813})^{-1} = 0.3245. \qquad \text{(c.3)}$$

By substituting Eqs. (c.1) and (c.2) into Eq. (11.3C.11),

$$\ln\hat{\theta}_W = \frac{1.774 \cdot \ln 2.963 + 3.8392 \cdot \ln 2.7108 + 3.8813 \cdot ln 1.2363}{1.774 + 3.8392 + 3.8813}$$

$$= 0.692879 \approx 0.6929.$$

Or equivalently, the point estimator for θ is

$$\hat{\theta}_W = \exp(0.6929) = 1.999463 \approx 1.9995. \qquad \text{(c.4)}$$

By substituting Eqs. (c.3) and (c.4) into Eq. (11.3C.11), 95% confidence interval for θ is

$$\exp(0.6929 - 1.96 \cdot 0.3245) \leq \theta \leq \exp(0.6929 + 1.96 \cdot 0.3245)$$

$$\Rightarrow 1.0218 \leq \theta \leq 3.9126. \qquad \text{(c.5)}$$

Remarks

1. Although Mantel–Haenszel's estimator $\hat{\theta}_{MH} = 1.9918$ in part (b) is close to Woolf's estimator $\hat{\theta}_W = 1.9995$ in part (c), the 95% confidence interval of Eq. (c.5) is very different from that of Eq. (b.4), namely, Eq. (c.5) does not include the number one, but Eq. (b.4) includes the number one.

2. If the zero second-order interaction is not established, it means that there is no common odds ratio among K 2×2 subtables. As a result, it is pointless to use the Mantel–Haenszel estimator to estimate it. Yet, Woolf's estimator is still applicable, regardless whether the zero second-order interaction is valid. However, the interpretation for Woolf's estimator is not an estimator for the common odds ratio. Rather it is the estimation of the population odds ratio from using the odds ratio from empirical heterogeneous subpopulations. See Example 11.3D-1 for clarification.

D. *Simpson's Paradox*

EP Simpson[54] presented a paradox in 1951 to warn us that an association may be reversed when we collapse the $2 \times 2 \times K$ tables with respect to the Z variable. Simpson attributed his observational result back to a well- known result on p. 317 in Kendall's book[30] published in 1945. However, Good and Mittal[25] gave a historical account by tracing back from Kendall to Yule and then from Yule to Pearson. It is, therefore, fair to regard it as the Pearson–Yule–Kendall–Simpson paradox.

Y Mittal[44] gave a classification of this kind of paradoxical behavior involving the use of odds ratio into the following three types. The first two comes from Yule,[62] whereas the third from Good and Mittal.[25]

Definition 11.3D.1. A paradoxical phenonmenon is said to be Yule's association paradox (YAP) if and only if the following statement holds significantly:

$$\hat{\theta}_{2 \times 2}^{(k)} \equiv n_{11k} n_{22k} / n_{12k} n_{21k} = 1, \quad k = 1, 2, \ldots, K,$$

but

$$\tilde{\theta}_{2 \times 2}^{(Z+)} \equiv \left(\sum_{k=1}^{K} n_{11k} \cdot \sum_{k=1}^{K} n_{22k} \right) \bigg/ \left(\sum_{k=1}^{K} n_{12k} \cdot \sum_{k=1}^{K} n_{21k} \right) \neq 1, \quad (11.3D.1)$$

where $\tilde{\theta}_{2\times2}^{(Z+)}$ is the odds ratio for the 2 × 2 table of X and Y, given that Z is pooled.

Definition 11.3D.2. A paradoxical phenonmenon is said to be Yule's reversal paradox (YRP) if and only if the following statement holds significantly:

$$\hat{\theta}_{2\times2}^{(Z+)} > 1(< 1), \quad k = 1, 2, \dots, K,$$

but

$$\tilde{\theta}_{2\times2}^{(Z+)} < 1(> 1), \tag{11.3D.2}$$

where $\hat{\theta}_{2\times2}^{(k)}$ and $\tilde{\theta}_{2\times2}^{(Z+)}$ are defined in Eq. (11.3D.1).

Definition 11.3D.3. A paradoxical phenonmenon is said to be the amalgamation paradox (AMP) if and only if the following statement holds significantly:

$$\tilde{\theta}_{2\times2}^{(Z+)} < \min_k \hat{\theta}_{2\times2}^{(k)}, \quad k = 1, 2, \dots, K,$$

or

$$\tilde{\theta}_{2\times2}^{(Z+)} < \max_k \hat{\theta}_{2\times2}^{(k)}, \quad k = 1, 2, \dots, K, \tag{11.3D.3}$$

where $\hat{\theta}_{2\times2}^{(k)}$ and $\tilde{\theta}_{2\times2}^{(Z+)}$ are defined in Eq. (11.3D.1).

Remarks

1. YRP is popularly known nowadays as Simpson's paradox.
2. Note that $YAP \Rightarrow YCP \Rightarrow AMP$.
3. PS Bandyoapdhyay *et al.*[6] recently presented three important questions relating to Simpson's paradox and gave a formal answer to the first two, but argued that the third question "how to proceed for a final answer when the data has exhibited Simpson's paradox" did not have a unique answer. It depends on the expert's subject matter knowledge (see my remark below Example 11.3D-1.)

Example 11.3D-1

The data in Table 11.3D-1 is taken from Ref. 4. In 1972–1974 a survey largely concerned with thyroid and/or heart diseases was carried out in Whickham, United Kingdom. Twenty years later a follow-up study was conducted. Some of the results presented dealt with smoking habits as reported in the original survey and whether or not the individual survived until the second survey. For simplicity, the data in Table 11.3D-1 refer to 1314 women who were classified either as current or nonsmokers. It is presented as a three-way ($2 \times 2 \times 7$) table in which both X (living) and Y (smoking) has two levels, while Z (age group) has seven levels.

By ignoring the 7th 2×2 subtable that has zero in the second row (see my first remark), let us calculate the estimated odds ratio $\hat{\theta}_{2\times2}^{(k)}$ for the first six 2×2 tables:

$$\hat{\theta}_{2\times2}^{(1)} = (2 \cdot 61)/(1 \cdot 53) = 2.301887 \approx 2.3019,$$

$$\hat{\theta}_{2\times2}^{(2)} = (3 \cdot 152)/(5 \cdot 121) = 0.753719 \approx 0.7537,$$

Table 11.3D-1. **The sample data of X (living), Y (smoking) and Z (age group)**

	Age group (Z)					
	18–24		25–34		35–44	
	Smoker (Y)					
	Yes	No	Yes	No	Yes	No
Dead (X = 1)	2	1	3	5	14	7
Alive (X = 2)	53	61	121	152	95	114

	Age group (Z)							
	45–54		55–64		65–74		75+	
	Smoker (Y)							
	Yes	No	Yes	No	Yes	No	Yes	No
Dead (X = 1)	27	12	51	40	29	101	13	64
Alive (X = 2)	103	66	64	81	7	28	0	0

$$\hat{\theta}_{2\times2}^{(3)} = (14 \cdot 114)/(7 \cdot 95) = 2.4,$$

$$\hat{\theta}_{2\times2}^{(4)} = (27 \cdot 66)/(12 \cdot 103) = 1.441748 \approx 1.4417,$$

$$\hat{\theta}_{2\times2}^{(5)} = (51 \cdot 81)/(40 \cdot 64) = 1.613672 \approx 1.6137, \tag{1}$$

$$\hat{\theta}_{2\times2}^{(6)} = (29 \cdot 28)/(101 \cdot 7) = 1.148515 \approx 1.1485.$$

From Eq. (1), the estimated odds ratios for almost all age groups except for the 25–34 category are greater than one. It implies that the odds of dying for smokers is greater than for nonsmokers.

Next, let us calculate the overall average odds ratio from the first six groups. Thus,

$$w_1 = (2^{-1} + 61^{-1} + 1^{-1} + 53^{-1})^{-1} = 0.65135489 \approx 0.6514,$$

$$w_2 = (3^{-1} + 152^{-1} + 5^{-1} + 121^{-1})^{-1} = 1.824229 \approx 1.8242,$$

$$w_3 = (14^{-1} + 114^{-1} + 7^{-1} + 95^{-1})^{-1} = 4.28111588 \approx 4.2811,$$

$$w_4 = (27^{-1} + 66^{-1} + 12^{-1} + 103^{-1})^{-1} = 6.885600135 \approx 6.8856, \tag{2}$$

$$w_5 = (51^{-1} + 81^{-1} + 40^{-1} + 64^{-1})^{-1} = 13.77818079 \approx 13.7782,$$

$$w_6 = (29^{-1} + 28^{-1} + 101^{-1} + 7^{-1})^{-1} = 4.485206 \approx 4.4852.$$

By substituting Eqs. (1) and (2) into Eq. (11.3C.11),

$$\ln\hat{\bar{\theta}}_{2\times2} = \frac{0.6514 \cdot \ln 2.3019 + \cdots + 4.4852 \cdot \ln 1.1485}{0.6514 + \cdots + 4.4852} \approx 0.4234$$

or equivalently, the point estimator for $\bar{\theta}_{2\times2}$ is

$$\hat{\bar{\theta}} = \exp(0.4234) = 1.527127 \approx 1.53. \tag{3}$$

By substituting Eqs. (2) and (3) into Eqs. (11.3C.11) and (11.3C.12), the 95% confidence interval for $\bar{\theta}_{2\times2}$ is

$$\exp(0.4234 - 1.96 \cdot 0.177) \le \bar{\theta}_{2\times2} \le \exp(0.4234 + 1.96 \cdot 0.177),$$

$$\Rightarrow 1.0794 \le \bar{\theta}_{2\times2} \le 2.1606. \tag{4}$$

From Eq. (3), the overall odds of dying for smokers is 53% significantly higher than that for nonsmokers.

Table 11.3D-2. The data of Table 11.3D-1 after Z is pooled

	Smoker	
	Yes	No
Dead	139	230
Alive	443	502

If Z is pooled, Table 11.3D-1 is collapsed to become Table 11.3D-2.

Let $\hat{\theta}_{2\times2}^{(Z+)}$ be the estimated odds ratio for Table 11.3D-2. Thus, the point estimator for $\theta_{2\times2}^{(Z+)}$ is

$$\ln\hat{\theta}_{2\times2}^{Z+} = \ln[(139\cdot502)/(230\cdot443)] = \ln0.684837 \approx -0.3786. \quad (5)$$

Also,

$$\hat{\sigma}(\ln\hat{\theta}_{2\times2}^{(Z+)}) = \sqrt{139^{-1} + 230^{-1} + 443^{-1} + 502^{-1}} \approx 0.1257. \quad (6)$$

By using Eq. (11.1B.7) with Eqs. (5) and (6), the 95% confidence interval for $\theta_{2\times2}^{(Z+)}$ is

$$\exp(-0.3786 - 1.96\cdot0.1257) \le \theta_{2\times2}^{(Z+)} \le \exp(-0.3786 + 1.96\cdot0.1237),$$

$$\Rightarrow 0.5353 \le \theta_{2\times2}^{(Z+)} \le 0.8761. \quad (7)$$

From Eq. (5), it implies that the odds of dying for smokers is 32% less than that for nonsmokers and Eq. (7) implies that the beneficial effect of smoking is significant at the level of significance 0.05. However, this contradicts what we have concluded from the estimated overall average odds ratio given by Eq. (3). It makes more sense to take the overall average estimated odds ratio as a final solution.

Remarks

1. There are two ways to handle the zero cell entries in the 7th 2×2 subtable: either combine the 6th and 7th subtable into one table of 65+ or add 0.5 to every cell in the 7th subtable.[49]

2. We take the overall average odds ratio rather than the pooled odds ratio as our answer to the analysis of this data set. However, this is not always the case. The univariate analysis of pooled data shows that the association between antibiotic prophylaxis and urinary tract infections has a relative risk < 1, whereas the stratified analysis shows that the association between antibiotic prophylaxis and urinary tract infections has a relative risk > 1 in all strata. Yet, the "true" association (considering the findings of clinical trials to be the gold standard) is thus given by the unstratified analysis.[50]

3 Since Eq. (5) is less than the smallest odds ratio given in Eq. (1), the paradoxical type of this data set is of an AMP (see Definition 11.3D.3).

4. By plotting the numerator and denominator of the odds ratio as the x- and y-coordinate of a point $P(n_{12k}n_{21k}, n_{11k}n_{22k})$ in a plane,[53] the odds ratio can be viewed as the slope of the line connecting the origin $O(0, 0)$ and the P. This representation establishes the line as an equivalent class for K 2×2 subtables exhibiting a common odds ratio. Thus, the assumption that the odds ratio $\theta_{2\times2}^k$ does not depend on k is translated into the collinearity of the K points $P_1, P_2, \ldots$ and P_k. As a result, a simple representation of the conditions under which collapsing preserves a conditional constant relationship, that is, a necessary and sufficient condition for the collapsibility that does not vary among the K 2×2 subtables.

11.4   Exercises

1. Show that the null hypothesis in both Eqs. (11.1A.3) and (11.1B.3) are equivalent, namely, if $p_{ij} = p_{i+}p_{+j}$ holds, then $\theta_{2\times2} = \frac{p_{11}p_{22}}{p_{12}p_{21}}$ holds too; and vice versa.

2. Find the 95% confidence interval for $\theta_{2\times2}$ in Example 11.1B-1 by using Eq. (11.1B.8).

3. In Example 11.1C-1, show that $\Pr(n_{11} = 5) > \Pr(n_{11} = 1)$.

4. Show in Eq. (11.1D.1) that $p_A = p_{11} + p_{12}$ and $p_B = p_{11} + p_{21}$.

5. By using the properties of the multinomial distribution: $\sigma^2(\hat{p}_{ij}) = n^{-1}p_{ij}q_{ij}$ and $\text{cov}(\hat{p}_{ij}, \hat{p}_{ji}) = -n^{-1}p_{ij}p_{ji}$ if $i \neq j$, where $q_{ij} = 1 - p_{ij}$, $i, j = 1, 2$, show that Eq. (11.1D.5) holds.

6. By substituting $p_{10} = \psi p_{01}$ and $p_{00} = 1 - p_{11} - (1 + \psi)p_{01}$ into the likelihood function associated with the multinomial distribution, we have

$$L(p_{11}, p_{01}, \psi | n) = C p_{11}^{a_{11}} p_{01}^{a_{10}+a_{01}} \psi^{a_{10}} [1 - p_{11} - (1 + \psi)p_{01}]^{a_{00}},$$

(11.1E.15)

   where C is constant. By equating to zero the partial derivative of the natural logarithm function of Eq. (11.1E.15) with respect to p_{11}, p_{01}, and ψ, show that $\hat{p}_{11} = \frac{a_{11}}{n}$, $\hat{p}_{01} = \frac{a_{01}}{n}$, and $\hat{\psi} = \frac{a_{10}}{a_{01}}$.

7. With Table 11.2A.2, apply Yates' test to see if there exists a linear trend among the row marginal probabilities of the teacher's rating by taking the five column scores as $v_1 = +2$, $v_2 = +1$, $v_3 = 0$, $v_4 = -1$ and $v_5 = -2$.

8. Redo Example 11.2D-1 by dropping the second term $\hat{\eta}_2$ from consideration in forming Eq. (11.2D.7) instead of the third term $\hat{\eta}_3$.

9. Apply Kendall's test to the data in Table 11.2D-2.

10. Apply Pearson's test to analyze the independence between Y_A and Y_B in Table 11.2D-2.

11. For a comparison with the Wilcoxon–Mann–Whitney's test, apply Stuart's test in Sec. 11.2D to Table 11.2F-2.

12. With the data given in Table 11.3B-2, test at the level of significance 0.05 if there exists a zero first-order interaction between Y and Z (or Z and X), given that X (or Y) is pooled.

13. First, let us recognize Eq. (11.3C.5) is a nonlinear function in 2K independent variables, that is,

$$g(\vec{P}^T) \equiv \theta_{MH} = \frac{\sum_{k=1}^{K} p_{1k}q_{2k}}{\sum_{k=1}^{K} p_{2k}q_{1k}},$$

(1)

   where $\vec{P} = (p_{11}, p_{21}, \ldots, p_{1k}, p_{2k}, \ldots, p_{1K}, p_{2K})^T$. Note that Eq. (11.3C.6) is just $\hat{\theta}_{MH} = g(\hat{\vec{P}})$, where $\hat{\vec{P}} = (\hat{p}_{11}, \hat{p}_{11}, \ldots,$

$\hat{p}_{1K}, \hat{p}_{2K})^T$. Show that for $k = 1, 2, \ldots, K$,

$$c_{1k} = \frac{\partial g}{\partial p_{1k}} = \frac{q_{2k} + \theta_{MH} p_{2k}}{\sum_{k=1}^{K} p_{2k} q_{1k}}, \qquad (2)$$

and

$$c_{1k} = \frac{\partial g}{\partial p_{2k}} = \frac{p_{1k} + \theta_{MH} q_{1k}}{\sum_{k=1}^{K} p_{2k} q_{1k}}. \qquad (3)$$

By applying Eq. (14.4) in Ref. 2, the variance of Eq. (11.3C.6) is

$$\sigma^2(\hat{\theta}_{MH}) = \sqrt{n^{-1} \vec{C} \Sigma \vec{C}} = \sqrt{n^{-1}} \sum_{k=1}^{K} \sum_{i=1}^{2} c_{ik}^2 \sigma^2(\hat{p}_{ik}), \qquad (4)$$

where $\vec{C} = (c_{11}, c_{21}, \ldots, c_{1k}, c_{2k}, \ldots, c_{1K}, c_{2K})^T$, $c'_{ik} S$ are given by Eqs. (2) and (3), and Σ is a matrix of size $2K \times 2K$ consisting of K blocks of diagonal matrix of size 2×2 and given by

$$\Sigma = [\ldots, diag(\sigma^2(\hat{p}_{1k}), \sigma^2(\hat{p}_{2k})), \ldots]_{2K \times 2K},$$

$$\sigma^2(\hat{p}_{ik}) = n_{ik} p_{ik} q_{ik}, \ i = 1, 2, \ k = 1, 2, \ldots, K, \qquad (5)$$

$$\text{and } n = \sum_{k=1}^{K} \sum_{i=1}^{2} n_{ik}.$$

14. By adding one more 2×2 subtable to Table 11.3C-1:

Age ≥ 60	Alcohol	Yes	Smoker	Yes	199	126
				No	10	35

(a) Test at the level of significance 0.05 if this new table has a zero second-order ineraction.
(b) If the answer to (a) is yes, use the Mantel–Haenszel estimator to estimate the common odds ratio among the four 2×2 subtables; otherwise, detect that there exists any type of paradoxical behavior defined in Sec. 11.3D.

References

1. Agresti A. (1983) Testing marginal homogeneity for ordinal categorical variables. *Biometrics* **39**: 505–510.
2. Agresti A. (2002) *Categorical Data Analysis*, 2nd ed. Wiley, New York.
3. Agresti A. (2010) *Analysis of Ordinal Categorical Data*, 2nd ed. Wiley, New York.
4. Appleton DR, French JM, Vanderpump MPJ. (1996) Ignoring a covariate: An example of Simpson's paradox. *Am Statist* **50**: 340–341.
5. Armitage P. (1955) Tests for linear trend in proportions and frequencies. *Biometrics* **11**: 375–386.
6. Bandyoapdhyay PS, Nelson D, Greenwood M, *et al.* (2011) The logic of Simpson's paradox. *Synthese* **181**: 185–208.
7. Bartlett MS. (1935) Contingency table interactions. *J R Statist Soc* Supple. **2**: 248–252.
8. Birch MW. (1963) Maximum likelihood in three-way contingency tables. *J R Statist Soc B* **25**: 220–233.
9. Birch MW. (1964) The detection of partial association, I: The 2 × 2 case. *J R Statist Soc B* **26**: 313–324.
10. Bishop YM, Fienberg SE, Holland PW. (1975) *Discrete Multivariate Analysis*. The MIT Press, Boston, MA.
11. Casagrande JT, Pike MC, Smith PG. (1978) The power function of the "exact" test for comparing two binomial distributions. *Appl Statist* **27**: 176–180.
12. Cormack RS, Mantel N. (1991) Fisher's exact test: The margin totals as seen from two different angles. *Statistician* **40**: 27–34.
13. Crane J, Pearce N, Flatt A, *et al.* (1989) Prescribed fenoterol and death from asthma in New Zealand, 1981–1983: Case-control study. *Lancet* 29 April.
14. Darroch JN. (1962) Interactions in multi-factor contingency tables. *J R Statist Soc B* **24**: 251–263.
15. Darroch JN. (1974) Multiplicative and additive interaction in contingency tables. *Biometrika* **61**: 207–214.
16. Edwards AL. (1948) Note on the "correction to continuity" in testing the significance of the difference between correlated proportions. *Psychometrika* **13**: 185–187.
17. Ejigou A, McHugh R. (1977) Estimation of relative risk from matched pairs in epidemiologic research. *Biometrics* **33**: 552–556.
18. Ejigou A, McHugh R. (1981) Relative risk estimation under multiple matching. *Biometrika* **68**: 85–91.
19. Fienberg SE. (1980) *The Analysis of Cross-Classified Categorical Data*, 2nd ed. The MIT Press, Cambridge, MA.

20. Fisher RA. (1935) The logic of inductive inference. *J R Statist Soc* **98**: 39–82.
21. Fleiss JL. (1979) Confidence intervals for the odds ratio in case-control studies: The state of the art. *J Chron Dis* **32**: 69–77.
22. Fleiss JL, Levin B, Paik MC. (2003) *Statistical Methods for Rates and Proportions*, 3rd ed. John Wiley & Sons, Inc, New York.
23. Freeman GH, Halton JH (1951) Note on an exact treatment of contingency, goodness-of-fit and other problems of significance. *Biometrika* **38**: 141–149.
24. Gart JJ. (1962) On the combination of relative risks. *Biometrics* **18**: 601–610.
25. Good IJ, Mittal Y. (1987) The amalgamation and geometry of two-by-two contingency tables. *Ann Statist* **15**: 694–711.
26. Haldane JBS. (1956) The estimation and significance of the logarithm of a ratio of frequencies. *Ann Hum Genet* **20**: 309—311.
27. Hauck WW. (1979) The large sample variance of the Mantel-Haenszel estimator of a common odds ratio. *Biometrics* **35**: 817–819.
28. Irwin JO. (1935) Tests of significance for differences between between percentages based on small numbers. *Metron* **12**: 83–94.
29. Kastenbaum MA, Lamphiear DE. (1959) Calculation of chi-square to test the no. three factor interaction hypothesis. *Biometrics* **15**: 107–115.
30. Kendall MG. (1945) *The Advanced Theory of Statistics, Vol. I*. Griffin.
31. Killion RA, Zahn DA. (1976) A bibliography of contingency table literature: 1900–1974. *Int Statist Rev* **44**: 71–112.
32. Lancaster HO. (1951) Complex contingency tables treated by the partition. *J R Statist Soc B* **13**: 242–249.
33. Lancaster HO. (1961) Significance tests in discrete distributions. *J Am Statist Assoc* **56**: 223–234.
34. Lancaster HO. (1971) The multiplicative definition of interaction. *Austral J Statist* **13**: 36–44.
35. Lee T-S. (2015) *College Algebra: Historical Notes*. Applied Math Press, Atlanta, GA.
36. Lewis BN. (1961) On the analysis of interaction in multi-dimensional contingency tables. *J Roy Statist A* **125**: 88–117.
37. Mantel N, Haenszel W. (1959) Statistical aspects of the analysis of data from retrospective studies of disease. *J National Cancer Institute* **22**: 719–748.
38. Mantel N. (1963) Chi-square tests with one degree of freedom: Extensions of the Mantel–Haenszel procedure. *J Amer Statist Assoc* **58**: 690–700.
39. McNemar Q. (1947) Note on the sampling error of the difference between correlated proportions or percentages. *Psychometrika* **12**: 153–157.
40. Miettinen OS. (1969) Individual matching with multiple controls in the case of all-or-none responses. *Biometrics* **25**: 339–355.

41. Miettinen OS. (1970) Estimation of relative risk from individually matched series. *Biometrics* **26**: 75–86.
42. Miettinen OS. (1976) Estimability and estimation in case-referent studies. *Am J Epidemiol* **103**: 226–235.
43. Mirkin B. (2001) Eleven ways to look at the chi-squared coefficient for contingency tables. *Am Statist* **55**: 111–120.
44. Mittal Y. (1991) Homogeneity of subpopulations and Simpson's paradox. *J Am Statist Assoc* **86**: 167–172.
45. Mosteller F. (1952) Some statistical problems in measuring the subjective response to drugs. *Biometrics* **8**: 220–226.
46. Norton HW. (1945) Calculation of chi-square for complex contingency tables. *J Am Statist Assoc* **40**: 251–258.
47. Patefield WM. (1982) Exact tests for trend in ordered contingency tables. *Appl Statist* **31**: 32–43.
48. Pearson K. (1900) On a criterion that a given system of deviations from the probable in the case of correlated system of variables is such that it can be reasonably supposed to have arisen from random sampling. *Philos Mag Ser* **5**: 157–175.
49. Plackett RL. (1962) A note on interactions in contingency tables. *J R Statist Soc B* **24**: 162–166.
50. Reintjes R, de Boer A, van Pelt W, Mintjes-de Groot J. (2000): Simpson's paradox: An example from hospital epidemiology. *Epidemiology* **11**: 81–83.
51. Roy SN, Kastenbaum MA. (1956) On the hypothesis of no "interaction" in a multiway contingency table. *Ann Math Statist* **27**: 749–757.
52. Rothman KJ. (1976) The estimation of synergy or antagonism. *Am J Epidemiol* **103**: 506–511.
53. Shapiro SH. (1982) Collapsing contingency tables — A\ geometric approach. *Am Statist* **36**: 43–46.
54. Simpson EH. (1951) The interpretation of interaction in contingency tables. *J R Statist Soc B* **13**: 238–241.
55. Stuart A. (1953) The estimation and comparison of strengths of association in contingency tables. *Biometrika* **40**: 105–110.
56. Stuart A. (1955) A test for homogeneity of the marginal distributions in a two-way classification. *Biometrika* **42**: 412–416.
57. Tallis GM. (1962) The maximum likelihood estimation of correlation from contingency tables. *Biometrics* **18**: 342–353.
58. Wilks SS. (1935) The likelihood test of independence in contingency tables. *Ann Math Statist* **6**: 190–196.
59. Woolf B. (1955) On estimating the relation between blood group and disease. *Ann Hum Genet* **19**: 251–253.

60. Yates F. (1934) Contingency tables involving small numbers and the chi-square test. *J Roy Statis Soc Suppl* **1**: 217–235.
61. Yates F. (1948) The analysis of contingency tables with groupings based on quantitative characters. *Biometrika* **35**: 176–181.
62. Yule GU. (1903) Notes on the theory of association of attributes in statistics. *Biometrika* **2**: 121–134.

12 Survival Analysis

In this chapter we are going to learn statistical methods for analyzing the survival data.

12.0 A Brief History of Survival Analysis

The history for statistical analysis of survival data can be dated back to 1693 when British astronomer Halley published his article on the population life table. Many early publications are in the fields of actuary science and demography. It remained silent until 1950. Then the interest was arosed by a publication of Kaplan and Meier on the product limit estimator for the survival curve in 1958. Other key contributions include Gehan's generalization of the Wilcoxon test to survival data and Cox's proportional hazard model, which opened up the whole field of regression to survival analysts.[9]

12.1 Introduction

Survival data have a peculiar property, namely, they are oftentimes censored. There are at least two types of censored data.

Definition 12.1.1. A random sample of survival data is said to be of type I censored if some of the data are observed to be less than while the remaining data are known to survive beyond a predetermined time point.

Definition 12.1.2. A random sample of survival data is said to be of type II censored if only the smallest k observations of n items are observed to die, where k is a fixed integer $(1 \le k \le n)$.

Remarks

1. A type I censored sample is also called censoring on the right, which is often encountered in clinical trials, while a type II censored sample is frequently met in life testing of the reliability of industry mass production.
2. There are other types of censoring including progressive type II censoring and random censoring. For details, please refer to Lawless' book.[22]

Before mentioning some important basic concepts related to the survival data, let us first see an example.

Example 12.1-1

The data in Table 12.1-1 is taken from Table 10 in Ref. 16 for $n = 18$ pairs. There were 11 institutions participating in testing the effect of 6-Mercaptopouring (6-MP) on the duration of steroid-induced remissions in acute leukemia. A restricted (closed) sequential procedure[1] was used to compare the lengths of remission maintained on the case group treated by using 6-MP and the placebo group in phase II. The patients at each institution were paired according to remission status (complete or partial), with one patient to have 6-MP and the other a placebo by random allocation. As the patients relapsed from remission, a preference was recorded for either the 6-MP or placebo, depending on which therapy resulted in a longer remission. The trial was designed to be sensitive when the proportion of preferences reached 0.75 favoring either therapy. After 18 preferences were recorded and 15 were favoring the 6-MP, the trial was halted in April 1960.

In Table 12.1-1 there are 9 uncensored and 9 censored observations for 6-MP, whereas all 18 observations are uncensored for the

Table 12.1-1. **The sample data of the remission of Leukemia patients treated by drug 6-MP or placebo**

Group	Lengths of Remission (Weeks)
Drug-6MP	6, 6, 6, 7, 10, 11*, 13, 16, 17*, 19*, 20*, 22, 23, 25*, 32* ,3 2*, 34*, 35*
Placebo	1, 2, 2, 3, 4, 5, 5, 8, 8, 8, 11, 11, 12, 12, 15, 17, 22, 23

*Censored

placebo. We will use the exponential random variable to model the lengths of remission in the next example.

Remarks

1. The reason why Table 12.1-1 has only 18 observations for both groups is that, according to the original restricted sequential design, the trial should be terminated at $n = 18$ pairs because the sample path crosses the upper boundary (see Fig. 8 in Ref. 16). But due to the data collected every three months just prior to the committee meeting, the trial was not stopped until it reached $n = 21$ pairs.
2. A detailed description on the effect of 6-MP on the duration of steroid-induced remissions in acute leukemia was already covered in Example 10.4-2.

   Now we are ready to learn some basic concepts in survival analysis. First, let T be a continuous nonnegative random variable defined over $[0, +\infty)$ representing the lifetime of individuals in a population. Let $F(t)$ and $f(t)$ denote the (cumulative) distribution function and probability density function (p.d.f.) of T, respectively. Thus,

$$F(t) = \int_0^t f(s)ds, \qquad (12.1.1)$$

and

$$f(t) = F'(t) \equiv dF/dt, \qquad (12.1.2)$$

where $F'(t)$ is the first derivative of $F(t)$. The survivor function $S(t)$ represents the probability of an individual who has survived beyond time t given by

$$S(t) = \Pr(T \geq t) = 1 - F(t). \qquad (12.1.3)$$

The hazard function $h(t)$ represents the instantaneous rate of change of the death of an individual who survives beyond time t given by

$$h(t) = \lim_{\Delta t \to 0} \frac{\Pr(t \leq T < t + \Delta t | T \geq t)}{\Delta t} = \frac{F'(t)}{S(t)} = \frac{f(t)}{S(t)},$$
$$(12.1.4)$$

where $f(t)$ and $S(t)$ are defined by Eqs. (12.1.2) and (12.1.3), respectively.

Remarks

1. It can be shown (see Exercise 12.6-1) that the relationship between the hazard function $h(t)$ and the survivor function $S(t)$ is given by

$$S(t) = \exp(-h(t)). \qquad (12.1.5)$$

2. If the p.d.f. of T is an exponential distribution given by Eq. (3.2B.1), then its survivor function $S(t)$ and hazard function $h(t)$ are given respectively by (see Exercise 12.6-2)

$$S(t) = \exp(-\xi t) \quad \text{and} \quad h(t) = \xi. \qquad (12.1.6)$$

The exponential distribution is the only probability distribution in which its hazard function is a constant ξ (Eq. (12.1.6)).

Next, let us learn how to express the associated likelihood function for the survival data under type I censoring. Suppose that there are n individuals under study and that the ith individual has a lifetime T_i and a fixed censoring time C_i. Assume that all the T_is are i.i.d. (independently identically distributed) with the same p.d.f. $f(t)$ and survivor function $S(t)$. Thus, the ith observation is expressed by a pair of two random variables (r.v.s) (T_i, η_i) defined by

$$T_i = t_i \quad \text{if} \quad \eta_i = 1; T_i = C_i \quad \text{if} \quad \eta_i = 0, \quad \text{otherwise.} \qquad (12.1.7)$$

Assume that n pairs (T_i, η_i) of observations are independent. Then, its associated likelihood function is

$$L = \prod_{i=1}^{n} f(t_i)^{\eta_i} S(C_i)^{1-\eta_i}. \qquad (12.1.8)$$

When all the T_is are exponential random variables with their p.d.f. given by Eq. (3.2B.1), Eq. (12.1.8) becomes (see Exercise 12.6-3)

$$L(\xi) = \xi^r \exp(-\xi T^*), \qquad (12.1.9)$$

where $r = \sum_{i \in D} \eta_i$, $T^* = \sum_{i \in D} t_i + \sum_{i \in D} C_i$, and D and C denote respectively the sets of individuals whose observed lifetimes are uncensored and censored. The maximum likelihood estimator for ξ is (see Exercise 12.6-4)

$$\hat{\xi} = r / T^*. \qquad (12.1.10)$$

The estimated mean lifetime of the exponential random variable is

$$\hat{\mu}_T = \hat{\xi}^{-1} = T^* / r. \qquad (12.1.11)$$

Remarks

1. Only Eq. (12.1.11) has a practical interpretation, that is, it represents the estimated average lifetime of T, while Eq. (12.1.10) does not.
2. In Eq. (12.1.10) r is tacitly assumed to be > 0. For a sufficiently large sample size n the probability of $r = 0$ is negligible.
3. In principle the variance of the maximum likelihood estimator is $\hat{\xi}$ obtained as the expected information in the sample,[24] that

is,

$$\sigma^2(\hat{\xi}) = [E(I(\xi))]^{-1} \equiv [E(-L''(\xi))]^{-1} = \xi^2 / E(r), \qquad (12.1.12)$$

where $E(r) = \sum_{i \in D} (1 - e^{-\xi t_i})$ and $L''(\xi) \equiv d^2 L / d\xi^2$ is the second derivative of Eq. (12.1.9) with respect to ξ. Consequently, the estimated standard error of $\hat{\xi}$ is

$$\hat{\sigma}(\hat{\xi}) = \hat{\xi} / \sqrt{\hat{E}(r)}, \qquad (12.1.13)$$

where $\hat{E}(r)$ is defined by

$$\hat{E}(r) \equiv E(r)|_{\xi = \hat{\xi}} = \sum_{i \in D} \left(1 - e^{-\hat{\xi} t_i}\right). \qquad (12.1.14)$$

The $100(1 - \alpha)\%$ confidence interval for ξ is

$$\hat{\xi} - z_{1-\frac{\alpha}{2}} \hat{\sigma}(\hat{\xi}) \leq \xi \leq \hat{\xi} + z_{1-\frac{\alpha}{2}} \hat{\sigma}(\hat{\xi}). \qquad (12.1.15)$$

4. It can be shown[32] that Eq. (12.1.13) is a rather poor approximation to make the sampling distribution of $(\hat{\xi} - \xi)/\hat{\sigma}(\hat{\xi})$ behave like a standard normal random variable unless the sample size n is fairly large. A better approximation is to take the cubic root transformation of the parameter ξ in the exponential distribution, namely, first finding the $100(1 - \alpha)\%$ confidence interval for $\omega = \sqrt[3]{\xi}$:

$$\hat{\omega} - z_{1-\frac{\alpha}{2}} \hat{\sigma}(\hat{\omega}) \leq \omega \leq \hat{\omega} - z_{1-\frac{\alpha}{2}} \hat{\sigma}(\hat{\omega}), \qquad (12.1.16)$$

where $\hat{\omega} = \sqrt[3]{\hat{\xi}}$ and $\hat{\sigma}(\hat{\omega}) = 3\hat{\omega}\sqrt{[\hat{E}(r)]^{-1}}$, and $\hat{E}(r)$ is defined by Eq. (12.1.14) (see Exercise 12.6-5). To find the desired confidence interval, convert Eq. (12.1.15) back for the original ξ by using $\xi = \omega^3$.

5. When the sample data are of type II censored, the estimate of ξ in the exponential distribution has the same form of Eq. (12.1.10), except that r is a fixed constant rather than a random variable for the type I censored data.[22]

Example 12.1-2

Assume that the exponential distribution with its p.d.f. given by Eq. (3.2B.1) with the parameter ξ_A is an appropriate model for the lengths of remission of patients in the case group who were treated with drug 6-MP.

(a) Use Eqs. (12.1.10) and (12.1.15) to find respectively the point and 95% interval estimators for the unkown parameter ξ_A.
(b) For a comparison find the 95% interval estimators for the unknown parameter ξ_A by using Eq. (12.1.14).

Solution

(a) From Table 12.1-1, we have $r = 9$ and $n = 18$. By using Eq. (12.1.9),

$$T^* = \sum_{i \in D} t_i + \sum_{i \in C} C_i$$

$$= (6 + 6 + 6 + 7 + 10 + 13 + 16 + 22 + 23)$$

$$+ (11 + 17 + 19 + 20 + 32 + 32 + 34 + 35)$$

$$= 109 + 225 = 334. \tag{a.1}$$

By substituting Eq. (a.1) into Eqs. (12.1.10) and (12.1.11),

$$\hat{\xi}_A = 9/334 = 0.026946 \approx 0.027, \tag{a.2}$$

or

$$\hat{\mu}_A = \hat{\xi}_A^{-1} = 334/9 = 37.11111 \approx 37.1. \tag{a.3}$$

Before calculating Eq. (12.1.13), let us first calculate Eq. (12.1.14):

$$\hat{E}(r) = \left(1 - e^{-0.027 \cdot 6}\right) + \left(1 - e^{-0.027 \cdot 6}\right) + \left(1 - e^{-0.027 \cdot 6}\right)$$

$$+ \cdots + \left(1 - e^{-0.027 \cdot 23}\right) = 2.414796 \approx 2.415. \tag{a.4}$$

By substituting Eq. (a.4) into Eq. (12.1.13),

$$\hat{\sigma}\left(\hat{\xi}_A\right) = 0.027 \Big/ \sqrt{2.415} \approx 0.017. \tag{a.5}$$

By substituting Eqs. (a.2) and (a.5) into Eq. (12.1.14),

$$0.027 - 1.96 \cdot 0.017 \le \xi_A \le 0.027 + 1.96 \cdot 0.017, \text{ or}$$
$$-0.006 \le \xi_A \le 0.06. \tag{a.6}$$

The 95% confidence interval for ξ_A is [–0.006, 0.06]. Incidentally, Eq. (a.3) indicates that the average lifetime for patients in the case group is 37.1 weeks.

(b) Since $\hat{\omega}_A = \sqrt[3]{\hat{\xi}_A}$, we have by using Eq. (a.2)

$$\hat{\omega}_A = \sqrt[3]{0.027} = 0.3. \tag{b.1}$$

By using Eqs. (a.4) and (b.1),

$$\hat{\sigma}\left(\hat{\omega}_A\right) = 3 \cdot 0.3 \Big/ \sqrt{2.415} = 0.579141 \approx 0.58. \tag{b.2}$$

By substituting Eqs. (b.1) and (b.2) into Eq. (12.1.17) (see Exercise 12.6-5), the 95% confidence interval for ω_A is

$$0.3 - 1.96 \cdot 0.58 \le \omega_A \le 0.3 + 1.96 \cdot 0.58, \text{ or}$$
$$-0.837 \le \omega_A \le 1.437. \tag{b.3}$$

By taking the cubic power on both sides of Eq. (b.3), the 95% confidence interval for ξ_A is

$$-0.586 \le \xi_A \le 2.966. \tag{b.4}$$

Remarks

1. Although Eq. (b.4) is wider than Eq. (a.6), Eq. (b.4) is in theory superior to Eq. (a.6) since the sample size $n = 18$ is less than 30.
2. However, it was pointed out in Ref. 33 that large sample normal approximation depends on more than merely the size of the sample.

3. Both Eqs. (12.1.10) and (12.1.15) are obtained for the fixed sample size n. However, the sample size for Table 12.1-1 that was determined by the stopping rule of sequential procedure is random rather than fixed. There is not much problem with a point estimator because the likelihood function is independent of the stopping rule. However, there is a serious bias in the 95% confidence interval of Eq. (a.6).[35]

Example 12.1-3

Assume that the exponential distribution with its p.d.f. given by Eq. (3.2B.1) with the parameter ξ_B is an appropriate model for the lengths of remission of patients in the control group who were treated with a placebo. By using Eq. (12.1.10), find the point and 95% interval estimator for ξ_B and also the sample average remission length for patients in the control group.

Solution

Since there are no censored observations in the control group, $r = n = 18$. By computing T^* in Eq. (12.1.9),

$$T^* = \sum_{i=1}^{18} t_i = 1 + 2 + 2 + 3 + 4 + 5 + 8 + 8 + 8 + 11 + 11$$
$$+ 12 + 12 + 15 + 17 + 22 + 23 = 169. \tag{1}$$

By substituting Eq. (1) into Eq. (12.1.10),

$$\hat{\xi}_B = 18/169 = 0.106507 \approx 0.107. \tag{2}$$

By using Eq. (12.1.11), the sample average remission length for patients in the control group is

$$\hat{\mu}_B = \hat{\xi}_B^{-1} = 1/0.107 = 9.3888889 \approx 9.4. \tag{3}$$

By substituting Eq. (2) into Eq. (12.1.14),

$$\hat{E}(r) = \sum_{i=1}^{18}(1 - e^{-\hat{\xi}_B t_i}) = (1 - e^{-0.107 \cdot 1}) + (1 - e^{-0.107 \cdot 2})$$

$$+ \cdots + (1 - e^{-0.107 \cdot 23}) = 9.949956 \approx 9.95. \tag{4}$$

By substituting Eqs. (2) and (4) into Eq. (12.1.13),

$$\hat{\sigma}(\hat{\xi}_B) = 0.107 \big/ \sqrt{9.95} = 0.033925 \approx 0.034. \tag{5}$$

By substituting Eqs. (2) and (5) into Eq. (12.1.15), the 95% confidence interval for ξ_B is

$$0.107 - 1.96 \cdot 0.034 \le \xi_B \le 0.107 + 1.96 \cdot 0.034.$$

$$\text{or} \quad 0.04 \le \xi_B \le 0.17. \tag{6}$$

Remark

The same remark as the remark in Example 12.1-2 is applicable here.

12.2 Estimates of the Survivor Function

Depending on whether the collected data are grouped or ungrouped, there are two ways to estimate the survivor function: (1) the life table method and (2) the Kaplan–Meier method.

A. *The Life Table Method for Grouped Data*

The life table can be viewed as an extension of the relative frequency table in Sec. 1.4 to the case of censored data. Here we emphasize the estimation of the conditional probability of death in a time interval, given survival at the start of the interval and the probability of surviving past the end of the interval.

Assume that the time axis is divided into $K + 1$ intervals $I_k = (t_{k-1}, t_k], k = 1, 2, \ldots, K + 1$, with $t_0 = 0, t_K = t^*$ and $t_{K+1} = +\infty$, where t^* is an upper limit on observation. Let $S(t)$ be the survivor function of lifetimes for the population under study. For $k = 1, 2, \ldots, K + 1$, we define

$$s_k = \Pr(\text{an individual survives beyond } I_k) = S(t_k),$$

$$\varphi_k = \Pr(\text{an individual survives beyond } I_k | \text{he survives}$$
$$\text{beyond } I_{k-1}), \quad (12.2A.1)$$

$$\psi_k = \Pr(\text{an individual dies in } I_k | \text{he survives beyond } I_{k-1})$$
$$= 1 - \varphi_k.$$

From Eq. (12.2A.1), s_k can be written as

$$s_k = \varphi_k \cdot s_{k-1} = \varphi_k \varphi_{k-1} s_{k-2} = \cdots = \varphi_k \varphi_{k-1} \cdots \varphi_1. \quad (12.2A.2)$$

Note that $s_0 = 1, s_{K+1} = 0$ and $\Psi_{K+1} = 1$. It is easier to estimate Ψ_k as

$$\hat{\Psi}_k = d_k / n_k^*, \quad (12.2A.3)$$

where $n_k(> 0) = $ number of individuals at risk, that is, alive and uncensored at time $t_{k-1}, d_k = $ number of deaths that falls into I_k, $u_k = $ number of individual lost to follow-up, $w_k = $ number of withdrawals (censored observation) in I_k, and n_k^* is the effective number of individuals at risk in I_k given by

$$n_k^* = n_k - \frac{1}{2} u_k - \frac{1}{2} w_k. \quad (12.2A.4)$$

Note that $\hat{\Psi}_k = 1$ if $n_k^* = 0$.

Once Ψ_k is estimated by Eq. (12.2A.3), φ_k is thus estimated as $\hat{\varphi}_k = 1 - \hat{\Psi}_k$. As a result, s_k of Eq. (12.2A.2) is estimated as

$$\hat{s}_k = \hat{\varphi}_k \hat{s}_{k-1}. \quad (12.2A.5)$$

Thus, the life table estimator of the survivor function $S(t)$ is

$$\hat{S}_{LT}(t) = \hat{s}_k, \quad \text{if } t \in I_k = (t_{k-1}, t_k], \quad (12.2A.6)$$

where $\hat{s}_k$ is given by Eq. (12.2A.5).

The estimated standard error of $\hat{s}_k$ is given by[16]

$$\hat{\sigma}(\hat{s}_k) = \hat{s}_k \sqrt{\sum_{j=1}^{k} [\hat{\Psi}_j (n_j^* \hat{\varphi}_j)^{-1}]}, \qquad (12.2A.7)$$

where n_j^* is given by Eq. (12.2A.4). Here it is supposed that a withdrawn indidual is at risk for half the interval.

It can be shown that the sampling distribution of $\hat{s}_k / \hat{\sigma}(\hat{s}_k)$ is a standard normal distribution. Therefore, the $100(1 - \alpha)\%$ confidence interval for s_k of Eq. (12.2A.1) is given by

$$\hat{s}_k - z_{1-\frac{\alpha}{2}} \cdot \hat{\sigma}(\hat{s}_k) \leq s_k \leq \hat{s}_k + z_{1-\frac{\alpha}{2}} \cdot \hat{\sigma}(\hat{s}_k), \qquad (12.2A.8)$$

where $\hat{s}_k$ and $\hat{\sigma}(\hat{s}_k)$ are given by Eqs. (12.2A.5) and (12.2A.7), respectively.

Remarks

1. Equation (12.2A.5) is also called the "standard" life table (or actuarial) estimator by Breslow and Crowly[6] and it points out that the constant $1/2$ in Eq. (12.2A.4) was modified by Littell[26] in order to improve the approximation in certain circumstances.
2. Equation (12.2A.5) is not a consistent estimator for the unknown survivor function $S(t)$. A necessary and sufficient condition for Eq. (12.2A.5) to be a consistent estimator was given in Ref. 6 under random censorship.
3. In practical applications, the life table may be organized in intervals of varying length. For example, when a large number of deaths occur in the first year, it may be desirable to record experience during the first year in monthly intervals and the experience thereafter in annual intervals.

Example 12.2A-1

A group of male kidney patients living in the State of Connecticut entering observation continuously from 1 January 1946 to 31 December 1951 was studied. The purpose of the study was to

Table 12.2A-1. The life-table estimator for male kidney patients living in Connecticut

The kth Year Interval	n_k	d_k	u_k	w_k	n_k^*	$\hat{s}_k$	$\hat{\sigma}(\hat{s}_k)$
(0, 1]	126	47	4	15	116.5	0.597	0.045
(1, 2]	60	5	6	11	51.5	0.539	0.048
(2, 3]	38	2	0	15	30.5	0.503	0.051
(3, 4]	21	2	2	7	16.5	0.442	0.06
(4, 5]	10	0	0	6	7.0	0.442	0.06
(5, 6]	4	0	0	4	0	0.0	0.06

analyze the survival experience of these patients to obtain a 5-year survival rate.

Table 12.2A-1 is taken from Table III in Ref. 13, which is in fact the pooled table of six cohorts of male kidney patients who were diagnosed in 1946–1950 and 1951, respectively. The first column of Table 12.2A-1 represents the year interval after diagnosis and the values in the second to the fifth columns were recorded to represent the number of patients at risk (n_k), deaths (d_k), lost to follow-up (u_k), and withdrawal alive during the kth year interval (w_k), while the values of n_k^* in the 6th column of Table 12.2A-1 is obtained by calculation using Eq. (12.2A.4).

(a) Based on the data given in Table 12.2A-1, find the life-table estimator for the survivor function s_k.
(b) Find the 95% confidence interval for the 5-year survival rate for the male kidney patients living in the State of Connecticut.

Solution

(a) Before using Eq. (12.2A.5) to find the life-table estimate for $\hat{s}_k$ recursively, we need to first calculate $\hat{\Psi}_1$ of Eq. (12.2A.3) for the 1st year interval (0, 1]. From the first row of Table 12.2A-1, $d_1 = 47$ and $n_1^* = 116.5$. By using Eq. (12.2A.3),

$$\hat{\Psi}_1 = 47/116.5 = 0.403433 \approx 0.403. \qquad (a.1)$$

From Eq. (a.1),

$$\hat{\varphi}_1 = 1 - \hat{\Psi}_1 = 1 - 0.403 = 0.597. \qquad (a.2)$$

Since $\hat{s}_0 = 1$, we have by using Eq. (12.2A.5)

$$\hat{s}_1 = \hat{\varphi}_1 \cdot \hat{s}_0 = 0.597 \cdot 1 = 0.597. \qquad (a.3)$$

Next, let us calculate $\hat{\Psi}_2$ for the 2nd year interval $(1, 2]$ by using Eq. (12.2A.3)

$$\hat{\Psi}_2 = d_2 / n_2^* = 5/51.5 = 0.097087 \approx 0.097. \qquad (a.4)$$

From Eq. (a.4),

$$\hat{\varphi}_2 = 1 - \hat{\Psi}_2 = 1 - 0.097 = 0.903. \qquad (a.5)$$

By substituting Eqs. (a.3) and (a.5) into Eq. (12.2A.5),

$$\hat{s}_2 = \hat{\varphi}_2 \cdot \hat{s}_1 = 0.903 \cdot 0.597 = 0.539091 \approx 0.539. \qquad (a.6)$$

Similarly, let us calculate $\hat{\Psi}_3$ for the 3rd year interval $(2, 3]$ by using Eq. (12.2A.3)

$$\hat{\Psi}_3 = d_3 / n_3^* = 2/30.5 = 0.065574 \approx 0.066. \qquad (a.7)$$

From Eq. (a.7),

$$\hat{\varphi}_3 = 1 - \hat{\Psi}_3 = 1 - 0.066 = 0.934. \qquad (a.8)$$

By substituting Eqs. (a.6) and (a.8) into Eq. (12.2A.5),

$$\hat{s}_3 = \hat{\varphi}_3 \cdot \hat{s}_2 = 0.934 \cdot 0.539 = 0.503426 \approx 0.503. \qquad (a.9)$$

Continuously, let us calculate $\hat{\Psi}_4$ for the 4th year interval $(3, 4]$ by using Eq. (12.2A.3):

$$\hat{\Psi}_4 = d_4 / n_4^* = 2/16.5 = 0.121212 \approx 0.121. \qquad (a.10)$$

From Eq. (a.10),

$$\hat{\varphi}_4 = 1 - \hat{\Psi}_4 = 1 - 0.121 = 0.879. \qquad (a.11)$$

By substituting Eqs. (a.9) and (a.11) into Eq. (12.2A.5),

$$\hat{s}_4 = \hat{\varphi}_4 \cdot \hat{s}_3 = 0.879 \cdot 0.503 = 0.442137 \approx 0.442. \qquad (a.12)$$

Again, let us calculate $\hat{\Psi}_5$ for the 5th year interval $(4, 5]$ by using Eq. (12.2A.3):

$$\hat{\Psi}_5 = d_5 / n_5^* = 0/7.0 = 0.0. \tag{a.13}$$

From Eq. (a.13),

$$\hat{\varphi}_5 = 1 - \hat{\Psi}_5 = 1 - 0.0 = 1. \tag{a.14}$$

By substituting Eqs. (a.12) and (a.14) into Eq. (12.2A.5),

$$\hat{s}_5 = \hat{\varphi}_5 \cdot \hat{s}_4 = 1 \cdot 0.442 = 0.442. \tag{a.15}$$

Since $n_6^* = 0$ in Table 12.2A-1, $\hat{\Psi}_6 = 1$. As a result,

$$\hat{\varphi}_6 = 1 - \hat{\Psi}_6 = 1 - 1 = 0. \tag{a.16}$$

By substituting Eqs. (a.15) and (a.16) into Eq. (12.2A.5),

$$\hat{s}_6 = 0 \cdot 0.442 = 0. \tag{a.17}$$

The values of $\hat{s}_k$ given by Eqs. (a.3), (a.6), (a.9), (a.12), (a.15) and (a.17) are listed in the 7th column of Table 12.2A-1.

The life table estimator for the survivor function of kidney patients is

$$\hat{S}_{LT}(t) = \begin{cases} 0.597, & 0 < t \leq 1 \\ 0.539, & 1 < t \leq 2 \\ 0.503, & 2 < t \leq 3 \\ 0.442, & 3 < t \leq 4 \\ 0.442, & 4 < t \leq 5 \\ 0, & 5 < t \leq 6 \end{cases} \tag{a.18}$$

(b) From Eq. (a.18), the 5-year survival rate for the kidney patients in Connecticut is

$$\hat{s}_5 = \hat{S}_{LT}(t | 4 < t \leq 5) = 0.442. \tag{b.1}$$

Before applying Eq. (12.2A.8) to find the 95% confidence interval for the true unknown 5-year survival rate s_5, we need to calculate the estimated standard error of $\hat{s}_5$. By using Eq. (12.2A.7),

$$\hat{\sigma}(\hat{s}_5) = \hat{s}_5 \sqrt{\sum_{j=1}^{5} \frac{\hat{\Psi}_j}{n_j^* \hat{\varphi}_j}}$$

$$= 0.442 \cdot \sqrt{\frac{0.403}{116.5 \cdot 0.597} + \frac{0.097}{51.5 \cdot 0.903}}$$

$$\sqrt{+ \frac{0.066}{30.5 \cdot 0.934} + \frac{0.121}{16.5 \cdot 0.879} + \frac{0}{7 \cdot 1}} = 0.06. \qquad \text{(b.2)}$$

By substituting Eqs. (b.1) and (b.2) into Eq. (12.2A.8),

$$0.442 - 1.96 \cdot 0.06 \le s_5 \le 0.442 + 1.96 \cdot 0.06$$

$$\Rightarrow 0.32 \le s_5 \le 0.56. \qquad \text{(b.3)}$$

Therefore, the 95% confidence interval for the true unknown 5-year survival rate s_5 is [0.32, 0.56].

Remarks

1. The 5-year survival rate has no special virtue to evaluate the survival of cancer patients. For some cancers like leukemia (see Example 12.1-1), the 24-week survival rate is more suitable to serve as a measure. Nevertheless, examining the survival experience beyond 5 years is desirable in order to provide a basis for interpreting the significance of 5-year survival rates and insight into the meaning of survival rates in general.[14]
2. The life table, with its amplifications in the form of multiple decrements and the select table was applied in the analysis of problems in public health, clinical medicine and population characteristics (marriage, growth, labor force, and the money value of a man to his dependents).[31]

B. *The Kapla–Meier Method for Ungrouped Data*

Given the sample of survival data of size n, assume that there are K distinct uncensored observations ($K \le n$) $0 < \tau_1 < \tau_2 < \cdots < \tau_K$

and let d_k be the number of deaths at t_k. Kaplan–Meier's estimator for the survivor function $S(t)$ is[20]

$$\hat{S}_{KM}(t) = \prod_{\{k|\tau_k < t\}} (n_k - d_k) n_k^{-1}, \qquad (12.2B.1)$$

where n_k is the number of individuals at risk at τ_k, namely, the number of individuals alive and uncensored just prior to τ_k. If a recorded censored observation happens to equal the uncensored death time τ_k, it is not counted into the number of deaths, but rather it is counted into n_k.

The estimated standard error of $\hat{S}_{KM}(t)$ is given by[20]

$$\hat{\sigma}(\hat{S}_{KM}(t)) = \hat{S}_{KM}(t) \sqrt{\sum_{\{k|\tau_k < t\}} d_k [n_k (n_k - d_k)]^{-1}}. \qquad (12.2B.2)$$

It can be shown[20] that the sampling distribution of $[\hat{S}_{KM}(t) - S(t)]/\hat{\sigma}(\hat{S}_{KM})$ at a time point $t = t_0$ is a standard normal random variable. As a result, the $100(1 - \alpha)\%$ confidence interval for $S(t_0)$ is

$$\hat{S}_{KM}(t_0) - z_{1-\frac{\alpha}{2}} \hat{\sigma}(\hat{S}_{KM}(t_0)) \leq S(t_0) \leq \hat{S}_{KM}(t_0)$$

$$+ z_{1-\frac{\alpha}{2}} \hat{\sigma}(\hat{S}_{KM}(t_0)). \qquad (12.2B.3)$$

where $\hat{S}_{KM}(t_0)$ and $\hat{\sigma}(\hat{S}_{KM}(t_0))$ are given respectively by Eqs. (12.2B.1) and (12.2B.2) that are evaluated at $t = t_0$.

Remarks

1. Equation (12.2B.1) is called the product limit estimate because it is the limiting case of the life table estimator Eq. (12.2A.4).[9]
2. If the largest observation is censored, Eq. (12.2B.1) never reaches zero. In addition, an anomalous feature of the Kaplan–Meier estimator is that certain estimated survival probabilities can be decreased when the data are perturbed in a way that improves the overall group survival.[28]

3. Since $\hat{S}_{KM}(t)$ has a jump at the uncensored observation, Eq. (12.2B.1) can be calculated recursively as

$$\hat{S}_{KM}(\tau_k+) = \hat{S}_{KM}(\tau_{k-1}+) \cdot (n_k - d_k) n_k^{-1}. \qquad (12.2B.4)$$

4. If the data set of size n contains no censored observation, the Kaplan–Meier estimator reduces to the empirical survivor function given by

$$\hat{S}_{ES}(t) = (\text{number of observations} \geq t)/n, \ t \geq 0. \qquad (12.2B.5)$$

Example 12.2B-1

With Table 12.1-1, find:

(a) The Kaplan–Meier estimate for the survivor function associated with the case group of 6-MP drugs.
(b) The 95% confidence interval for $S(12)$, the survival probability of a leukemia patient at the 12th week.

Solution

Let us list the information of τ_k, n_k, and d_k in Table 12.2B-1 by using the data in Table 12.1-1 and then calculate the Kaplan–Meier estimator by using Eq. (12.2B.3).

Table 12.2B-1. The sample information of τ_k, n_k, d_k in Table 12.1-1.

	Case Group (Drug 6-MP)			
k	τ_k	n_k	d_k	$\hat{S}_{KM}(\tau_k+)$
1	6	18	3	0.833
2	7	15	1	0.778
3	10	14	1	0.722
4	13	12	1	0.662
5	16	11	1	0.602
6	22	8	1	0.527
7	23	7	1	0.451

From the last column of Table 12.2B-1, the Kaplan–Meier estimator is a step function given by

$$\hat{S}_{KM}(t) = \begin{cases} 1, & 0 < t \leq 6 \\ 0.833, & 6 < t \leq 7 \\ 0.778, & 7 < t \leq 10 \\ 0.722, & 10 < t \leq 13 \\ 0.662, & 13 < t \leq 16 \\ 0.602, & 16 < t \leq 22 \\ 0.527, & 22 < t \leq 23 \\ 0.451, & 23 < t \leq 35 \end{cases} \tag{a.1}$$

(b) By using Eq. (a.1) with $t_0 = 12$,

$$\hat{S}_{KM}(12) = 0.722. \tag{b.1}$$

Before applying Eq. (12.2B.3), let us calculate $\hat{\sigma}(\hat{S}_{KM}(12))$ by using Eq. (12.2B.2). Thus,

$$\hat{\sigma}(\hat{S}_{KM}(12)) = \sum_{k=1}^{3} \frac{d_k}{n_k(n_k - d_k)} = \frac{3}{18(18 - 3)}$$

$$+ \frac{1}{15(15 - 1)} + \frac{1}{14(14 - 1)} = 0.106. \tag{b.2}$$

By substituting Eqs. (b.1) and (b.2) into Eq. (12.2B.3),

$$0.722 - 1.96 \cdot 0.106 \leq S(12) \leq 0.722 + 1.96 \cdot 0.106$$
$$\Rightarrow 0.51 \leq S(12) \leq 0.93. \tag{b.3}$$

From Eq. (b.3), the 95% confidence interval for $S(12)$ is $[0.51, 0.93]$.

Remarks

1. Since the largest observation (35) is censored data, $\hat{S}_{KM}(t)$ is undefined for the interval $(35, +\infty)$.

Table 12.2B-2. The Kaplan-Meier estimator reduces to the empirical survivor function of Eq. (12.2B.5)

		Control Group (Placebo)		
k	τ_k	n_k	d_k	$\hat{S}_{ES}(\tau_k+)$
1	1	18	1	0.944
2	2	17	2	0.833
3	3	15	1	0.778
4	4	14	1	0.722
5	5	13	2	0.611
6	8	11	3	0.444
7	11	8	2	0.333
8	12	6	2	0.222
9	15	4	1	0.167
10	17	3	1	0.111
11	22	2	1	0.056
12	23	1	1	0.0

2. Although the methods for obtaining the confidence band — either by the Kolmogorov–Smirnov test for censored data[5] or by assuming the random censorship model — are available to be applicable to the Kaplan–Meier estimator,[18] its formulas are based upon the fixed sample size. Yet the sample size obtained in Table 12.1-1 was based the sequential probability ratio test. Therefore, strictly speaking, it is not applicable to the data of the drug 6-MP group, because intervals obtained from the usual fixed-sample-size formula will not yield the nominal confidence coefficients in repeated sampling with sequential stopping rule.

Example 12.2B-2

Since the placebo group in Table 12.1-1 has no censored observation, find:

(a) The empirical survival function $\hat{S}_{ES}(t)$ of Eq. (12.2B.5);
(b) The 95% Kolmogorov's confidence band for the empirical survival function $\hat{S}_{ES}(t)$ obtained in (a).

Solution

(a) Let us find the the empirical survival function $\hat{S}_{ES}(t)$ for the placebo group by listing the uncensored (death) time point, the number of patients at risk, and the number of deaths from using Table 12.1-1 in the 2nd, 3rd and 4th column of Table 12.2B-2, while the 1st column merely represents the index. Then we calculate the value of Table 12.2B-2 according to Eq. (12.2B.1).

From the last column of Table 12.2B-2, the empirical survival function for the placebo group is a step function given by

$$
\hat{S}_{ES}(t) = \begin{cases}
1, & 0 < t \leq 1, \\
0.944, & 1 < t \leq 2, \\
0.833, & 2 < t \leq 3, \\
0.778, & 3 < t \leq 4, \\
0.722, & 4 < t \leq 5, \\
0.611, & 5 < t \leq 8, \\
0.444, & 8 < t \leq 11, \\
0.333, & 11 < t \leq 12, \\
0.222, & 12 < t \leq 15, \\
0.167, & 15 < t \leq 17, \\
0.111, & 17 < t \leq 22, \\
0.056, & 22 < t \leq 23, \\
0.0, & 23 < t < +\infty.
\end{cases}
\tag{a.1}
$$

(b) By using Table A-4 in the appendix with $n = 18$ and $\alpha = 0.05$, we have

$$
d_{18;0.95} = 0.3094 \approx 0.309
\tag{b.1}
$$

By substituting Eq. (b.1) into Eqs. (8.4A.8) and (8.4A.9),

$$S_L(t) = \begin{cases} 0.691, & 0 < t \le 1 \\ 0.635, & 1 < t \le 2 \\ 0.524, & 2 < t \le 3 \\ 0.469, & 3 < t \le 4 \\ 0.413, & 4 < t \le 5 \\ 0.302, & 5 < t \le 8 \\ 0.135, & 8 < t \le 11 \\ 0.024, & 11 < t \le 12 \\ 0 & t > 12 \end{cases} \tag{b.2}$$

and

$$S_U(t) = \begin{cases} 1, & 0 < t \le 5 \\ 0.920, & 5 < t \le 8 \\ 0.753, & 8 < t \le 11 \\ 0.642, & 11 < t \le 12 \\ 0.531, & 12 < t \le 15 \\ 0.476, & 15 < t \le 17 \\ 0.420, & 17 < t \le 22 \\ 0.365, & 22 < t \le 23 \\ 0.309, & t > 23 \end{cases} \tag{b.3}$$

The lower and upper band of 95% Kolmogorov–Smirnov's confidence interval for the survival function $S(t)$ are given by $S_L(t)$ (Eq. b.2) and $S_U(t)$ (Eq. b.3), respectively.

12.3 Methods for Comparing Two Survival Curves

A. *The Maximum Likelihood Method*

In a clinical trial, let n_i be the number of patients in group i being treated with drug i, $i = A, B$. We make the following two assumptions:

(i) During the interval $(0, t^*)$ patients enter the trial at a contant rate n_i/t^*.

(ii) The survival time distributions for two groups are exponential, the probability of deaths before time t after being treated with drugs A and B given respectively by

$$F_A(t) = 1 - \exp(-\xi_A t), \qquad (12.3A.1)$$

and

$$F_B(t) = 1 - \exp(-\xi_B t),$$

where $\xi_i > 0, i = A, B$. We wish to test the following pair of hypothesis

$$H_0 : \xi_A = \xi_B \quad \text{versus} \quad H_1 : \xi_A \neq \xi_B. \qquad (12.3A.2)$$

Equation (12.3A.2) can be re-expressed as

$$H_0 : \delta = 0 \quad \text{versus} \quad H_1 : \delta \neq 0, \qquad (12.3A.3)$$

where $\delta = \xi_B - \xi_A$.

Suppose that the jth patient in group i has a lifetime T_{ij} and a fixed censoring time C_{ij}. Thus, the observation of the jth patient in group i is expressed by a pair of two random variables (T_{ij}, η_{ij})

defined by

$$T_{ij} = \tau_{ij} \quad \text{if } \eta_{ij} = 1; T_{ij} = C_{ij} \quad \text{if } \eta_{ij} = 0, \qquad (12.3A.4)$$

where τ_{ij} is the death time of the jth patient in group i. By following Eq. (12.1.10), the maximum likelihood estimator of δ is

$$\hat{\delta} = \hat{\xi}_B - \hat{\xi}_A, \qquad (12.3A.5)$$

where for $i = A, B$ $\hat{\xi}_i$ is given by

$$\hat{\xi}_i = r_i / T_i^*, \qquad (12.3A.6)$$

$r_i = \sum_{j \in D_i} \eta_{ij}$, $T_i^* = \sum_{j \in D_i} \tau_{ij} + \sum_{j \in C_i} C_{ij}$, D_i and C_i denote respectively the set of patients in group i whose lifetimes are uncensored and censored. It can be shown (see Exercise 12.6-7) that the estimated standard error of $\hat{\delta}$ of Eq. (12.3.5) is

$$\hat{\sigma}(\hat{\delta}) = \sqrt{\sum_{i=A}^{B} \frac{\hat{\xi}_i^2}{n_i \{1 - (\hat{\xi}_i t^*)^{-1} [1 - \exp(-\hat{\xi}_i t^*)]\}}}. \qquad (12.3A.7)$$

Thus, the test statistic for of Eq. (12.3A.3) is

$$\chi_{mle} = [\hat{\delta} / \hat{\sigma}(\hat{\delta})]^2. \qquad (12.3A.8)$$

where $\hat{\delta}$ and $\hat{\sigma}(\hat{\delta})$ are given by Eqs. (12.3A.5) and (12.3A.7), respectively. It is easily shown that the asymptotic sampling distribution of Eq. (12.3A.8) is a chi-squared distribution with one degree of freedom. The decision rule for testing Eq. (12.3A.3) is given as follows.

Decision Rule 12.3A-1 (Comparing two exponential survival curves)

Reject H_0 of Eq. (12.3A.3) at the level of significance α if the computed χ_{mle} of Eq. (12.3A.8) is greater than the critical value $\chi_{1;1-\alpha}^2$. Otherwise, do not reject H_0.

Example 12.3A-1

Assume that both the distributions of the remission length of the leukemia patients for the case (6-MP drug) and the control (placebo) groups are exponential. By using Eq. (12.3A.8), test at the significance level of 0.05 if the survival curves are different from each other.

Solution

Let the 6-MP and the placebo denote drugs A and B, respectively. From Examples 12.1-2 and 12.1-3, the maximum likelihood estimators of ξ_A and ξ_B are

$$\hat{\xi}_A = 0.027 \quad \text{and} \quad \hat{\xi}_B = 0.107. \tag{1}$$

Although the duration for the 6-MP trial was one year long, the sequential trial only begun in phase II, four weeks after phase I ended. Hence, the total duration for Table 12.1-1 is 48 weeks long, namely, $t^* = 48$.

By substituting Eq. (1) into Eq. (12.3A.5),

$$\hat{\delta} = 0.027 - 0.107 = -0.08. \tag{2}$$

By substituting Eq. (1), $n_A = n_B = 18$ and $t^* = 48$ into Eq. (12.3A.7),

$$\hat{\sigma}(\hat{\delta}) = \sqrt{\frac{0.027^2}{18 \cdot \{1 - (0.027 \cdot 48)^{-1}(1 - e^{-0.027 \cdot 48})}}$$
$$+ \sqrt{\frac{0.107^2}{18 \cdot \{1 - (0.107 \cdot 48)^{-1}(1 - e^{-0.107 \cdot 48})}}$$
$$= 0.029567 \approx 0.03. \tag{3}$$

By substituting Eqs. (2) and (3) into Eq. (12.3A.8),

$$\chi_{mle} = (0.08/0.03)^2 = 7.11111 \approx 7.11. \tag{4}$$

Since the computed χ_{mle} of Eq. (4) is greater than the critical value $\chi^2_{1;0.95} = 3.841$, H_0 of Eq. (12.3A.3) is rejected at the significance level of 0.05.

Remarks

1. Fixed-sample-size analysis of sequential observations was criticized by Anscombe.[4]

2. Since DR 12.3A-1 is derived for the case of fixed sample size and the sample size is random in Table 12.1-1, we are obliged to hold reservation whether DR 12.3A-1 is applicable to the data in Table 12.1-1.

B. *Armitage's "Preference" Method*

Suppose that patients enter the trial over the period $(0, t^*)$ in pairs at a constant rate of n/t^* per unit time and that members of each pair are allocated to be treated with drugs A or B. Let t_A and t_B be the survival times for patients on drugs A and B, respectively. The following definition specifies which drug is preferred.

Definition 12.3B.1. A pair of patients is said to be of (i) "A-preference" if $t_A > t_B$; (ii) "B-preference" if $t_A < t_B$; and (iii) "no preference" if $t_A = t_B$ or $t_A > t^*$ and $t_B > t^*$.

Again, assume that the survival time distributions for two groups on drugs A and B are exponential given by Eq. (12.3A.1). Thus, the probability that an A-preference occurring at time t after treatment is[2]

$$v = \frac{f_B(t)S_A(t)}{f_A(t)S_B(t) + f_B(t)S_A(t)} = \frac{\xi_B}{\xi_A + \xi_B}. \tag{12.3B.1}$$

Equation (12.3A.2) can be written as

$$H_0: v = \frac{1}{2} \quad \text{versus} \quad H_1: v \neq \frac{1}{2}. \tag{12.3B.2}$$

Now the hypothesis that $\xi_A = \xi_B$ may be tested at time t^* by testing the difference between the observed proportion $\hat{v}$ of A-preferences and its null value $\frac{1}{2}$, where $\hat{\xi}$ is given by

$$\hat{v} = \hat{\xi}_B / (\hat{\xi}_A + \hat{\xi}_B), \tag{12.3B.3}$$

where $\hat{\xi}_A$ and $\hat{\xi}_B$ are given by Eq. (12.3A.6).

The expected proportion of A-preference is (see Exercise 12.6-8)

$$E(\hat{v}) = \frac{\xi_B}{\xi_A + \xi_B} = \frac{1}{2} + \frac{\delta}{4\xi_B} + o(\delta), \tag{12.3B.4}$$

where $\delta = \xi_B - \xi_A$. It can be shown[2] that the estimated standard error of $\hat{v}$ is

$$\hat{\sigma}(\hat{v}) = \frac{1}{2}\left\{\sqrt{n\left[1 - \left(1 - e^{-2t^*\hat{\zeta}_A}\right)/\left(2t^*\hat{\xi}_A\right)\right]}\right\}^{-1}. \tag{12.3B.5}$$

The test statistic for Eq. (12.3B.2) is

$$\chi_{Armi} = \left[\frac{\hat{v} - \frac{1}{2}}{\hat{\sigma}(\hat{v})}\right]^2 = \left[\frac{\hat{\delta}}{4\hat{\xi}_B \cdot \hat{\sigma}(\hat{v})}\right]^2, \tag{12.3B.6}$$

where $\hat{\delta}$ and $\hat{\sigma}(\hat{v})$ are given by Eq. (12.3A.5) and Eq. (12.3B.5), respectively.

Decision Rule 12.3B-1 (Armitage's preference method for comparing two exponential survival curves)
Reject H_0 of Eq. (12.3B.2) at the level of significance α if the computed χ_{Armi} of Eq. (12.3B.6) is greater than the critical value $\chi^2_{1;1-\alpha}$. Otherwise, do not reject H_0.

Remarks

1. Since Armitage's sign method[2] is very different from the ordinary nonparametric sign test, I change its name to the preference method to avoid confusion.
2. Armitage's preference method is applicable to any two distributions in the Lehmann family, that is, their survivor functions satisfying

$$S_A(t) = S_B^k(t). \tag{12.3B.7}$$

Exponential distributions of Eq. (12.3A.1) are in the Lehmann family because they satify Eq. (12.3B.7).

Example 12.3B-1

Assume that both the distributions of the remission length of the leukemia patients for the case (6-MP drug) and the control (placebo) groups are exponential. By using Eq. (12.3B.6), test Eq. (12.3B.2) at the significance level of 0.05 if the survival curves for two groups are different from each other.

Solution

First, by substituting Eq. (1) in the solution of Example 12.3A-1 into Eq. (12.3B.3),

$$\hat{\upsilon} = 0.107/(0.027 + 0.107) = 0.798507 \approx 0.8. \tag{1}$$

By substituting $\hat{\xi}_A = 0.027$ and $t^* = 48$ into Eq. (12.3B.5),

$$\hat{\sigma}(\hat{\upsilon}) = \frac{1}{2}\left\{\sqrt{18\left[1 - (1 - e^{-2 \cdot 48 \cdot 0.027})/(2 \cdot 48 \cdot 0.027)\right]}\right\}^{-1} \approx 0.147. \tag{2}$$

By substituting Eqs. (1) and (2) with $\hat{\delta} = -0.08$ and $\hat{\xi}_B = 0.107$ into Eq. (12.3B.6)

$$\chi_{Armi} = [-0.08/(4 \cdot 0.107 \cdot 0.147)]^2 = 1.616805 \approx 1.617. \tag{3}$$

Since the computed χ_{Armi} of Eq. (3) is less than the critical value $\chi^2_{1;0.95} = 3.841$, H_0 of Eq. (12.3B.2) is not rejected at the significance level of 0.05.

Remarks

1. The testing result in this example contradicts Example 12.3A-1. We are not sure which one is more accurate.
2. In fact, we are not sure whether the assumption that both the lifetime distributions of the 6-MP drug and the placebo are exponential is correct. As a result, the use of DR 12.3A-1 and DR 12.3B-1 is questionable.

C. Wald's Sequential Sign Test

In a clinical trial, pairs of patients are randomly treated with drug $j, j = A, B$, respectively. Let T_A and T_B be two lifetime random variables for patients treated with drugs A and B, respectively. Let U be a random variable that is the sign of difference between T_A and T_B, namely,

$$u_i = 1 \quad \text{if } u_i > 0 \quad \text{or} \quad u_i = 0 \quad \text{if } u_i < 0, \qquad (12.3\text{C}.1)$$

where $u_i \equiv t_{Ai} - t_{Bi}$, t_{Ai} and t_{Bi} ($t_{Ai} \neq t_{Bi}$ for all i) are the observations of T_A and T_B for the ith pair of patients. Assume that U is a Bernoulli random variable with the distribution given by Eq. (3.1A.1), namely,

$$\Pr(U = u) = p^u q^{1-u}, \quad u = 1, 0, \quad q = 1 - p. \qquad (12.3\text{C}.2)$$

Then the likelihood of obtaining a sample equal to the observed $(u_1, u_2, \ldots, u_k)$ is given by

$$L\left(u_1, u_2, \ldots, u_k; p\right) = p^{\lambda_k} q^{k - \lambda_k}, \qquad (12.3\text{C}.3)$$

where λ_k is the number of positive signs among $\{u_i\}_{i=1}^{k}$.

If there is no difference in the therapeutic effect of drugs A and B, we wish to test the following pairs of hypotheses

$$\text{H}_0: p = p_0 = 0.5 \quad \text{versus} \quad \text{H}_1: p = p_1 > 0.5. \qquad (12.3\text{C}.4)$$

The natural logarithm of the ratio of the likelihood of Eq. (12.3C.3) under H_1 versus under H_0 of Eq. (12.3C.4) is

$$\ln \frac{L(u_1, u_2, \ldots, u_k; p_1)}{L(u_1, u_2, \ldots, u_k; p_0)} = \lambda_k \ln \frac{p_1}{q_1} + k \ln(2q_1), \qquad (12.3\text{C}.5)$$

where $q_1 = 1 - p_1$.

The clinical trial is continued as long as Eq. (12.3C.5) satisfies[34]

$$\ln \frac{\beta}{1-\alpha} < \ln \frac{L(u_1, u_2, \ldots, u_k; p_1)}{L(u_1, u_2, \ldots, u_k; p_0)} < \ln \frac{1-\beta}{\alpha}, \tag{12.3C.6}$$

where α and β denote type I and II errors, respectively. By substituting Eq. (12.3C.5) into Eq. (12.3C.6) and simplifying it,

$$\ell_0(k) < \lambda_k < \ell_1(k), \tag{12.3C.7}$$

where $\ell_0(k)$ and $\ell_1(k)$ are given respectively by

$$\ell_0(k) = a_0 + b_0 k \equiv \frac{\ln \frac{\beta}{1-\alpha}}{\ln \frac{p_1}{q_1}} - \frac{\ln (2q_1)}{\ln \frac{p_1}{q_1}} k, \tag{12.3C.8}$$

and

$$\ell_1(k) = a_1 + b_0 k \equiv \frac{\ln \frac{1-\beta}{\alpha}}{\ln \frac{p_1}{q_1}} - \frac{\ln (2q_1)}{\ln \frac{p_1}{q_1}} k. \tag{12.3C.9}$$

Define two integer functions as follows:

$$c_k = \text{the largest integer} < \ell_0(k), \tag{12.3C.10}$$

and

$$d_k = \text{the smallest integer} > \ell_1(k), \tag{12.3C.11}$$

A stopping rule for the clinical trial is given as follows: H_0 is accepted if we have at the kth trial

$$\lambda_k \le c_k, \tag{12.3C.12}$$

or H_0 is rejected if we have at the kth trial

$$\lambda_k \ge d_k, \tag{12.3C.13}$$

where c_k and d_k are given by Eqs. (12.3C.10) and (12.3C.11), respectively.

Remarks

1. By treating k as the x-variable and λ_k as the y-variable in the xy-plane, two parallel straight lines $L_0: \lambda_k = \ell_0$ and $L_1: \lambda_k = \ell_1$ divide the first quardrant of the plane into three regions: (i) the region lying above the straight line L_1 is a rejection region; (ii) the region lying between two straight lines L_0 and L_1 are the continuation region; and (iii) the region lying below L_0 is an acceptance region. Wald's sequential sign test for any sequential clinical trial proceeds graphically as follows: with given values α, β and p_1 plot the two straight lines L_0 and L_1 first. Then plot the points (k, λ_k), $k = 1, 2, \ldots$ where λ_k is collected from the outcome of the cinical trial. Once the point (k, λ_k) for some k crosses either lines, L_0 or L_1, the trial is stopped and a decision is made accordingly.

2. Wald's sequential sign test is an "open" procedure, that is, it does not provide any definite upper bound for the random sample size n. It is sometimes desirable to set a definite upper bound n_0 for n. A truncated sequential sign test is set up as follows: H_0 is accepted if

$$\lambda_{n_0} < \frac{1}{2}(c_{n_0} + d_{n_0}) \quad \text{or} \quad H_0 \quad \text{is rejected if} \quad \lambda_{n_0} \geq \frac{1}{2}(c_{n_0} + d_{n_0}).$$

The operating characteristic (OC) curve $L(p)$ of Wald's sequential sign test is given by

$$L(p) = \frac{[(1-\beta)/\alpha]^h - 1}{[(1-\beta)/\alpha]^h - [\beta/(1-\alpha)]^h}, \tag{12.3C.14}$$

where h is determined by

$$p = \frac{1 - (2q_1)^h}{2^h(p_1^h - q_1^h)}. \tag{12.3C.15}$$

Also, its average sample number (ASN) is

$$E_p(n) = \frac{L(p) \ln \frac{\beta}{1-\alpha} + [1 - L(p)] \ln \frac{1-\beta}{\alpha}}{p \ln \frac{p_1}{q_1} + \ln(2q_1)}, \tag{12.3C.16}$$

where $L(p)$ is given by Eq. (12.3C.14).

Remarks

1. Equations (12.3C.14) to (12.3C.16) are obtained from substituting $p_0 = 0.5$ into Eqs. (5.19), (5.20) and (5.23) in Ref. 34.
2. To compute the OC curve of Eq. (12.3C.14), it is not necessary to solve Eq. (12.3C.15) for h. All we have to do is to compute the values of p and $L(p)$ from Eqs. (12.3C.14) and (12.3C.15) for various values of h in the range of $(-\infty, +\infty)$. The point $(p, L(p))$ computed in this way will be a point on the OC curve. As a result, the OC curve can be plotted for a sufficiently large number of points $(p, L(p))$ corresponding to various values of h (see Fig. 12.3C-1).
3. When $h = 0$, both Eqs. (12.3C.14) and (12.3C.15) are undefined. However, it can be shown[34] that

$$\lim_{h \to 0} L(p) = L(b_0) = \frac{a_1}{a_1 + |a_0|}, \qquad (12.3C.17)$$

and

$$\lim_{h \to 0} p = b_0, \qquad (12.3C.18)$$

where a_0, a_1 and b_0 are given by Eqs. (12.3C.8) and (12.3C.9), respectively.

Example 12.3C-1

The data in Table 12.3C-1 is taken from Table 10 in Ref. 16 for $n = 18$ pairs. Let drug A = 6-MP, drug B = placebo and u_i be defined by Eq. (12.3C.1).

Applying the stopping rule of Eqs. (12.3C.12) and (12.3C.13) with $\alpha = 0.05$ and $\beta = 0.1$, find

(a) the random sample size n to test H_0: $p = p_0 = 0.5$ against H_1: $p = p_1 = 0.7$.
(b) the OC curve for the sequential sign test applied to Table 12.3C-1.
(c) the ASN for the sequential sign test applied to Table 12.3C-1.

Table 12.3C-1.   Length of Remission for Patients with Leukemia

i^{th} trial	1st	2nd	3rd	4th	5th	6th
t_{Ai} : 6-MP	10	7	32+	23	22	6
t_{Bi} : Placebo	1	22	3	12	8	17
u_i	1	0	1	1	1	0
i^{th} trial	7th	8th	9th	10th	11th	12th
t_{Ai} : 6-MP	16	34+	32+	25+	11+	20+
t_{Bi} : Placebo	2	11	8	12	2	5
u_i	1	1	1	1	1	1
i^{th} trial	13th	14th	15th	16th	17th	18th
t_{Ai} : 6-MP	19+	6	17+	35+	6	13
t_{Bi} : Placebo	4	15	8	23	5	11
u_i	1	0	1	1	1	1

Solution

(a) By using Eqs. (12.3C.3, 8) to (12.3C.11) to compute the values of $\lambda_k, \ell_0(k), \ell_1(k)$, c_k and d_k for $k = 1, 2, \ldots, 18$, their values are given in Table 12.3C-2. At the 17th trial, we have for the first time that $d_{17} = \lambda_{17} = 14$. Hence the random sample size is $n = 17$. Also, H_0 is rejected at the significance level of $\alpha = 0.05$ with $\beta = 0.1$. A plot of Table 12.3C-2 is given in Fig. 12.3C-1.

(b) By using Eqs. (12.3C.14) and (12.3C.15), the values of p and $L(p)$ are computed for various values of $h = -10, -5, -4, -3, -2.6, -2.56, -2.5, -2, -1, 1, 5$ and 10, which are given in Table 12.3C-3. After plotting the points $(p, L(p))$, the OC curves is given in Fig. 12.3C-2.

The true unknown p of the Bernoulli random variable U is estimated by

$$\hat{p} = d_{17}/n = 14/17 = 0.823529 \approx 0.824. \qquad \text{(b.1)}$$

From Table 12.3C-3,

$$L(\hat{p}) = L(0.824) = 0.003. \qquad \text{(b.2)}$$

Table 12.3C-2. Values of c_k, λ_k, and d_k

k^{th} Trial	1st	2nd	3rd	4th	5th	6th
c_k	−3	−2	−1	−1	0	0
λ_k	1	1	2	3	4	4
d_k	5	5	6	6	7	8
k^{th} Trial	7th	8th	9th	10th	11th	12th
c_k	1	2	2	3	3	4
λ_k	5	6	7	8	9	10
d_k	8	9	9	10	11	11
k^{th} Trial	13th	14th	15th	16th	17th	18th
c_k	5	5	6	6	7	8
λ_k	11	11	12	13	14	15
d_k	12	12	13	14	14	15

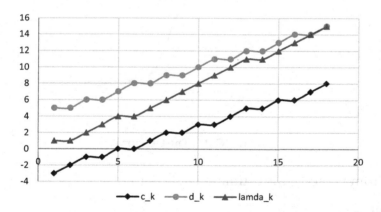

Fig. 12.3C-1. A plot of Table 12.3C.2.

Equation (b.2) is the p-value of Eq. (b.1) that is 0.003.

(c) By substituting $p = \hat{p}$ (Eq. (b.1)) with $\alpha = 0.05$, $\beta = 0.1$, $p_1 = 0.7$ and $q_1 = 0.3$ into Eq. (12.3C.16),

$$E_{\hat{p}}(n) = \frac{0.003 \cdot \ln\frac{0.1}{0.95} + (1 - 0.003) \cdot \ln\frac{0.9}{0.05}}{0.824 \cdot \ln\frac{0.7}{0.3} + \ln(2 \cdot 0.3)} = 15.35 \approx 16. \qquad (c.1)$$

Table 12.3C-3.   Values of h, p and $L(p)$

h	-10	-5	-4	-3	-2.6	-2.56	-2.55
p	0.994	0.936	0.901	0.851	0.826	0.824	0.823
$L(p)$	1.7×10^{-10}	1.3×10^{-5}	0.0001	0.001	0.003	0.003	0.003

h	-2	-1	0	1	2	5	10
p	0.7844	0.7	0.603	0.5	0.4	0.174	0.034
$L(p)$	0.011	0.1	0.562	0.95	0.997	1.0	1.0

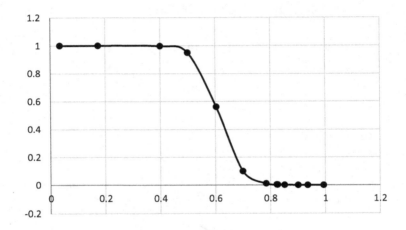

Fig. 12.3C-2.   The OC curve.

From Eq. (c.1), the estimated ASN is 16.

Remarks

1. Wald's sequential sign test depends on the values of α, β and p_1. For fixed p_1, the smaller the values of α and β, the larger the random sample size n. For fixed α and β, the larger the value of p_1, the smaller the random sample size n (see Exercise 12.6-9).
2. When $h = 0$, we have to use Eqs. (12.3C.17) and (12.3C.18) to compute the values of $L(p)$ and p in Fig. 12.3C-2.

D. *Armitage's Restricted Sequential Test*

In a clinical trial, pairs of patients are randomly treated with drug $j, j = A, B$, respectively. Let T_A and T_B be two continuous lifetime random variables for patients treated respectively with drugs A and B. Let U^* be a discrete random variable that takes the values of ± 1 defined by

$$u_i^* = 1 \quad \text{if} \quad u_i^* > 0 \quad \text{or} \quad u_i^* = -1 \quad \text{if} \quad u_i^* < 0, \qquad (12.3D.1)$$

where $u_i^* \equiv t_{Ai} - t_{Bi}$, t_{Ai} and t_{Bi} are the observations of T_A and T_B for the ith pair of patients. Since T_A and T_B are two continuous lifetime random variables, the probability that $t_{Ai} = t_{Bi}$ is almost zero. Hence, it is reasonable to assume that $t_{Ai} \neq t_{Bi}$ for all i.

According to Definition 12.3B.1, the pair of patients is said to be of A-preference if $u_i^* = 1$ and of B-preference if $u_i^* = -1$. If the preference rates for drugs A and B in a single pair of patients occurring at any time point t are denoted by p_A and p_B, respectively. Thus, we have

$$p_B = 1 - p_A. \qquad (12.3D.2)$$

To test that $P_A = P_B$ is equivalent to testing the following hypotheses:

$$\text{H}_0: p_A = p_0^* = \frac{1}{2} \quad \text{versus} \quad \text{H}_1: p_A = p_1^* \neq \frac{1}{2}. \qquad (12.3D.3)$$

Among the first k pairs of patients, let k_1 and k_2 denote the number of A-preference and B-preference, respectively, where $k = k_1 + k_2$. Define

$$\lambda_k^* = \sum_{i=1}^{k} u_i^* = k_1 - k_2. \qquad (12.3D.4)$$

The likelihood function of the first k pair of patients is

$$L(\vec{u}^*; p_A) = p_A^{k_1} q_A^{k_2}, \qquad (12.3D.5)$$

where $\vec{u}^* = (u_1^*, u_2^*, \ldots, u_k^*)$, u_i^*s are defined by Eq. (12.3D.1). The natural logarithm of the ratio of Eq. (12.3D.5) under H_1 to H_0 of Eq. (12.3D.3) is

$$\ln \frac{L(\vec{u}^*; p_1^*)}{L(\vec{u}^*; p_0^*)} = \frac{1}{2}\lambda_k^* \ln \frac{p_1^*}{q_1^*} + \frac{1}{2}k\ln\left[4p_1^*q_1^*\right]. \qquad (12.3D.6)$$

Armitage's restricted (or closed) sequential test is defined as follows: The clinical trial is continued if λ_k^* lies between two straight lines,[1] the upper and lower boundaries $\ell_1^*(k)$ and $\ell_0^*(k)$, namely,

$$\ell_0^*(k) \le \lambda_k^* \le \ell_1^*(k), \qquad (12.3D.7)$$

where $\ell_1^*(k)$ and $\ell_0^*(k)$ are defined respectively by

$$\ell_0^*(k) = -a_0^* - b_0^* k, \qquad (12.3D.8)$$

and

$$\ell_1^*(k) = a_0^* + b_0^* k, \qquad (12.3D.9)$$

where a_0^* and b_0^* are defined respectively by

$$a_0^* = 2\ln[(1-\beta)/\alpha]/\ln(p_1^*/q_1^*), \qquad (12.3D.10)$$

and

$$b_0^* = -\ln\left(4p_1^*q_1^*\right)/\ln(p_1^*/q_1^*). \qquad (12.3D.11)$$

The clinical trial is stopped as follows: H_0 is accepted if we have at the kth trial

$$\lambda_k^* \le c_k^*, \qquad (12.3D.12)$$

or H_0 is rejected if we have at the kth trial

$$\lambda_k^* \ge d_k^*, \qquad (12.3D.13)$$

where c_k^* and d_k^* are given respectively by

$$c_k^* = \text{the largest integer} < \ell_0^*(k), \qquad (12.3D.14)$$

and

$$d_k^* = \text{the smallest integer} > \ell_1^*(k). \tag{12.3D.15}$$

Note that Eq. (12.3D.4) is a random walk. It will therefore be approximated by a diffusion process with a drift $\mu - b_0^*$ per unit time, growth in variance at a rate σ^2, and at an absorbing barrier at a_0^*, where μ and σ^2 are given respectively by[1]

$$\mu = 2p^* - 1 \quad \text{and} \quad \sigma^2 = 4p^*q^*, \tag{12.3D.16}$$

where p^* is defined by Eq. (12.3D.2). If $\Pr(\mu, N_1)$ is the probability of absorption on the upper boundary $\ell_1^*(k)$ in less than N_1 observations, with no other boundary having previously been reached, N_1 is chosen such that $\Pr(\mu_1, N_1) = 1 - \beta$, where $\mu_1 = 2p_1^* - 1, p_1^*$ is defined in H_1 of Eq. (12.3D.3), it follows that $\Pr(0, N_1) = \alpha$ if overshooting the boundaries is neglected. The value of β is required to satisfy

$$\beta = \Phi\left(\frac{a_0^* - m_1 N_1}{\sigma_1 \sqrt{N_1}}\right) - \exp\left(\frac{2a_0^* m_1}{\sigma_1^2}\right) \Phi\left(-\frac{a_0^* + m_1 N_1}{\sigma_1 \sqrt{N_1}}\right),$$

$$\tag{12.3D.17}$$

where $\Phi(z) = \int_{-\infty}^{z} \frac{1}{\sqrt{2\pi}} \exp(-\frac{1}{2}x^2)dx, m_1 = \mu_1 - b_0^*, \sigma_1^2 = 4p_1^* q_1^*, a_0^*$ and b_0^* are given Eqs. (12.3D.10) and (12.3D.11). Since α, β and p_1^* are known, Eq. (12.3D.17) may be solved for N_1 by successive approximation (see Example 12.3D-1(b)).

The clinical trial is terminated eventually at the middle boundary $M : k = N_1$, a vertical line if neither Eq. (12.3D.12) nor Eq. (12.3D.13) are satisfied at the N_1^{th} trial.

Remarks

1. Equation (12.3D.6) is obtained by a simplification after solving k_1 and k_2 in Eq. (12.3D.4) in terms of k and λ_k^*, namely, $k_1 = \frac{1}{2}\lambda_k^* + \frac{1}{2}k$ and $k_2 = \frac{1}{2}k - \frac{1}{2}\lambda_k^*$ and substituting them into Eq. (12.3D.6).

2. The right side $\ell_1^*(k)$ of Eq. (12.3D.7) is obtained by solving Eq. (12.3D.6) being less than or equal to $\ln[(1 - \beta)/\alpha]$. The left side $\ell_0^*(k)$ of Eq. (12.3D.7) is obtained by using the symmetric design of Armitage's restricted sequential test.
3. Since the value N_1 solved by Eq. (12.3D.17) for the middle boundary is possibly greater than the ASN of Wald's open sequestial test, Armitage's restricted sequential test is modified by replacing the middle boundary M by two wedged lines of inner boundaries[3]

$$\text{Upper wedged line } M_U: \ell_1^{**}(k) = a_0^{**} - N_1 + k,$$

$$(12.3D.18)$$

and

$$\text{lower wedged line } M_L: \ell_0^{**}(k) = N_1 - a_0^{**} - k,$$

$$(12.3D.19)$$

where a_0^{**} is given by

$$a_0^{**} \equiv [\ell_1^*(N_1)] = \text{the largest integer} \le \ell_1^*(N_1).$$

$$(12.3D.20)$$

Example 12.3D-1

Use the data in the first three rows of Table 12.3C-1, the last row u_i is replaced by u_i^*, namely, the three entries with value 0 need to be replaced by -1. Applying the stopping rule of Eqs. (12.3D.12) and (12.3D.13) with $\alpha = 0.025$ and $\beta = 0.05$, find:

(a) the stopping sample size k to test $H_0: p^* = p_0^* = 0.5$ against H_1: $p^* = p_1^* = 0.75$.
(b) Find the value N_1 of the middle boundary M in Armitage's restricted sequential test.
(c) Using Eqs. (12.3D.18) to (12.3D.20), find the two wedged lines for the inner boundaries in Armitage's modified restricted sequential test.

Table 12.3D-1. Values of c_k^*, λ_k^* and d_k^*

k^{th} Trial	1st	2nd	3rd	4th	5th	6th
c_k^*	-7	-8	-8	-8	-8	-9
λ_k^*	1	0	1	2	3	2
d_k^*	7	8	8	8	8	9
k^{th} Trial	7th	8th	9th	10th	11th	12th
c_k^*	-9	-9	-9	-10	-10	-10
λ_k^*	3	4	5	6	7	8
d_k^*	9	9	9	10	10	10
k^{th} Trial	textbf13th	14th	15th	16th	17th	18th
c_k^*	-11	-11	-11	-11	-12	-12
λ_k^*	9	10	9	10	11	12
d_k^*	11	11	11	11	12	12

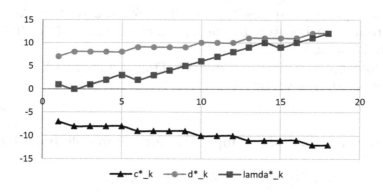

Fig. 12.3D-1. A plot of Table 12.3D-1.

Solution

(a) By using Eqs. (12.3D.4) and (12.3D.8) to (12.3D.15) to compute the values of λ_k^*, $\ell_0^*(k)$, $\ell_1^*(k)$, c_k^* and d_k^* for $k = 1, 2, \ldots, 18$, their values are given in Table 12.3D-1. At the 18th trial, we have the first time that $d_{18}^* = \lambda_{18}^* = 12$. Hence the stopping sample size is $n = 18$. Also, H$_0$ is rejected at the significance level of $\alpha = 0.025$ with $\beta = 0.05$. A plot of Table 12.3D-1 is given in Fig. 12.3D-1.

Table 12.3D-2.   A search for the root of $g(x)$ of Eq. (b.1)

x	62	63	64	65	66	67
$g(x)$	0.0089	0.0059	0.0031	0.0004	-0.0021	-0.0045

(b) Let N_1 be the sample size for the middle boundary corresponding to $\alpha = 0.025$, $\beta = 0.05$ and $p_1^* = 0.75$. By letting

$$g(x) = \Phi\left(\frac{a_0^* - m_1 x}{\sigma_1\sqrt{x}}\right) - \exp\left(\frac{2a_0^* m_1}{\sigma_1^2}\right)\Phi\left(-\frac{a_0^* + m_1 x}{\sigma_1\sqrt{x}}\right) - \beta. \quad \text{(b.1)}$$

where x is defined by

$$x = N_1. \quad \text{(b.2)}$$

To solve Eq. (12.3D.17) for the value of N in the middle boundary is equivalent to solving Eq. (b.1) for the root x. We find the root x for Eq. (b.1) by successive evaluations of Eq. (b.1) in Table 12.3D-2.

From $g(65)=0.0004$ in Table 12.3D-2, the root to Eq. (b.1) is approximately given by

$$x = 65. \quad \text{(b.3)}$$

From Eq. (b.3), the sample size for the middle boundary is $N_1 = 65$.

(c) By using Eqs. (12.3D.10) and (12.3D.11),

$$a_0^* = 2\ \ln(0.95/0.025)/\ln(0.75/0.25) = 6.622147 \approx 6.622, \quad \text{(c.1)}$$

and

$$b_0^* = -\ln(4 \cdot 0.75 \cdot 0.25)/(\ln(0.75/0.25) = 0.26186 \approx 0.262. \quad \text{(c.2)}$$

By substituting Eqs. (c.1) and (c.2) into Eq. (12.3D.9),

$$\ell_1^*(k) = 6.622 + 0.262k. \quad \text{(c.3)}$$

By substituting Eq. (b.3) for k into Eq. (c.3),

$$\ell_1^*(65) = 6.622 + 0.262 \cdot 65 = 23.652. \quad \text{(c.4)}$$

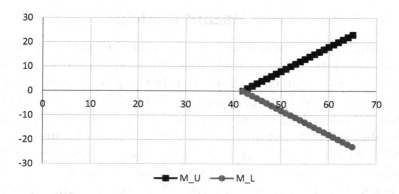

Fig. 12.3D-2. Two inner boundaries for Example 12.3D-1(c).

By substituting Eq. (c.4) into Eq. (12.3D.20),

$$a_0^{**} = [23.652] = 23 \tag{c.5}$$

By substituting Eqs. (b.3) and (c.5) into Eqs. (12.3D.18) and (12.3D.19), the two inner boundaries in Armitage's modified restricted sequential test are

$$M_U : \ell_1^{**}(k) = -42 + k, \tag{c.6}$$

and

$$M_L : \ell_0^{**}(k) = 42 - k, \tag{c.7}$$

A plot of Eqs. (c.6) and (c.7) for k = 42,...,50 is given in Fig. 12.3D-2.

Remarks

1. The stopping sample size is $n = 18$. It confirms what was stated in Example 12.3A-1. Also, Fig. 12.3D-2 is exactly the same as Fig. 8 in Ref. 16.
2. In a medical experiment, the traditional significance test of choosing $\alpha = 0.05$ is not very realistic. I Bross[7] suggested to relax to $\alpha = 0.10$ or even to $\alpha = 0.20$.

12.4 Proportional Hazard Models

The usual regression model specifies that the survival times or some transform such as their logarithms are equal to a linear combination of the concomitant variables plus a random error term. Unfortunately, to generalize such models for use with censored data is awkward and computationally involved. Thus considerable interest was aroused by Cox[10, 11] when he proposed a model formulated in terms of the regression variables on the instaneous death rates rather than on times of death.

Cox's model is defined in terms of the hazard function h(t|$\vec{z}$) for an individual having a p-dimensional vector of covariates $\vec{z} = (z_1, z_2, \ldots, z_p)^T$ given by

$$h(t|\vec{z}) = \exp(\vec{\beta}^T \vec{z}) h_0(t) \tag{12.4.1}$$

where $\vec{\beta} = (\beta_1, \beta_2, \ldots, \beta_p)^T$ is a p-dimensional vector of unknown parameters, and $h_0(t)$ is the unknown death rate function for an individual at the baseline $\vec{z} = \vec{0}$. Equation (12.4.1) is called the proportional hazard model. The relative risk is a useful measure of association between a chronic disease and suspected risk factors. Use of this measure involves the implicit assumption that the relative risk is a constant with respect to age and other personal characteristics. Cox's model of Eq. (12.4.1) gives a proability formulation for the constant relative risk concept.

To estimate the unknown regression parameters of $\vec{\beta}$, a random sample of data from n individuals has to be collected in which there are K distinct observed lifetimes and n−K censored observations. The K observed lifetimes are denoted by $t_{(1)} < t_{(2)} < \cdots < t_{(K)}$ and $R_k = R(t_{(k)})$ is the risk set at time $t_{(k)}$, which is the set of individuals alive and uncensored just prior to $t_{(k)}$. In the absence of knowledge of $h_0(t)$, the conditional likelihood function of $\vec{\beta}$ is given by

$$L(\vec{\beta}) = \prod_{k=1}^{K} \frac{\exp(\vec{\beta}^T \vec{z}_{(k)})}{\sum_{\ell \in R_k} \exp(\vec{\beta}^T \vec{z}_{(\ell)})}, \tag{12.4.2}$$

where $\vec{z}_{(k)}$ is the regression vector of covariates associated with the individual observed to die at $t_{(k)}$. Note that Eq. (12.4.2) is obtained under the condition that all observed lifetimes $t_{(k)}$, $k = 1,\ldots,K$, are distinct. If there are ties among $\{t_{(k)}\}$, Eq. (12.4.2) has to be replaced

$$L(\vec{\beta}) = \prod_{k=1}^{K} \frac{\exp\left(\vec{\beta}^T \vec{s}_{(k)}\right)}{\left[\sum_{\ell \in R_k} \exp\left(\vec{\beta}^T \vec{z}_\ell\right)\right]^{d_k}}, \tag{12.4.3}$$

where d_k is the number of tied lifetimes at $t_{(k)}$ and $\vec{s}_{(k)} = \sum_{\ell \in D_k} \vec{z}_\ell$, D_k is the set of individuals who die at $t_{(k)}$. Equation (12.4.3) reduces to Eq. (12.4.2), provided that there are no ties.

The natural logarithm of Eq. (12.4.3) is given by

$$\ln(L(\vec{\beta})) = \sum_{k=1}^{K} \vec{\beta}^T \vec{s}_{(k)} - \sum_{k=1}^{K} d_k \ln\left(\sum_{\ell \in R_k} \exp\left(\vec{\beta}^T \vec{z}_\ell\right)\right), \tag{12.4.4}$$

and the first derivatives of Eq. (12.4.4) are for $i = 1,\ldots,p$

$$\frac{\partial \ln\left(L(\vec{\beta})\right)}{\partial \beta_i} = \sum_{k=1}^{K} s_{ki} - \frac{d_k \sum_{l \in R_k} z_{li} \exp(\vec{\beta}^T \vec{z}_l)}{\sum_{l \in R_k} \exp(\vec{\beta}^T \vec{z}_l)}, \tag{12.4.5}$$

where s_{ki} is the ith component of $\vec{s}_{(k)} = (s_{k1}, s_{k2},\ldots,s_{kp})^T$. By setting Eq. (12.4.5) equal to zero, the maximum likelihood estimator $\hat{\vec{\beta}}$ can be obtained by applying the Newton–Raphson method to solve $\frac{\partial \ln(L(\vec{\beta}))}{\partial \beta_i} = 0$ for $\vec{\beta}$.

The information matrix $I(\vec{\beta})$ of Eq. (12.4.4) is obtained by adding the minus sign of the second partial derivative to

Eq. (12.4.4) for $i, j = 1, \ldots, p$

$$I_{ij}(\vec{\beta}) = -\frac{\partial^2 \ln(L(\vec{\beta}))}{\partial \beta_i \partial \beta_j} = \sum_{k=1}^{K} d_k \left\{ \frac{\sum_{\ell \in R_k} z_{\ell i} z_{\ell j} \exp\left(\vec{\beta}^T \vec{z}_\ell\right)}{\sum_{\ell \in R_k} \exp\left(\vec{\beta}^T \vec{z}_\ell\right)} \right.$$
$$\left. - \frac{\left[\sum_{\ell \in R_k} z_{\ell i} \exp\left(\vec{\beta}^T \vec{z}_\ell\right)\right] \left[\sum_{\ell \in R_k} z_{\ell j} \exp\left(\vec{\beta}^T \vec{z}_\ell\right)\right]}{\left[\sum_{\ell \in R_k} \exp\left(\vec{\beta}^T \vec{z}_\ell\right)\right]^2} \right\}$$

$$(12.4.6)$$

To make inferences about $\vec{\beta}$ we have to rely on large-sample procedures. Computation of the expected value of $I_{ij}(\vec{\beta})$ given by Eq. (12.4.6) is impossible without detailed knowledge of the censoring mechanism. The simplest way is to treat $\hat{\vec{\beta}}$ as a normal distribution with mean $\vec{\beta}$ and variance-covariance matrix $[I(\hat{\vec{\beta}})]^{-1}$. Inference can also be based on likelihood ratio methods.

Let us learn how to apply the proportional hazard model to the two sample test problems. Suppose that we would like to test whether populations 1 and 2 have the same survivor functions, that is,

$$H_0 : S_1(t) = S_2(t), \qquad (12.4.7)$$

where $S_i(t)$ denotes the survivor function of the lifetime variable of population $i, i = 1, 2$. Assume that their corresponding hazard functions $h_1(t)$ and $h_2(t)$ satisfy the proportional hazard model assumption with the dummy variable z signifying that an observation is from population 1 ($z = 0$) or from population 2 ($z = 1$). As a consequence,

$$h_1(t) = h_0(t) \quad \text{and} \quad h_2(t) = h_0(t)e^{\beta}. \qquad (12.4.8)$$

This is equivalent to that $S_1(t)$ and $S_2(t)$ are related by

$$S_2(t) = [S_1(t)]^{\gamma}, \qquad (12.4.9)$$

where $\gamma = e^{\beta}$. Under the assumption of proportional hazard the null hypothesis H_0 of Eq. (12.4.7) is equivalent to testing $\beta = 0$ and the alternative hypothesis of Eq. (12.4.7) becomes

$$H_1 : \beta \neq 0, \tag{12.4.10}$$

where $\beta \neq 0$ is equivalent to $\gamma \neq 1$. If the survivor functions of populations 1 and 2 satisfy Eq. (12.4.10), their lifetime random variables are said to be of the Lehmann family.[24]

Suppose that observations are randomly collected on n_1 individuals from population 1 and n_2 individuals from population 2. Some observations may be censored. By combining these two samples of n_1 and n_2 observations as a single sample, let $t_{(1)} < t_{(2)} < \cdots < t_{(K)}$ denote the K distinct observed lifetimes in the combined sample and let $d_k = d_{1k} + d_{2k}$ represent the number of deaths at $t_{(k)}$, and $n_k = n_{1k} + n_{2k}$ the number of individuals in the risk set R_k, where d_{ik} and n_{ik} denote respectively the number of deaths and individuals in population $i, i = 1, 2$ at $t_{(k)}$.

Under this setup Eq. (12.4.4) becomes

$$\ln(L(\beta)) = \delta_2 \beta - \sum_{k=1}^{K} [d_k \ln(n_{1k} + n_{2k}, e^{\beta})] \tag{12.4.11}$$

where $\delta_2 = \sum_{k=1}^{K} d_{2k}$ is the total number of deaths in population 2. The first derivative, called the score function, and the negative of the second derivative of Eq. (12.4.11) are given respectively by

$$U(\beta) = \frac{\partial \ln(L(\beta))}{\partial \beta} = \delta_2 - \sum_{k=1}^{K} \frac{d_k n_{2k} e^{\beta}}{n_{1k} + n_{2k} e^{\beta}}, \tag{12.4.12}$$

and

$$I(\beta) = -\frac{\partial^2 \ln(L(\beta))}{\partial \beta^2} = \sum_{k=1}^{K} \frac{d_k n_{1k} n_{2k} e^{\beta}}{(n_{1k} + n_{2k} e^{\beta})^2}. \tag{12.4.13}$$

The maximum likelihood estimator $\hat{\beta}$ can be obtained by setting Eq. (12.4.12) equal to zero and solving for β. The sampling statistics to test Eq. (12.4.7) against Eq. (12.4.10) is given by

$$z = \frac{\hat{\beta}}{\sqrt{I(\hat{\beta})}}, \tag{12.4.14}$$

where $I(\hat{\beta})$ is obtained by evaluating Eq. (12.4.13) at $\beta = \hat{\beta}$.

The decision rule for testing Eq. (12.4.7) is given as follows.

Decision Rule 12.4-1 (A test for the equality of two survivor functions)

The level of significance for the test statistics of Eq. (12.4.14) is α. The null hypothesis H_0 of Eq.(12.4.7) ($\beta = 0$) is rejected if the computed value of z in Eq. (12.4.14) is greater than $z_{1-\frac{\alpha}{2}}$ or less than $z_{\frac{\alpha}{2}}$. Otherwise, do not reject H_0.

Example 12.4-1

By using the data given by Table 12.1-1 and the proportional hazard model, test at the level of significance 0.05 if the survivor functions for the length of remission from the patients treated by drug 6-MP and the placebo group are of the Lehmann family by using DR 12.4-1.

Solution

First, list the length of remission time according to the order of its magnitude for each sample in columns 1 and 2 in Table 12.4-1. By counting the number of rows in Table 12.4-1, we have K = 17.

By using the data in Table 12.4-1, we have from Eq. (12.4.12)

$$U(\beta) = 18 - \left\{ \frac{1 \times 18e^{\beta}}{18 + 18e^{\beta}} + \frac{2 \times 17e^{\beta}}{18 + 17e^{\beta}} + \cdots + \frac{2 \times 2e^{\beta}}{7 + 2e^{\beta}} + \frac{2 \times e^{\beta}}{6 + 1 \times e^{\beta}} \right\}.$$

(4)

To obtain the maximum likelihood estimator $\hat{\beta}$, we solve for β by setting Eq. (4) to zero, namely

$$U(\beta) = 0.$$

(5)

Since Eq. (5) is nonlinear in β, we apply the Newton–Raphson method to Eq. (5) iteratively for m = 0, 1, 2, ...

$$\beta_{m+1} = \beta_m - \frac{U(\beta_m)}{U'(\beta_m)},$$

(6)

Table 12.4-1. The list in the risk sets of samples 1 (6-MP) and 2 (placebo)

Length of Remission Time		No. in Risk Set			
Sample 1 (6-MP)	Sample 2 (Placebo)	n_{1k}	n_{2k}	d_{1k}	d_{2k}
	1	18	18	0	1
	2, 2	18	17	0	2
	3	18	15	0	1
	4	18	14	0	1
	5, 5	18	13	0	2
6, 6, 6		18	13	3	0
7		15	13	1	0
	8, 8, 8	14	11	0	3
10		14	8	1	0
	11, 11	13	8	0	2
	12, 12	12	6	0	2
13		12	4	1	0
	15	11	4	0	1
16		11	3	1	0
	17	10	3	0	1
22	22	7	2	1	1
23	23	6	1	1	1

where $U'(\beta)$ is the first derivative of Eq. (4) given by using Eq. (12.4.13)

$$U'(\beta) = -\left\{ \frac{1 \times 18 \times 18e^\beta}{(18 + 18e^\beta)^2} + \frac{2 \times 18 \times 17e^\beta}{(18 + 17e^\beta)^2} + \cdots + \frac{2 \times 7 \times 2e^\beta}{(7 + 2e^\beta)^2} \right.$$

$$\left. + \frac{2 \times 6 \times 1 \times e^\beta}{(6 + 1 \times e^\beta)^2} \right\}. \tag{7}$$

The numerical results obtained from the iterative use of Eq. (6) is given in Table 12.4-2.

It takes only five iterations for the value of the score function $U(\beta_3)$ to reach 2.65×10^{-6} (see Table 12.4-2). Hence, the maximum likelihood estimator is

$$\hat{\beta} = \beta_2 = 1.346479. \tag{8}$$

Table 12.4-2.   The iterative calculation of Eq. (6)

m	β_m	$U(\beta_m)$	$U'(\beta_m)$	β_{m+1}
0	0	8.27138	−5.93362	1.393984
1	1.393984	−0.26544	−5.55877	1.346233
2	1.346233	0.001387	−5.64281	1.346479
3	1.346479	2.65×10^{-6}	−5.64239	1.346479

By substituting Eq. (8) into Eq. (12.4.13), we have

$$I(1.346479) = 5.64239. \tag{9}$$

By applying Eq. (12.4.14),

$$z = \frac{\hat{\beta}}{\sqrt{I(\hat{\beta})}} = \frac{1.346479}{\sqrt{5.64239}} = 0.56685 \approx 0.5669. \tag{10}$$

Since the computed z-value of Eq. (10) is less than the standard normal critical value $z_{0.975} = 1.96$, the null hypothesis H_0 of Eq. (12.4.7) is not rejected at the significance level of 0.05, that is, the survivor functions for the 6-MP and the placebo groups are of the Lehmann family.

Remarks

1. The remark given by using Eq. (7.2.13) in the Lawless' book[22] as a testing statistic without the need to compute $\hat{\beta}$ seems incorrect, as shown by this example. The values of $U(0) = 7.692$ and $I(0) = 5.641$ give the z-value $\left(\frac{U(0)}{\sqrt{I(0)}} \right) = 3.2386$, which contradicts Eq. (10).
2. The calculation of Table 12.4-2 is done on an EXCEL spreadsheet.

12.5   The Log-Rank Test

In this section we present a nonparametric test for testing whether two independent survival functions S_1 and S_2 of a lifetime random variable (r.v.) T equal one another, that is,

$$H_0 : S_1(t) = S_2(t) \quad \text{versus} \quad H_1 : S_1(t) \neq S_2(t). \tag{12.5.1}$$

Suppose that there are n_1 and n_2 individuals in groups 1 and 2, respectively. Also, suppose that group 1 has s_1 right-censored observations and $n_1 - s_1$ death times, while group 2 has s_2 right-censored observations and $n_2 - s_2$ death times. The log-rank test is based on a set of scores $\{w_i\}$, which are functions of the logarithm of the survival function, assigned to various observations.

Let $t_{(1)} < \cdots < t_{(K)}$ be the distinct ordered death times in the total combined observations of two groups together and $m_{(i)}$ be the number of death times at $t_{(i)}$. Furthermore, let R(t) be the risk set at time t, that is, the set of individuals whose death or censoring times are at least t. The log-rank test is based on the sum ζ of the w scores in one of the two groups, say, group 2, given by

$$\zeta = n_2 - s_2 - \sum_{i=1}^{K} m_{(i)} A_{(i)}, \tag{12.5.2}$$

where $r_{(i)} \equiv n\left(R_{t_{(i)}}\right)$ = the number of observations in the risk set $R_{t_{(i)}}$, and $A_{(i)}$ is the proportion of $r_{(i)}$ that belong to group 2. The variance of Eq. (12.5.1) is given by[23]

$$V = \frac{n_1 n_2}{(n_1 + n_2)(n_1 + n_2 - 1)} \sum_{j=1}^{K} \frac{m_{(j)}(r_{(j)} - m_{(j)})}{r(j)}. \tag{12.5.3}$$

It can be shown[23] that the following testing statistics

$$z_{LR} = \frac{\zeta}{\sqrt{V}} \tag{12.5.4}$$

is distributed as a standard normal r.v. Z. A decision rule is set up as follows.

Decision Rule 12.5-1 (The log-rank test)
For the test below the significance level is α:

A two-tailed test for Eq. (12.5.1) is to reject H_0 if the computed z_{LR} of Eq. (12.5.4) is greater than $z_{1-\frac{\alpha}{2}}$ or less than $z_{\frac{\alpha}{2}}$. Otherwise, do not reject H_0.

Remarks

1. Another alternative estimator $\hat{\sigma}^2_{MP}$ for the variance of Eq. (12.5.2) is based on the Mantel–Haenszel approach. A comparison of $\hat{\sigma}^2_{MP}$ and V of Eq. (12.5.3) is done in Brown.[8]
2. The powers of several nonparametric tests for the two-sample problem with censored data are compared by simulation.[21] It was noticed that the sample sizes, censoring mechanism, and distribution of the random variables all influenced the relative performance of the test statistics. The log-rank test appears to be the best when the random variables are exponential or Weibull.

Example 12.5-1

With the data given in Table 12.5-1 test Eq. (12.5.1) at the level of significance of 0.05 by applying DR 12.5-1 (the log-rank test).

Solution

The combined data of the treatment (6-MP) group (G1) and the placebo group (G2) in Table 12.1-1 are listed in descending order in the first and second columns of Table 12.5-1.

Since there are no censored observation in G2, $s_2 = 0$. By substituting $n_2 = 18$ and the values of $m_{(i)}$ and $A_{(i)}$ in the 6th and 7th columns in Table 12.5-1 into Eq. (12.5.2),

$$\zeta = 18 - 0 - \{2 \cdot 0.1429 + 2 \cdot 0.2222 + 1 \cdot 0.2308 + \cdots$$

$$+ 1 \cdot 0.4545 + 2 \cdot 0.48571 + 1 \cdot 0.5\} = 8.4327 \tag{1}$$

By substituting $n_1 = n_2 = 18$ and the values of $r_{(i)}$ and $m_{(i)}$ in the 5th and 6th columns in Table 12.5-1 into Eq. (12.5.3),

$$V = \frac{18 \cdot 18}{(18 + 18)(18 + 18 - 1)} \cdot \left\{ \frac{2 \cdot (7 - 2)}{7} + \frac{2 \cdot (9 - 2)}{9} + \cdots \right.$$

$$\left. + \frac{1 \cdot (36 - 1)}{36} \right\}$$

$$\approx 5.3319 \tag{2}$$

Table 12.5-1. The combined data of the treatment (6-MP) G2 and the placebo group G1 in Table 12.1-1

| Death Time $t_{(i)}$ | | Risk Set $R(t_{(i)})$ | | | | |
G1	G2	# in G1	# in G2	$r_{(i)}$	$m_{(i)}$	$A_{(i)}$
23	23	6	1	7	2	0.1429
22	22	7	2	9	2	0.2222
	17	10	3	13	1	0.2308
16		11	3	14	1	0.2143
	15	11	4	15	1	0.2667
13		12	4	16	1	0.25
	12, 12	12	6	18	2	0.3333
	11, 11	13	8	21	2	0.3810
10		14	8	22	1	0.3636
	8, 8, 8	14	11	25	3	0.44
7		15	11	26	1	0.4231
6, 6, 6		18	11	29	3	0.3793
	5, 5	18	13	31	2	0.4194
	4	18	14	32	1	0.4375
	3	18	15	33	1	0.4545
	2, 2	18	17	35	2	0.4857
	1	18	18	36	1	0.5

After substituting Eqs. (1) and (2) into Eq. (12.5.4),

$$z_{LR} = \frac{8.4327}{\sqrt{5.3319}} \approx 3.6520. \tag{3}$$

Since the computed z_{LR} of Eq. (3) is greater than $z_{0.975} = 1.96$, the null hypothesis H_0 in Eq. (12.5.1) is rejected, namely, the survival distributions of the treatment group (6-MP) and the placebo group are not the same.

12.6 Exercises

1. Show that Eq. (12.1.5) holds.
2. Show that Eq. (12.1.6) holds.
3. Show that Eq. (12.1.9) holds.

4. Show that Eq. (12.1.11) is obtained by setting $\frac{d\ln L(\xi)}{d\xi} = 0$, where $L(\xi)$ is given by Eq. (12.1.9).

5. (a) By substitutiing $\omega = \sqrt[3]{\xi}$ into Eq. (12.1.9), show that the likelihood function of ω becomes

$$L(\omega) = \omega^{3r} \exp(-\omega^3 T^*). \qquad (12.1.16)$$

(b) By using Eq. (12.1.15), show that

$$\sigma^2(\hat\omega) = \left[E\left(-\frac{d^2 \ln L(\omega)}{d\omega^2} \right) \right]^{-1} = 9\omega^2 [E(r)]^{-1}, \qquad (12.1.17)$$

where $E(r)$ is given in Eq. (12.1.12).

6. Repeat (a) and (b) in Example 12.1-2 for the placebo group.

7. Assume that the parameter ξ of an exponential survival distribution $F(t) = 1 - \exp(-\xi t), \xi > 0$ is estimated from the survival data of sample size n over the interval $(0, t^*)$ by $\hat\xi$, the maximum likelihood estimator. Show that the large sample variance of $\hat\xi$ is given by

$$\sigma^2(\hat\xi) = \left[E\left(-\frac{d^2 \ln L(\xi)}{d\xi^2} \right) \right]^{-1} = \frac{\xi^2}{n[1 - (\xi t^*)^{-1}(1 - e^{-\xi t^*})]}, \qquad (12.3A.9)$$

where $L(\xi)$ is given by Eq. (12.1.9).

8. After letting $k = \xi_A/\xi_B$, Show that Eq. (12.3B.4) is valid by expanding the function $g(k) \equiv E(\hat v) = (1 + k)^{-1}$ into a Taylor's series about $k = 1$.

9. Redo Example 12.3C-1 with the same values of α and β, but with different $p_1 = 0.8$.

10. Redo Example 12.3D-1 with $p_1 = 0.7$.

11. Survival data for 45 patients with high-grade gliomas are stratified with regard to patients aged less than or greater than 40 are given in Table 12.6-1.[29]

Test Eq. (12.5.1) at the level of significane 0.05 by applying the log-rank test of DR 12.5-1.

Table 12.6-1. Survival Tmes of Patients with High-Grade Gliomas

	Age	Survival Times (Months)
Group 1	< 40	1, 2, 3, 3, 3,3.5, 5, 5, 5, 7, 7+, 11, 12, 14+, 16.5+, 18, 18+, 18+, 18.5, 21, 22, 25+, 30+
Group 2	≥ 40	2, 3, 3, 3, 3, 3.5, 4, 5, 5.5, 6, 7,7.5, 8+,9, 11, 11, 12, 12, 13+, 19+, 24+, 32+

References

1. Armitage P. (1957) Restricted sequential procedures. *Biometrika* **44**: 9–26.
2. Armitage P. (1959) The comparision of survival curves. *J R Statist Soc A* **122**: 279–300.
3. Armitage P. (1975) *Sequential Medical Trials*, 2nd ed. A Halsted Press Book, John Wiley & Sons Inc., New York.
4. Anscombe FJ. (1954) Fixed-sample-size analysis of sequential observations. *Biometrics* **10**: 89–100.
5. Barr DR, Davidson TG. (1973) A Kolmogorov–Smirnov test for censored samples. *Technometrics* **15**: 739–757.
6. Breslow N, Crowley J. (1974) A large sample study of the lifetable and product limit estimates under random censorship. *Ann Statist* **2**: 437–453.
7. Bross I. (1952) Sequential medical plans. *Biometrics* **8**: 188–205.
8. Brown M. (1984) On the choice of variance for the log rank test. *Biometrika* **71**: 65–74.
9. Crowley J, Breslow N. (1984) Statistical analysis of survival data. *Ann Rev Publ Health* **5**: 385–411.
10. Cox DR. (1972) Regression models and life-tables. *J R Statist Soc B* **34**: 187–202.
11. Cox DR. (1975) Partial likelihood. *Biometrika* **62**: 269–276.
12. Cox DR, Oakes D. (1984) *Analysis of Survival Data.* Chapman & Hall, New York.
13. Cutler SJ, Ederer F. (1958) Maximum utilization of the life table method in analyzing survival. *J Chronic Dis* **8**: 699–712.
14. Cutler SJ, Griswold MH, Eisenberg H. (1957) An interpretation of survival rates: Cancer of the breast. *J National Cancer Institute* **19**: 1107–1117.
15. Dixon WJ, Mood AM. (1946) The statistical sign test. *J Am Stat Assoc* **41**: 557–566.
16. Freireich EJ, Gehan E, Frei E III, *et al.* (1963) The effect of 6-mercaptopurine on the duration of steroid-induced remissions in acute leukemia: A model for evaluation of other potentially useful therapy. *Blood* **21**: 699–716.

17. Greenwood M. (1926): *The Natural Duration Cancer*, Vol. 33. Her Majesty's Stationary Office, Reports of Public Health and Medical Subjects, London.
18. Hall WJ, Wellner JA. (1980) Confidence bands for a survival curve from censored data. *Biometrika* **67**: 133–143.
19. Kalbfleisch JD, Prentice RL. (1973) Marginal likelihoods based on Cox's regression and life model. *Biometrika* **60**: 267–278.
20. Kaplan EL, Meier P. (1958) Nonparametric estimation from the incomplete observations. *J Am Stat Assoc* **53**: 457–481.
21. Latta RB. (1981) A Monte Carlo study of some two-sample rank tests with censored data. *J Am Stat Assoc* **76**: 713–719.
22. Lawless JF. (1982) *Statistical Models and Methods for Lifetime Data.* Wiley, New York.
23. Lee ET, Desu MM, Gehan EA. (1975) A Monte Carlo study of the power of some two sample tests. *Biometrika* **62**: 425–432.
24. Lehman E, Romano JP. (2005) *Testing Statistical Hypotheses.* Springer, New York.
25. Lilliefors HW. (1969) On the Kolmogorov–Smirnov test for the exponential distribution with mean unknown. *J Am Stat Assoc* **64**: 387–389.
26. Littell AS. (1952) Estimation of the T-year survival rate from follow-up studies over a limited period of time. *Human Biol* **24**: 87–116.
27. Mantel N. (1966) Evaluation of survival data and two new rank order statistics arising in its observation. *Cancer Chemother Rep* **50**: 163–170.
28. Oakes D. (1993) A note on the Kaplan–Meier estimator. *Am Statist* **47**: 39–40.
29. Patronas NJ, Di Chiro G, Kufta C, *et al.* (1985) Prediction of survival in glioma patients by means of positronemission tomography. *J Neurosurg* **62**: 816–822.
30. Press WH, Teukolsky SA, Vetterling WT, Flannery BP. (1986) *Numerical Recipes: The Art of Scientific Computing.* Cambridge University Press, Cambridge, UK.
31. Spiegelman M. (1957) The versatility of the life table. *Am J Public Health* **47**: 297–304.
32. Sprott DA. (1973) Normal likelihood and relations to a large sample theory of estimation. *Biometrika* **60**: 457–465.
33. Sprott DA, Kalbfleisch JD. (1969) Examples of likelihoods and comparison with point estimates and large sample approximations. *J Am Stat Assoc* **64**: 468–484.
34. Wald A. (1947) *Sequential Analysis.* Dover Publications, Inc., New York.
35. Whitehead J. (1986) On the bias of maximum likelihood estimation following sequential test. *Biometrika* **73**: 573–581.

Appendix Tables

Table A-1. Standard Normal Distribution

$$\Pr(Z \le z) = \Phi(z) = \int_{-\infty}^{z} \frac{1}{\sqrt{2\pi}} e^{-x^2/2} dx$$

$$[\Phi(-z) = 1 - \Phi(z)]$$

z	0.00 0.05	0.01 0.06	0.02 0.07	0.03 0.08	0.04 0.09
0.0	0.5000 0.5199	0.5040 0.5239	0.5080 0.5279	0.5120 0.5319	0.5160 0.5359
0.1	0.5398 0.5596	0.5438 0.5636	0.5478 0.5675	0.5517 0.5714	0.5557 0.5753
0.2	0.5793 0.5987	0.5832 0.6026	0.5871 0.6064	0.5910 0.6103	0.5948 0.6141
0.3	0.6179 0.6368	0.6217 0.6406	0.6255 0.6443	0.6293 0.6480	0.6331 0.6517
0.4	0.6554 0.6736	0.6591 0.6772	0.6628 0.6808	0.6664 0.6844	0.6700 0.6879
0.5	0.6915 0.7088	0.6950 0.7123	0.6985 0.7157	0.7019 0.7190	0.7054 0.7224
0.6	0.7257 0.7422	0.7291 0.7454	0.7324 0.7486	0.7357 0.7517	0.7389 0.7549

(*Continued*)

Table A-1. (*Continued*)

z	0.00 0.05	0.01 0.06	0.02 0.07	0.03 0.08	0.04 0.09
0.7	0.7580	0.7611	0.7642	0.7673	0.7703
	0.7734	0.7764	0.7794	0.7823	0.7852
0.8	0.7881	0.7910	0.7939	0.7967	0.7995
	0.8023	0.8051	0.8078	0.8106	0.8133
0.9	0.8159	0.8186	0.8212	0.8238	0.8264
	0.8289	0.8315	0.8340	0.8365	0.8389
1.0	0.8413	0.8438	0.8461	0.8485	0.8508
	0.8531	0.8554	0.8577	0.8599	0.8621
1.1	0.8643	0.8665	0.8686	0.8708	0.8729
	0.8749	0.8770	0.8790	0.8810	0.8830
1.2	0.8849	0.8869	0.8888	0.8907	0.8925
	0.8944	0.8962	0.8980	0.8997	0.9015
1.3	0.9032	0.9049	0.9066	0.9082	0.9099
	0.9115	0.9131	0.9147	0.9162	0.9177
1.4	0.9192	0.9207	0.9222	0.9236	0.9251
	0.9265	0.9279	0.9292	0.9306	0.9319
1.5	0.9332	0.9345	0.9357	0.9370	0.9382
	0.9394	0.9406	0.9418	0.9429	0.9441
1.6	0.9452	0.9463	0.9474	0.9484	0.9495
	0.9505	0.9515	0.9525	0.9535	0.9545
1.7	0.9554	0.9564	0.9573	0.9582	0.9591
	0.9599	0.9608	0.9616	0.9625	0.9633
1.8	0.9641	0.9649	0.9656	0.9664	0.9671
	0.9678	0.9686	0.9693	0.9699	0.9706
1.9	0.9713	0.9719	0.9726	0.9732	0.9738
	0.9744	0.9750	0.9756	0.9761	0.9767
2.0	0.9772	0.9778	0.9783	0.9788	0.9793
	0.9798	0.9803	0.9808	0.9812	0.9817
2.1	0.9821	0.9826	0.9830	0.9834	0.9838
	0.9842	0.9846	0.9850	0.9854	0.9857

Table A-1. (*Continued*)

z	0.00 0.05	0.01 0.06	0.02 0.07	0.03 0.08	0.04 0.09
2.2	0.9861 0.9878	0.9864 0.9881	0.9868 0.9884	0.9871 0.9887	0.9875 0.9890
2.3	0.9893 0.9906	0.9896 0.9909	0.9898 0.9911	0.9901 0.9913	0.9904 0.9916
2.4	0.9918 0.9929	0.9920 0.9931	0.9922 0.9932	0.9925 0.9934	0.9927 0.9936
2.5	0.9938 0.9946	0.9940 0.9948	0.9941 0.9949	0.9943 0.9951	0.9945 0.9952
2.6	0.9953 0.9960	0.9955 0.9961	0.9956 0.9962	0.9957 0.9963	0.9959 0.9964
2.7	0.9965 0.9970	0.9966 0.9971	0.9967 0.9972	0.9968 0.9973	0.9969 0.9974
2.8	0.9974 0.9978	0.9975 0.9979	0.9976 0.9979	0.9977 0.9980	0.9977 0.9981
2.9	0.9981 0.9984	0.9982 0.9985	0.9982 0.9985	0.9983 0.9986	0.9984 0.9986
3.0	0.9987 0.9989	0.9987 0.9989	0.9987 0.9989	0.9988 0.9990	0.9988 0.9990
α	0.001 0.100	0.005 0.200	0.010 0.300	0.025 0.400	0.050
$z_{1-\frac{\alpha}{2}}$	3.291 1.645	2.807 1.282	2.576 1.036	2.240 0.842	1.960
$z_{1-\alpha}$	3.090 1.282	2.576 0.842	2.326 0.524	1.960 0.253	1.645

Table A-2. The t-Distribution

$$\Pr(T \le t) = \int_{-\infty}^{t} \frac{\Gamma(\frac{r+1}{2})}{\sqrt{\pi r}\,\Gamma(\frac{r}{2})(1 + \frac{u^2}{r})^{(r+1)/2}}\,du$$

$$[\Pr(T \le -t) = 1 - \Pr(T \le t)]$$

				α		
	0.25	0.10	0.05	0.025	0.01	0.005
r			$t_{r;1-\alpha}$			
1	1.000	3.078	6.314	12.706	31.821	63.657
2	0.816	1.886	2.920	4.303	6.965	9.925
3	0.765	1.638	2.353	3.182	4.541	5.841
4	0.741	1.533	2.312	2.776	3.747	4.604
5	0.727	1.476	2.015	2.571	3.365	4.032
6	0.718	1.440	1.943	2.447	3.143	3.707
7	0.711	1.415	1.895	2.365	2.998	3.499
8	0.706	1.397	1.860	2.306	2.896	3.355
9	0.703	1.383	1.833	2.262	2.821	3.250
10	0.700	1.372	1.812	2.228	2.764	3.169
11	0.697	1.363	1.796	2.201	2.718	3.106
12	0.695	1.356	1.782	2.179	2.681	3.055
13	0.694	1.350	1.771	2.160	2.650	3.012
14	0.692	1.345	1.761	2.145	2.624	2.997
15	0.691	1.341	1.753	2.131	2.602	2.947
16	0.690	1.337	1.746	2.120	2.583	2.921
17	0.689	1.333	1.740	2.110	2.567	2.898
18	0.688	1.330	1.734	2.101	2.552	2.878
19	0.688	1.328	1.729	2.093	2.539	2.861
20	0.687	1.325	1.725	2.086	2.528	2.845
21	0.686	1.323	1.721	2.080	2.518	2.831
22	0.686	1.321	1.717	2.074	2.508	2.819
23	0.685	1.319	1.714	2.069	2.500	2.807
24	0.685	1.318	1.711	2.064	2.492	2.797
25	0.684	1.316	1.708	2.060	2.485	2.787
26	0.684	1.315	1.706	2.056	2.479	2.779
27	0.684	1.314	1.703	2.052	2.473	2.771

Table A-2. (*Continued*)

	α					
	0.25	**0.10**	**0.05**	**0.025**	**0.01**	**0.005**
28	0.683	1.313	1.701	2.048	2.467	2.763
29	0.683	1.311	1.699	2.045	2.462	2.756
30	0.683	1.310	1.697	2.042	2.457	2.750
∞	0.674	1.282	1.645	1.960	2.326	2.576

Source: Adapted from Merrington M. (1942) Table of the percentage points of the t-distribution. *Biometrika* **32**: 300. It is published here with the kind permission of the Oxford University Press and Copyright Clearance Center.

Table A-3. The Chi-Squared Distribution

$$\Pr(X \le x) = \int_0^x \frac{1}{\Gamma(\frac{r}{2})2^{r/2}} u^{\frac{r}{2}-1} e^{-u/2} du$$

	α			
	0.010 **0.990**	**0.025** **0.975**	**0.050** **0.950**	**0.100** **0.900**
	$\chi^2_{r;1-\alpha}$			
r	$\chi^2_{r;.99}$ $\chi^2_{r;.01}$	$\chi^2_{r;.975}$ $\chi^2_{r;.025}$	$\chi^2_{r;.95}$ $\chi^2_{r;.05}$	$\chi^2_{r;.90}$ $\chi^2_{r;.10}$
1	0.000 2.706	0.001 3.841	0.004 5.024	0.016 6.635
2	0.020 4.605	0.051 5.991	0.103 7.378	0.211 9.210
3	0.115 6.251	0.216 7.815	0.352 9.348	0.584 11.34
4	0.297 7.779	0.484 9.488	0.711 11.14	1.064 13.28
5	0.554 9.236	0.831 11.07	1.145 12.83	1.610 15.09

(*Continued*)

Table A-3. (*Continued*)

	α			
	0.010 **0.990**	**0.025** **0.975**	**0.050** **0.950**	**0.100** **0.900**
6	0.872 10.64	1.237 12.59	1.635 14.45	2.204 16.81
7	1.239 12.02	1.690 14.07	2.167 16.01	2.833 18.48
8	1.646 13.36	2.180 15.51	2.733 17.54	3.490 20.09
9	2.088 14.68	2.700 16.92	3.325 19.02	4.168 21.67
10	2.558 15.99	3.247 18.31	3.940 20.48	4.865 23.21
11	3.053 17.28	3.816 19.68	4.575 21.92	5.578 24.72
12	3.571 18.55	4.404 21.03	5.226 23.34	6.304 26.22
13	4.107 19.81	5.009 22.36	5.892 24.74	7.042 27.69
14	4.660 21.06	5.629 23.68	6.571 26.12	7.790 29.14
15	5.229 22.31	6.262 25.00	7.261 27.49	8.547 30.58
16	5.812 23.54	6.908 26.30	7.962 28.84	9.312 32.00
17	6.408 24.77	7.564 27.59	8.672 30.19	10.08 33.41
18	7.015 25.99	8.231 28.87	9.390 31.53	10.86 34.80
19	7.633 27.20	8.907 30.14	10.12 32.85	11.65 36.19
20	8.260 28.41	9.591 31.41	10.85 34.17	12.44 37.57
21	8.897 29.62	10.28 32.67	11.59 35.48	13.24 38.93

Table A-3. (*Continued*)

	α			
	0.010 **0.990**	**0.025** **0.975**	**0.050** **0.950**	**0.100** **0.900**
22	9.542 30.81	10.98 33.92	12.34 36.78	14.04 40.29
23	10.20 32.01	11.69 35.17	13.09 38.08	14.85 41.64
24	10.86 33.20	12.40 36.42	13.85 39.36	15.66 42.98
25	11.52 34.38	13.12 37.65	14.61 40.65	16.47 44.31
26	12.20 35.56	13.84 38.88	15.38 41.92	17.29 45.64
27	12.88 36.74	14.57 40.11	16.15 43.19	18.11 46.96
28	13.56 37.92	15.31 41.34	16.93 44.46	18.94 48.28
29	14.26 39.09	16.05 42.56	17.71 45.72	19.77 49.59
30	14.95 40.26	16.79 43.77	18.49 46.98	20.60 50.89
40	22.16 51.80	24.43 55.76	26.51 59.34	29.05 63.69
50	29.71 63.17	32.36 67.50	34.76 71.42	37.69 76.15
60	37.48 74.40	40.48 79.08	43.19 83.30	46.46 88.38
70	45.44 85.53	48.76 90.53	51.74 95.02	55.33 100.4
80	53.34 96.58	57.15 101.9	60.39 106.6	64.28 112.3

Source: Adapted from Thompson, CM. (1941) Tables of the percentage points of the χ^2-distribution. *Biometrika* **31**: 188–189. It is published here with the kind permission of the Oxford University Press and Copyright Clearance Center.

Table A-4. Percentiles in Kolmogorov–Smirnov Statistics

$$\Pr(\sup_x |S_n(x) - F_0(x)| \le d_{n;1-\alpha}) = 1 - \alpha$$

			α		
	0.20	**0.10**	**0.05**	**0.02**	**0.01**
n			$d_{n;1-\alpha}$		
1	0.9000	0.9500	0.9750	0.9900	0.9950
2	0.6838	0.7764	0.8419	0.9000	0.9293
3	0.5648	0.6360	0.7076	0.7846	0.8290
4	0.4927	0.5652	0.6239	0.6889	0.7342
5	0.4470	0.5095	0.5633	0.6272	0.6685
6	0.4104	0.4680	0.5193	0.5774	0.6166
7	0.3815	0.4361	0.4834	0.5384	0.5758
8	0.3583	0.4096	0.4543	0.5065	0.5418
9	0.3391	0.3875	0.4300	0.4796	0.5133
10	0.3226	0.3687	0.4093	0.4566	0.4889
11	0.3083	0.3524	0.3912	0.4367	0.4677
12	0.2958	0.3382	0.3754	0.4192	0.4491
13	0.2847	0.3255	0.3614	0.4036	0.4325
14	0.2748	0.3142	0.3489	0.3897	0.4176
15	0.2659	0.3040	0.3376	0.3771	0.4042
16	0.2578	0.2947	0.3273	0.3657	0.3920
17	0.2504	0.2863	0.3180	0.3553	0.3809
18	0.2446	0.2785	0.3094	0.3457	0.3706
19	0.2374	0.2714	0.3014	0.3369	0.3612
20	0.2316	0.2647	0.2941	0.3287	0.3524
21	0.2262	0.2586	0.2872	0.3210	0.3443
22	0.2212	0.2528	0.2809	0.3139	0.3367
23	0.2165	0.2475	0.2749	0.3073	0.3295
24	0.2121	0.2424	0.2693	0.3010	0.3229
25	0.2079	0.2377	0.2640	0.2952	0.3166
26	0.2040	0.2332	0.2591	0.2896	0.3106
27	0.2003	0.2290	0.2544	0.2844	0.3050
28	0.1968	0.2250	0.2500	0.2794	0.2997
29	0.1935	0.2212	0.2457	0.2747	0.2947
30	0.1903	0.2176	0.2417	0.2702	0.2899
31	0.1873	0.2141	0.2379	0.2660	0.2853
32	0.1845	0.2109	0.2342	0.2619	0.2809

Table A-4. (*Continued*)

	0.20	0.10	0.05	0.02	0.01
33	0.1817	0.2077	0.2308	0.2580	0.2768
34	0.1791	0.2047	0.2274	0.2543	0.2728
35	0.1766	0.2019	0.2243	0.2507	0.2690
36	0.1742	0.1991	0.2212	0.2473	0.2653
37	0.1719	0.1965	0.2183	0.2440	0.2618
38	0.1697	0.1939	0.2154	0.2409	0.2584
39	0.1675	0.1915	0.2127	0.2379	0.2552
40	0.1655	0.1891	0.2101	0.2349	0.2521
41	0.1635	0.1869	0.2076	0.2321	0.2490
42	0.1616	0.1847	0.2052	0.2294	0.2461
43	0.1597	0.1826	0.2028	0.2268	0.2433
44	0.1580	0.1805	0.2006	0.2243	0.2406
45	0.1562	0.1786	0.1984	0.2218	0.2380
46	0.1546	0.1767	0.1963	0.2194	0.2354
47	0.1530	0.1748	0.1942	0.2172	0.2330
48	0.1514	0.1730	0.1922	0.2149	0.2306
49	0.1499	0.1713	0.1903	0.2128	0.2283
50	0.1484	0.1696	0.1884	0.2107	0.2260
51	0.1470	0.1680	0.1866	0.2086	0.2239
52	0.1456	0.1664	0.1848	0.2067	0.2217
53	0.1442	0.1648	0.1831	0.2048	0.2197
54	0.1429	0.1633	0.1814	0.2029	0.2177
55	0.1416	0.1619	0.1798	0.2011	0.2157
56	0.1404	0.1604	0.1782	0.1993	0.2138
57	0.1392	0.1591	0.1767	0.1976	0.2120
58	0.1380	0.1577	0.1752	0.1959	0.2102
59	0.1369	0.1564	0.1737	0.1943	0.2084
60	0.1357	0.1551	0.1723	0.1927	0.2067
61	0.1346	0.1539	0.1709	0.1911	0.2051
62	0.1336	0.1526	0.1696	0.1896	0.2034
63	0.1325	0.1514	0.1682	0.1881	0.2018
64	0.1315	0.1503	0.1669	0.1867	0.2003

(*Continued*)

Table A-4. (*Continued*)

			α		
	0.20	**0.10**	**0.05**	**0.02**	**0.01**
65	0.1305	0.1491	0.1657	0.1853	0.1988
66	0.1295	0.1480	0.1644	0.1839	0.1973
67	0.1286	0.1469	0.1632	0.1825	0.1958
68	0.1277	0.1459	0.1620	0.1812	0.1944
69	0.1268	0.1448	0.1609	0.1799	0.1930
70	0.1259	0.1438	0.1598	0.1786	0.1917
71	0.1250	0.1428	0.1586	0.1774	0.1903
72	0.1241	0.1418	0.1576	0.1762	0.1890
73	0.1233	0.1409	0.1565	0.1750	0.1878
74	0.1225	0.1399	0.1554	0.1738	0.1865
75	0.1217	0.1390	0.1544	0.1727	0.1853
76	0.1209	0.1381	0.1534	0.1716	0.1841
77	0.1201	0.1372	0.1524	0.1705	0.1829
78	0.1194	0.1364	0.1515	0.1694	0.1817
79	0.1186	0.1355	0.1505	0.1683	0.1806
80	0.1179	0.1347	0.1496	0.1673	0.1795
81	0.1172	0.1339	0.1487	0.1663	0.1784
82	0.1165	0.1331	0.1478	0.1653	0.1773
83	0.1158	0.1323	0.1469	0.1643	0.1763
84	0.1151	0.1315	0.1461	0.1633	0.1752
85	0.1144	0.1307	0.1452	0.1624	0.1742
86	0.1138	0.1300	0.1444	0.1614	0.1732
87	0.1131	0.1292	0.1436	0.1605	0.1722
88	0.1125	0.1285	0.1427	0.1596	0.1713
89	0.1119	0.1278	0.1420	0.1587	0.1703
90	0.1113	0.1271	0.1412	0.1579	0.1694
91	0.1106	0.1264	0.1404	0.1570	0.1685
92	0.1101	0.1257	0.1397	0.1562	0.1676
93	0.1095	0.1251	0.1389	0.1553	0.1667
94	0.1089	0.1244	0.1382	0.1545	0.1658

Table A-4.   (*Continued*)

	α				
	0.20	**0.10**	**0.05**	**0.02**	**0.01**
95	0.1083	0.1238	0.1375	0.1537	0.1649
96	0.1078	0.1231	0.1368	0.1529	0.1641
97	0.1072	0.1225	0.1361	0.1521	0.1632
98	0.1067	0.1219	0.1354	0.1514	0.1624
99	0.1062	0.1213	0.1347	0.1506	0.1616
100	0.1056	0.1207	0.1340	0.1499	0.1608

This table is taken from Table 1 in Miller LH. (1956) Table of percentage points of Kolmogorov statistics. *J Am Stat Assoc* **51**: 111–121.

Selected Answers to Exercises

Section 1.6

1. (a)

Intervals for FEV1	Frequency	Relative Frequency (%)
2.50–2.99	3	5.3
3.00–3.49	9	15.8
3.50–3.99	14	24.6
4.00–4.49	15	26.3
4.50–4.99	10	17.5
5.00–5.49	6	10.5

(b)

(i)

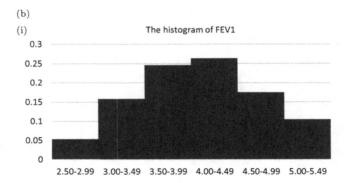

(ii)

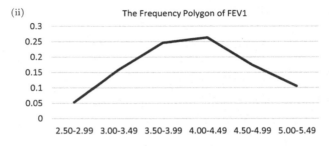

Section 2.5

4. For Table 2.4-4, $Se = \frac{55}{104} = 0.529$, $Sp = \frac{84}{91} = 0.923$, $PPV = \frac{55}{62} = 0.887$, $NPV = \frac{84}{133} = 0.632$; for Table 2.4-5, $Se = \frac{55}{104} = 0.529$, $Sp = \frac{478}{520} = 0.919$, $PPV = \frac{55}{97} = 0.567$, $NPV = \frac{478}{527} = 0.907$.

Section 3.4

7. $\Pr(X \geq 4{,}143) = \Pr(Z \geq 1.44) = 1 - \Pr(Z < 1.44) = 1 - 0.9251 = 0.0749 \approx 0.07$.

Section 8.6

3. Since $D_5(x) = 0.3257 < d_{5;0.95} = 0.5633$, H_0 is not rejected at the level of 0.05.
4. Since $D_{14,12}(x) = 0.5467 > d_{14,12;0.95} = 0.4815$, H_0 is rejected at the level of 0.05.

Section 9.6

1. $\alpha = 0.1$, $\sigma_X = 0.8$

δ	0.05	0.1	0.2	0.3	0.4	0.5
n	693	174	44	20	11	7

2. $\alpha = 0.1$, $\beta = 0.2$, $\sigma_X = 20$

η	5	10	15	20	25	30
n	99	25	11	7	4	3

3. $\alpha = 0.05$, $\sigma_X = 3$

δ	0.5	1	1.5	2	2.5	3
n	277	70	31	18	12	8

4. $\alpha = 0.05$, $\beta = 0.1$

p_D	0.1	0.2	0.3	0.4	0.5	0.6
n	527	132	59	33	22	15

5. $\alpha = 0.05$, $\beta = 0.1$

p_{XY}	0.01	0.05	0.1	0.3	0.5	0.7
n	104,972	4,196	1,046	113	38	17

Section 10.6

3. Since $\chi_{R_A} = 4.35 < \chi^2_{1;0.975} = 5.024$, two r.v.s "Diabetes" and "Cholecystitis" are independent. Yet, $\chi_{R_B} = 8.58 > \chi^2_{1;0.975} = 5.024$, "Diabetes" and "Cholecystitis" are not independent.

Section 11.4

2. $0.5664 \le \theta_{2 \times 2} \le 4.00$.
3. Since $\Pr(n_{11} = 5) = 0.1004$ and $\Pr(n_{11} = 1) = 0.065$, $\Pr(n_{11} = 5) > \Pr(n_{11} = 1)$
4. $p_A = \Pr(X_A = 1) = \Pr\{(X_A = 1) \cap [(X_B = 1) \cup (X_B = 2)]\}$
$= \Pr\{[(X_A = 1) \cap (X_B = 1)] \cup [(X_A = 1) \cap (X_B = 2)]\} = p_{11} + p_{12}$.
$p_B = p_{11} + p_{21}$ is proved in a similiar way.
5.

$$\sigma^2(\hat{\delta}) = \sigma^2(\hat{p}_{12} - \hat{p}_{21}) = \sigma^2(\hat{p}_{12}) + \sigma^2(\hat{p}_{21}) - 2\operatorname{cov}(\hat{p}_{12}, \hat{p}_{21})$$
$$= n^{-1}[p_{12}(1 - p_{12}) + p_{21}(1 - p_{21}) + 2p_{12}p_{21}]$$
$$= n^{-1}[p_{12} - p_{12}^2 + p_{21}^2 - p_{21}^2 + 2p_{12}p_{21}]$$
$$= n^{-1}[p_{12} + p_{21} - (p_{12}^2 - 2p_{12}p_{21} + p_{21}^2)]$$
$$= n^{-1}[p_{12} + p_{21} - (p_{12} - p_{21})^2]$$

6.

$$\frac{\partial \ell_n L}{\partial p_{11}} = \frac{a_{11}}{p_{11}} - \frac{a_{00}}{p_{00}} = 0 \Rightarrow \frac{a_{11}}{p_{11}} = \frac{a_{00}}{p_{00}}, \tag{1}$$

$$\frac{\partial \ell_n L}{\partial p_{01}} = \frac{a_{10} + a_{01}}{p_{01}} - \frac{a_{00}(\psi + 1)}{p_{00}} = 0 \Rightarrow \frac{a_{10} + a_{01}}{p_{01}} = \frac{a_{00}(\psi + 1)}{p_{00}},$$

$$(2)$$

$$\frac{\partial \ell_n L}{\partial \psi} = \frac{a_{10}}{\psi} - \frac{a_{00} p_{01}}{p_{00}} = 0 \Rightarrow \frac{a_{10}}{\psi} = \frac{a_{00} p_{01}}{p_{00}}.$$

$$(3)$$

By eliminating $\frac{a_{00}}{p_{00}}$ in Eqs. (1) and (3), we have

$$\frac{a_{11}}{p_{11}} = \frac{a_{10}}{\psi p_{01}} \Rightarrow \psi = \frac{a_{10}}{a_{11}} \cdot \frac{p_{11}}{p_{01}}.$$

$$(4)$$

By substituting Eq. (4) into Eq. (2) and simplifying,

$$\frac{p_{11}}{p_{01}} = \frac{a_{11}}{a_{01}}.$$

$$(5)$$

After substituting Eq. (5) into Eq. (4),

$$\hat{\psi} = \frac{a_{10}}{a_{01}}.$$

$$(6)$$

By substituting Eq. (6) into Eq. (3) and simplifying,

$$\hat{p}_{01} = \frac{a_{01}}{n}.$$

$$(7)$$

After substituting Eq. (7) into Eq. (5),

$$\hat{p}_{11} = \frac{a_{11}}{n}.$$

7. $\hat{b} = 0.0662$, $\hat{\sigma}^2 = 0.7478$, $\hat{\sigma}_{\hat{b}}^2 = 1.82 \cdot 10^{-6}$, $\chi_{Yates} = 2400.6$; H_0 is rejected, that is, it does not have a linear trend.

8. $\hat{\eta}_1 = 0.0837$, $\hat{\eta}_3 = 0.070485$, $\hat{\bar{\eta}} = [0.0837, 0.070485]^T$; $W = \begin{bmatrix} 87 & -9 \\ -9 & 106 \end{bmatrix}$, $V = W^{-1} = \begin{bmatrix} 0.011596 & 0.00098 \\ 0.00098 & 0.009518 \end{bmatrix}$, $\chi_{Stuart} = \hat{\bar{\eta}}^T V \hat{\bar{\eta}} = 0.00014 < 0.051$; hence H_0 is rejected, namely, no marginal homogeneity between the lambs of 1952 and 1953.

9. $\hat{\Delta} = 0.078635$, $\hat{\sigma}(\hat{\Delta}) = 0.035443$, $\chi_{kendall} = 4.922304 < \chi_{1,0.975}^2 = 5.024$; H_0 is not rejected, that is, there exists marginal homogeneity between the lambs of 1952 and 1953.

10. Since $\chi_{2-way} = 49.64 > \chi^2_{1,0.975} = 5.024$, H_0 is rejected, namely, Y_A and Y_B are not independent.

11. $\hat{\vec{\eta}} = [0.092283, 0.004547, -0.006821]^T$, $W = \begin{bmatrix} 843 & -500 & -241 \\ -500 & 1454 & -794 \\ -241 & -794 & 1419 \end{bmatrix}$, $V = W^{-1} = \begin{bmatrix} 0.002482 & 0.00156 & 0.001295 \\ 0.00156 & 0.001972 & 0.001368 \\ 0.001295 & 0.001368 & 0.00169 \end{bmatrix}$, $\chi_{Stuart} = \hat{\vec{\eta}}^T V \hat{\vec{\eta}} = 2.14 \cdot 10^{-7} < \chi^2_{3;0.025} = 0.216$; hence H_0 is rejected, left and right-eyes are not independent.

12. The first-order interaction does not exist between X and Y, given Z.

14. H_0 is rejected, that is, it has a nonzero second-order interaction. Hence, it does not have a common odds ratio. As a result, the Mantel–Haenszel estimator is not applicable.

Section 12.6

9. (a) random sample size n =15, (b) omitted, (c) $E_{\hat{p}(n)} = 12.328249 \approx 13$.

10. (a) $\mu_1 = 0.4$, $\sigma_1^2 = 0.84$

λ_k^*	1	0	1	2	...	13	14	15
c_k^*	−19	−19	−19	−19	...	−23	−23	−23
d_k^*	19	19	19	19	...	23	23	23

Since $c_k^* < \lambda_k^* < d_k^*$ for all k, the trial is not stopped, but it will continue.

(b) $N_1 = 54$ (c) $M_U(k) = -22 + k$, $M_L(k) = 22 - k$.

11. $\zeta = 3.60962$, $V = 7.377933$, $z_{LR} = 1.328906 < 1.96$.

Index

Printed in the United States
by Baker & Taylor Publisher Services